Rev'd 7/16

Primary Care in Obstetric and Gynecology

Second Edition

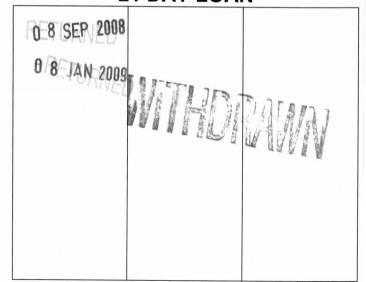

Primary Care in Obstetrics and Gynecology

A Handbook for Clinicians

Second Edition

Joseph S. Sanfilippo, MD, MBA

Professor, Department of Obstetrics, Gynecology, and Reproductive Sciences, University of Pittsburgh School of Medicine, Vice Chairman, Reproductive Sciences, Magee-Women's Hospital, Pittsburgh, Pennsylvania, USA

Roger P. Smith, MD

Professor, Vice Chair and Program Director, Department of Obstetrics and Gynecology, University of Missouri, Truman Medical Center, Kansas City, Missouri, USA

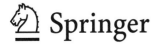 Springer

Joseph S. Sanfilippo, MD, MBA
Professor
Department of Obstetrics, Gynecology, and
    Reproductive Sciences
University of Pittsburgh School
    of Medicine
Vice Chairman
Reproductive Sciences
Magee-Women's Hospital
Pittsburgh, PA 15213
USA

Roger P. Smith, MD
Professor
Vice Chair and
    Program Director
Department of Obstetrics
    and Gynecology
University of Missouri
Truman Medical Center
Kansas City, MO 64108
USA

Drug Dosage Notice: The authors and editors of this book have checked carefully to ensure that drug dosage recommendations are precise and in agreement with accepted standards at the time of publication. Nevertheless, dosage schedules are changed periodically as research and clinical experience reveal new data. Therefore, you should check the manufacturer's recommendation for dosages of all medications, especially in instances when the drug is one which you use infrequently or with which you otherwise lack familiarity.

Library of Congress Control Number: 2006920204

ISBN: 978-0387-32327-5   e-ISBN: 978-0387-32328-2

Printed on acid-free paper.

Preface

"The obligation to promote the good of the patients is a basic presumption of medical care giving a defining feature of the physician's ethical responsibility. To promote the patient's good is to provide care in which benefits outweigh burdens or harms" [American College of Obstetricians & Gynecologists (ACOG) Committee Opinion #156, 1995].

How does the busy clinician balance this with the conflicting pressures of time, regulation, paperwork, increased costs, declining reimbursements, burnout, and ever-changing knowledge? These issues have affected us at all levels: the medical student, the resident, and the established practitioner. This second edition of this book has been designed to address the issue of changing knowledge and to touch on some of the other issues as well.

Let us begin with medical student training. More information, clinical application, problem-based learning (PBLs), and oftentimes short but succinct obstetrics and gynecology rotations are the current name of the game. How can we train our future physicians to think multisystem? The ability to collate all information and apply it to the specific clinical problem at hand remains a challenge. One objective of this book is to tie the gynecologic and the medical knowledge clinical application together and to apply them to the patient who is currently in front of us.

Residency training continues to stress exposure to primary and preventive ambulatory health care, i.e., internal medicine, critical care, geriatrics, and the emergency department. The book is designed to provide information that can integrate these disparate callings.

Primary care, as obstetricians and gynecologists are asked to provide, covers the spectrum from the pediatric-adolescent, to the reproductive-aged woman, to menopause and beyond. Adolescent and sexual development and awareness, along with psychological and cognitive development, all begin early and proceed rapidly into adulthood. When should the first pelvic examination be performed? How do we provide health guidance and counseling based on age? We attempt to provide guidelines to these questions in this second edition.

Periodic health assessment is important in our day-to-day clinical activities. How do we as clinicians provide primary and preventive care? How does a busy clinician identify the high-risk patient? For example, when is a lipid profile or colorectal screening indicated? What is the gynecologist's role in preconception counseling and genetic testing, hepatitis vaccination, human immunodeficiency (HIV) assessment, mammography, influenza, and human papilloma virus vaccinations? The list goes on.

The second edition of this book is designed to provide a succinct, immediately clinically applicable source of information. It is our sincere hope that everyone who has this new revised edition at his or her disposal can provide excellence in clinical care.

Joseph S. Sanfilippo, MD, MBA
Roger P. Smith, MD

Contents

---

†Deceased.

Contributors

Arnold P. Advincula, MD
Clinical Assistant Professor, Department of Obstetrics and Gynecology, Division of Gynecology, University of Michigan, Ann Arbor, MI 48109, USA

Hugh R.K. Barber, MD†
Emeritus Professor, New York University School of Medicine, Department of Obstetrics and Gynecology, Lenox Hill Hospital, New York, NY 10021, USA

Vasti L. Broadstone, MD
Southern Indiana Diabetes and Endocrinology Specialties, Joslin Diabetes Center, New Albany, IN 47150, USA

Jeffrey P. Callen, MD
Professor, Department of Medicine (Dermatology), Chief, Division of Dermatology, University of Louisville, Louisville, KY 40292, USA

Dayton W. Daberkow II, MD
Associate Professor, Department of Clinical Medicine, Internal Medicine Residency Program Director, Department of Internal Medicine, Louisiana State Health Sciences Center, New Orleans, LA 70112, USA

Freddie H. Fu, MD
Professor and Chairman, Department of Orthopedics, Center for Sports Medicine, University of Pittsburgh Medical Center, Pittsburgh, PA 15203, USA

Richard S. Guido, MD
Associate Professor, Department of Obstetrics, Gynecology, and Reproductive Sciences, Division of Gynecology Specialties, Magee-Women's Hospital, Pittsburgh, PA 15213, USA

---

†Deceased.

Tanya J. Hagen, MD
Assistant Professor, Department of Orthopedics, Center for Sports Medicine, University of Pittsburgh Medical Center, Pittsburgh, PA 15203, USA

Bryna Harwood, MD
Assistant Professor, Associate Director of Fellowship in Family Planning and Clinical Care Research, Department of Obstetrics, Gynecology, and Reproductive Sciences, University of Pittsburgh School of Medicine, Magee-Women's Hospital, Pittsburgh, PA 15213, USA

William H. Hindle, MD
Professor Emeritus, Department of Obstetrics and Gynecology, University of Southern California Keck School of Medicine, Founder, The William H. Hindle, M.D. Breast Diagnostic Center, Women's and Children's Hospital, Los Angeles County + USC Medical Center, Los Angeles, CA 90033, USA

Randall S. Hines, MD
Associate Professor and Director, Department of Obstetrics and Gynecology, Division of Reproductive Endocrinology and Infertility, University of Mississippi Medical Center, Jackson, MS 39216, USA

Mary Anne Jamieson, MD
Department of Obstetrics and Gynecology, Queen's University, Kingston, ON, Canada K7L 3N6

Jean D. Koehler, PhD
AASECT Certified Sex Therapist and Educator, Associate Professor of Psychiatry, University of Louisville Medical School, Louisville, KY 40207, USA

Mary Korytkowski, MD
Associate Professor, Department of Medicine, Division of Endocrinology, University of Pittsburgh, Medical Director, University of Pittsburgh Medical Center, Center for Diabetes and Endocrinology, Pittsburgh, PA 15213, USA

Haruko Akatsu Kuffner, MD
Associate Professor, Department of Medicine, Division of Endocrinology and Metabolism, University of Pittsburgh, Pittsburgh, PA 15213, USA

Joseph A. Lacy, MS, RD
Assistant Director, Department of Parenteral and Enteral Nutrition, University Hospital, Cincinnati, OH 45219, USA

Douglas W. Laube, MD
Professor and Chair, Department of Obstetrics and Gynecology, University of Wisconsin Medical School, Madison, WI 53792, USA

Mary Nan Mallory, MD
Department of Emergency Medicine, University of Louisville School of Medicine, Louisville, KY 40202, USA

Bernadette McIntire, MA, RD
Nutritionist, Dietician, Private Practice, Louisville, KY 40207, USA

Sri Prakash L. Mokshagundam, MD
Associate Professor, Department of Medicine, University of Louisville, Louisville, KY 40202, Southern Indiana Diabetes and Endocrinology Specialties, Joslin Diabetes Center, New Albany, IN 47150, USA

Amitasrigowri S. Murthy, MD
Assistant Director, Family Planning, Assistant Professor, Department of Obstetrics and Gynecology and Women's Health, Jacobi Medical Center, Albert Einstein College of Medicine, Bronx, NY 10461, USA

Thomas E. Nolan, MD
Abe Mickal Professor and Chair, Obstetrics and Gynecology, Louisiana State University Health Science Center, New Orleans, LA 70112, USA

Joseph S. Sanfilippo, MD, MBA
Professor, Department of Obstetrics, Gynecology, and Reproductive Sciences, University of Pittsburgh School of Medicine, Vice Chairman, Reproductive Sciences, Magee-Women's Hospital, Pittsburgh, PA 15213, USA

G. Randolph Schrodt, Jr., MD
Associate Professor, Department of Pathology, University of Louisville School of Medicine, Louisville, KY 40292, USA

Ruth Schwarz, MD[†]
Professor, Department of Obstetrics and Gynecology, University of Rochester – Strong Memorial Hospital, Rochester, NY 14642, USA

Roger P. Smith, MD
Professor, Vice Chair and Program Director, Department of Obstetrics and Gynecology, University of Missouri, Truman Medical Center, Kansas City, MO 64108, USA

Arleen Song, MD, MPH
Assistant Professor, Department of Obstetrics and Gynecology, University of Michigan Medical Center, Women's Hospital, Ann Arbor, MI 48109, USA

Nanette K. Wenger, MD
Professor, Department of Medicine, Division of Cardiology, Emory University School of Medicine, Chief of Cardiology, Grady Memorial Hospital, Atlanta, GA 30303, USA

[†]Deceased.

Primary Care and the Obstetrician-Gynecologist

1

Primary Care in Obstetrics and Gynecology: Health Maintenance and Screening

Douglas W. Laube

Background Information

Within a rapidly changing political and economic environment lies the fundamental need to provide continuity of patient care to decrease morbidity and mortality. Not all women need the same care and an attempt should be made by the clinician to focus on issues specific to high-risk categories and age-related variables (Tables 1.1–1.5). Additionally, scientific and economic documentation of the effectiveness of medical care has become an important issue in both clinical settings and policy-making situations. These concepts will also dictate physician reimbursement.

Periodic health maintenance implies the provision of health services generally considered to be part of primary care, but primary care must be differentiated from the confusing variety of other services, which are specialty specific. For example, "family care" would include a wide range of services to all family members regardless of age or sex and is characteristic of the practice of family medicine. "Comprehensive care" implies that all medical needs can be offered by a single provider, which is not a reasonable expectation. It is well recognized that all physicians who provide primary care services have limitations that depend on the content of their individual educational backgrounds and the scope of their subsequent practice experience. Periodic health maintenance for the gynecologist identifies a component of primary care that we can implement based on expertise acquired through our training as health care providers to women. Some of our health care provision may supersede issues of medical specialty, enabling us to provide for health maintenance and disease prevention.

Table 1.1. High-risk factors.

Intervention	High-risk factor
Bacteriuria testing	Diabetes mellitus
Colonoscopy	History of inflammatory bowel disease or colonic polyps; family history of familial polyposis coli, colorectal cancer, or cancer family syndrome
Fasting glucose test	Every 3–5 years for family history of diabetes mellitus (one first- or two second-degree relatives); marked obesity; history of gestational diabetes mellitus
Fluoride supplement	Live in area with inadequate water fluoridation (<0.7 ppm)
Genetic testing/ counseling	Exposure to teratogens; considering pregnancy at age 35 or older; patient, partner, or family member with history of genetic disorder or birth defect; African, Eastern European Jewish, Mediterranean, or Southeast Asian ancestry
Hemoglobin	Caribbean, Latin American, Asian, Mediterranean, or African ancestry; history of excessive menstrual flow
Hepatitis B vaccine	Intravenous drug use; current recipient of blood products; health-related job with exposure to blood or blood products; household or sexual contact with hepatitis B virus carriers; history of prostitution; history of sexual activity with multiple partners in last 6 months
Human immunodeficiency virus (HIV) testing	Seeking treatment for sexually transmissible diseases (STDs); drug use by injection; history of prostitution; past or present sexual partner who is HIV positive or bisexual or injects drugs; long-term residence or birth in an area with high prevalence of HIV infection; history of transfusion 1978 to 1985
Influenza vaccine	Resident in chronic care facility; chronic cardiopulmonary disorders; metabolic disease (e.g., diabetes mellitus, hemoglobinopathies, immunosuppression, or renal dysfunction)
Lipid profile	Elevated cholesterol level; history of parent or sibling with blood cholesterol of 240 mg/dl;

Table 1.1. *Continued.*

Intervention	High-risk factor
	history of sibling, parent, or grandparent with documented premature (<55 years) coronary artery disease; diabetes mellitus or smoking habit
Mammography	Age 35 and older with premenopausally diagnosed breast cancer in a first-degree relative
Measles, mumps, rubella (MMR)	Childbearing age and no evidence of immunity; a second measles immunization, preferably measles, mumps, rubella (MMR) vaccine, if no proof of immunity
Pneumococcal vaccine	Factors for influenza vaccine plus sickle cell disease, Hodgkin's disease, asplenia, alcoholism, cirrhosis, or multiple myeloma
STD testing	History of multiple sexual partners or a sexual partner with multiple contacts, sexual contact with persons with culture-proven STD, history of repeated episodes of STD, attendance at clinics for STDs
Skin	Increased recreational or occupational exposure to sunlight; family or personal history of skin cancer; clinical evidence of precursor lesions
Thyroid-stimulating hormone	Strong family history of thyroid disease; autoimmune disease (evidence of subclinical hypothyroidism may be related to unfavorable lipid profiles)
Tuberculosis (TB) skin test	HIV infection; close contact with persons known or suspected to have tuberculosis (TB); medical risk factors known to increase risk of disease if infected; born in country with high TB prevalence; medically underserved; low income; alcoholism; intravenous drug use; resident of long-term care facility (e.g., correctional institutions, mental institutions, nursing homes and facilities); health professional working in high-risk health care facilities

Source: Reproduced with permission from the American College of Obstetricians and Gynecologists, *Guidelines for Women's Health Care*, 2nd ed. Washington DC, © ACOG, 2002.

Table 1.2.   Guidelines for women's health care: ages 13–18 years.

Screening

History
Reason for visit
Health status: medical, surgical, family
Dietary/nutritional assessment
Physical activity
Tobacco, alcohol, other drugs
Abuse/neglect
Sexual practices

Physical examination
Height
Weight
Blood pressure
Secondary sexual characteristics (Tanner staging)
Pelvic examination (yearly when sexually active or by age 18)
Skin[a]

Laboratory tests
Periodic
Pap test (yearly when sexually active or by age 18)
Cholesterol, high-density lipoprotein cholesterol (every 5 years)

High-risk groups[a]
Hemoglobin
Bacteriuria testing
Sexually transmitted disease testing
Human immunodeficiency virus (HIV) testing
Genetic testing/counseling
Rubella titer
Tuberculosis skin test
Lipid profile
Fasting glucose

Evaluation and counseling

Sexuality
Development
High-risk behaviors
Preventing unwanted/unintended pregnancy
  Postponing sexual involvement
  Contraceptive options

Table 1.2. *Continued.*

Evaluation and counseling

Sexually transmitted diseases
   Partner selection
   Barrier protection

Fitness
Hygiene (including dental); fluoride supplementation
Dietary/nutritional assessment (including eating disorders)
Exercise: discussion of program

Psychosocial evaluation
Interpersonal/family relationships
Sexual identity
Personal goal development
Behavioral/learning disorders
Abuse/neglect

Cardiovascular risk factors
Family history
Hypertension
Dyslipidemia
Obesity
Diabetes mellitus

Health/risk behaviors
Injury prevention
   Safety belts and helmets
   Recreational hazards
   Firearms
   Hearing
Skin exposure to ultraviolet rays
Suicide: depressive symptoms
Tobacco, alcohol, other drugs

Immunizations

Periodic
Tetanus-diphtheria booster (once between ages 14 and 16)

High-risk groups[a]
Measles, mumps, rubella (MMR) vaccine
Hepatitis B vaccine

Continued.

Table 1.2. *Continued.*

Leading causes of death

Motor vehicle accidents
Homicide
Suicide
Leukemia

Leading causes of morbidity

Nose, throat, and upper respiratory conditions
Viral, bacterial, and parasitic infections
Sexual abuse
Musculoskeletal and soft tissue injuries
Acute ear infections
Digestive system and acute urinary conditions

[a]See Table 1.1.
Source: Reproduced with permission from the American College of Obstetricians and Gynecologists, *Guidelines for Women's Health Care*, 2nd ed. Washington DC, © ACOG, 2002.

Table 1.3. Guidelines for women's health care: ages 19–39 years.

Screening

History
Reason for visit
Health status: medical, surgical, family
Dietary/nutritional assessment
Physical activity
Tobacco, alcohol, other drugs
Abuse/neglect
Sexual practices

Physical examination
Height
Weight

Table 1.3. *Continued*.

Screening

Blood pressure
Neck: adenopathy, thyroid
Breasts
Abdomen
Pelvic examination
Skin[a]

Laboratory tests
Periodic
Pap test (physician and patient discretion after three consecutive normal
  tests if low risk)
Cholesterol, high-density lipoprotein cholesterol (every 5 years)

High-risk groups[a]
Hemoglobin
Bacteriuria testing
Mammography
Fasting glucose test
Sexually transmitted disease testing
Human immunodeficiency virus (HIV) testing
Genetic testing/counseling
Rubella titer
Tuberculosis skin test
Lipid profile
Thyroid-stimulating hormone

Evaluation and counseling

Sexuality
High-risk behaviors
Contraceptive options
  Genetic counseling
  Prevention of unwanted pregnancy
Sexually transmitted disease
  Partner selection
  Barrier protection
Sexual function

Continued.

Table 1.3.   *Continued.*

Evaluation and counseling

Fitness
Hygiene (including dental)
Dietary/nutritional assessment
Exercise: discussion of program

Psychosocial evaluation
Interpersonal/family relationships
Domestic violence
Job satisfaction
Life-style/stress
Sleep disorders

Cardiovascular risk factors
Family history
Hypertension
Dyslipidemia
Obesity/diabetes mellitus
Life-style

Health/risk behaviors
Injury prevention
    Safety belts and helmets
    Occupational hazards
    Recreational hazards
    Firearms
    Hearing
Breast self-examination
Skin exposure to ultraviolet rays
Suicide: depressive symptoms
Tobacco, alcohol, other drugs

Immunizations

Periodic
Tetanus–diphtheria booster (every 10 years)

***High-risk groups*[a]**
Measles, mumps, rubella (MMR) vaccine
Hepatitis B vaccine
Influenza vaccine
Pneumococcal vaccine

Table 1.3.   *Continued.*

Leading causes of death

Motor vehicle accidents
Cardiovascular disease
Homicide
Acquired immunodeficiency syndrome (AIDS)
Cerebrovascular disease
Cancer

Leading causes of morbidity

Nose, throat, and upper respiratory conditions
Musculoskeletal and soft tissue including back and upper and lower
  extremities

[a] See Table 1.1.
Source: Reproduced with permission from the American College of Obstetricians and Gynecologists, *Guidelines for Women's Health Care*, 2nd ed. Washington DC, © ACOG, 2002.

Table 1.4.   Guidelines for women's health care: ages 40–64 years.

Screening

History
Reason for visit
Health status: medical, surgical, family
Dietary/nutritional assessment
Physical activity
Tobacco, alcohol, other drugs
Abuse/neglect
Sexual practices

Physical examination
Height
Weight
Blood pressure

Continued.

Table 1.4. *Continued.*

Screening

Oral cavity
Neck: adenopathy, thyroid
Breasts, axillae
Abdomen
Pelvic and rectovaginal examination
Skin[a]

Laboratory tests
Periodic
Pap test (physician and patient discretion after three consecutive
   normal tests if low risk)
Mammography (every 1–2 years until age 50, yearly beginning
   at 50)
Cholesterol, high-density lipoprotein cholesterol (every 5 years)
Fecal occult blood test
Sigmoidoscopy (every 3–5 years after age 50)

High-Risk Groups[a]
Hemoglobin
Bacteriuria testing
Mammography
Fasting glucose test
Sexually transmitted disease testing
Human immunodeficiency virus (HIV) testing
Tuberculosis skin test
Lipid profile
Thyroid-stimulating hormone test
Colonoscopy

Evaluation and counseling

Sexuality
High-risk behaviors
Contraceptive options
   Genetic counseling
   Prevention of unwanted pregnancy

Table 1.4. *Continued.*

Evaluation and counseling

Sexually transmitted disease
   Partner selection
   Barrier protection
Sexual functioning

Fitness
Hygiene (including dental)
Dietary/nutritional assessment
Exercise: discussion of program

Psychosocial evaluation
Family relationships
Domestic violence
Job/work satisfaction
Retirement planning
Life-style/stress
Sleep disorders

Cardiovascular risk factors
Family history
Hypertension
Dyslipidemia
Obesity/diabetes mellitus
Life-style

Health/risk behaviors
Hormone replacement therapy
Injury prevention
   Safety belts and helmets
   Occupational hazards
   Recreational hazards
   Sports involvement
   Firearms
   Hearing
Breast self-examination
Skin exposure to ultraviolet rays
Suicide: depressive symptoms
Tobacco, alcohol, other drugs

Continued.

Table 1.4. *Continued.*

Immunizations

Periodic
Tetanus–diphtheria booster (every 10 years)
Influenza vaccine (annually beginning at age 55)

High-risk groups[a]
Measles, mumps, rubella (MMR) vaccine
Hepatitis B vaccine
Influenza vaccine
Pneumococcal vaccine

Leading causes of death

Coronary artery disease
Breast, lung, colorectal, and ovarian cancer
Cerebrovascular disease
Obstructive pulmonary disease

Leading causes of morbidity

Nose, throat, and upper respiratory conditions
Osteoporosis
Arthritis
Hypertension
Orthopedic deformities, including back and upper and lower
extremities
Heart disease
Hearing and vision impairments

[a] See Table 1.1.
Source: Reproduced with permission from the American College of
Obstetricians and Gynecologists, *Guidelines for Women's Health Care*, 2nd
ed. Washington DC, © ACOG, 2002.

Table 1.5.   Guidelines for women's health care: age 65 years and older.

Screening

History
Reason for visit
Health status: medical, surgical, family
Dietary/nutritional assessment
Physical activity
Tobacco, alcohol, other drugs, concurrent medications
Abuse/neglect
Sexual practices

Physical examination
Height
Weight
Blood pressure
Oral cavity
Neck: adenopathy, thyroid
Breasts, axillae
Abdomen
Pelvic and rectovaginal examination
Skin[a]

Laboratory tests
Periodic
Pap test (physician and patient discretion after three consecutive normal
     tests)
Urinalysis/dipstick
Mammography
Cholesterol, high-density lipoprotein cholesterol (every 3–5 years)
Fecal occult blood test
Sigmoidoscopy (every 3–5 years)
Thyroid-stimulating hormone test (every 3–5 years)

High-risk groups[a]
Hemoglobin
Fasting glucose test
Sexually transmitted disease testing
Human immunodeficiency virus (HIV) testing
Tuberculosis skin test
Lipid profile

Continued.

Table 1.5. *Continued.*

Evaluation and counseling

Sexuality
Sexual functioning
Sexual behaviors
Sexually transmitted diseases

Fitness
Hygiene (general and dental)
Dietary/nutritional assessment
Exercise: discussion of program

Psychosocial evaluation
Neglect/abuse
Life-style/stress
Depression/sleep disorders
Family relationships
Job/work/retirement satisfaction

Cardiovascular risk factors
Hypertension
Dyslipidemia
Obesity
Diabetes mellitus
Sedentary life-style

Health/risk behaviors
Hormone replacement therapy
Injury prevention
   Safety belts and helmets
   Occupational hazards
   Recreational hazards
   Firearms
Visual acuity/glaucoma
Hearing
Breast self-examination
Skin exposure to ultraviolet rays
Suicide: depressive symptoms
Tobacco, alcohol, other drugs

Table 1.5. *Continued.*

Immunizations

Periodic
Tetanus–diphtheria booster (every 10 years)
Influenza vaccine (annually)
Pneumococcal vaccine (once)

High-risk groups[a]
Hepatitis B vaccine

Leading causes of death

Cardiovascular disease
Coronary artery disease
Cerebrovascular disease
Pneumonia/influenza
Obstructive lung disease
Colorectal, lung, and breast cancer
Accidents

Leading causes of morbidity

Nose, throat, and upper respiratory conditions
Osteoporosis
Arthritis
Hypertension
Urinary incontinence
Heart disease
Musculoskeletal and soft tissue injuries
Hearing and vision impairment
Colonoscopy

[a] See Table 1.1.

Source: Reproduced with permission from the American College of Obstetricians and Gynecologists, *Guidelines for Women's Health Care*, 2nd ed. Washington DC, © ACOG, 2002.

The necessary provision of periodic health maintenance by the gynecologist should include all matters pertaining to the female reproductive system and nongynecologic care that may be related to disorders of the female reproductive system. For example, thyroid dysfunction, although not generally considered a gynecologic entity, may relate directly to an aberration in menstrual interval. Likewise, hypercholesterolemia and cholesterol metabolism are generally considered under the purview of other medical specialties. However, the relationship of cholesterol to hormone replacement in the menopausal patient gives it a higher priority in the gynecologist's periodic health care of women in appropriate age groups. Commonly included practices of gynecologic care such as cervical cytology, breast examination, and mammographic screening coupled with nongynecologic periodic health maintenance complete a wide range of services that can be timed according to individual need and age.

As the number of older women in the United States increases, the focus of women's health care must change as well. There will be less need for obstetric and surgical care and more demand for preventive health care. Additional surgical and obstetric training is less important for this most rapidly growing segment of society than a more comprehensive knowledge of matters relating to the morbidities of aging.

As the first proposals for health care reform were explained in 1993, the leadership of the American College of Obstetricians and Gynecologists (ACOG) was concerned that the proposed "gatekeeper" concept could undermine women's unrestricted, direct access to their obstetrician-gynecologist. It became clear that the only way to achieve this goal was to ensure that obstetrician-gynecologists are classified as primary care providers by insurance and managed-care entities. Survey data by the ACOG as well as data generated by the National Ambulatory Health Care Council suggest that both patients and practitioners view obstetrician-gynecologists as primary care physicians. This, coupled with the realization that the specialty has to accommodate to the managed care environment, has led to the only viable option of seeking designation as primary care providers.

It should be understood that there are many obstetrician-gynecologists both in the generalist ranks as well as subspecialists who do not want to function as primary care providers and who will not do so. Certainly this group of physicians should not provide primary care services and should be encouraged to function in the more traditional consultant role. However, a large number of obstetrician-gynecologists prefer the designation of primary care provider to preserve their patients' unrestricted access to care. Another aspect relative to the delivery of more broad-based health care services relates to the type and training of the health care practitioner. It is clear that the restructuring of health care financing and health care access using various managed care delivery systems is necessitating a reconsideration of our practice partners for the future. More consideration will be given in the future to physician collaboration with nonphysician health care providers for a variety of economically driven reasons. To provide comprehensive nongynecologic health care, the obstetrician-gynecologist may benefit from employing non-physician health care providers who can provide cost-effective primary care or expand management or clinical services not available within his or her own practice. This allows the obstetrician-gynecologist to gain access to a larger group of patients and to reduce the cost of providing existing services. The net effect is to stabilize revenue at a time when managed care reimbursement is shrinking per unit of service. Additionally, the obstetrician-gynecologist partners of the future may include physicians in other specialties, particularly family physicians and general internists. The ebb and flow of patient-related services in this type of arrangement is evident and potentially beneficial to all groups with the net effect of building a larger patient base. To accommodate to changes and provide appropriate educational foundations, a number of changes in the preparation of the provider for women's health care services will be necessary. It is anticipated that changes should begin early enough to provide the upper-level medical school undergraduate with the foundations for a more broad-based approach to women's health care/primary care.

The Association of Professors of Gynecology and Obstetrics (APGO) and the Council on Residency Education in Obstetrics and Gynecology (CREOG) are collaborating in designing a general fourth-year medical school curriculum to serve as a basis for guiding students interested in women's health care fields. It is thought that by focusing on these generally accepted areas, the future resident will already have sound educational underpinnings. Currently, funding limitations in many states are being discussed for medical schools that are not committed to the production of larger numbers of primary care providers. In the foreseeable future, limits will be imposed on the number of specialists and subspecialists that medical schools are able to train. Many states are considering legislation to mandate a higher percentage of primary care providers, offering funding only to the schools that are willing to meet this requirement.

Similarly, federal mandates will begin to change the number of residency positions through limits that are placed on monies allocated to hospitals to pay for postgraduate education. In addition, federal and state legislatures will probably increase their demands for larger numbers of nonphysician health care provider education. This will include physician assistants, advanced nurse-practitioners, and certified nurse-midwives as well as other allied health care professionals such as social workers and/or psychologists.

As the scope and responsibilities of the specialty change, so do the procedures and requirements by which physicians must be trained. An important aspect of the new special requirements promulgated by the Residency Review Committee in Obstetrics and Gynecology is to ensure that obstetrics and gynecology training programs respond to recent changes in medical practice. Under the new requirements, residency programs must provide training in primary and preventive care for at least 6 months of the 4-year residency. They must emphasize ambulatory care of patients, which includes both knowledge and skills in the areas of health maintenance, disease prevention, risk assessment, counseling, and the use of consultants and community resources. Some of these specific areas include comprehensive history taking (medical, nutritional, sexual, family, genetic, and social behavior); complete physical examination; appropriate use of laboratory studies and diagnostic techniques; patient education and counseling; immunization; and diagnosis and treatment of nonreproductive illnesses commonly affecting women. Included in this time frame is a requirement for at least 1 month of training in the care of geriatric patients as this is the largest growing segment of our patient population. Additionally, emphasis is given to requiring that our educational process will ensure physician competency as well as sufficient knowledge.

The probability of a greater degree of multidisciplinary training is evident in specialties with significant overlap for women's health care provision. This includes internal medicine and family practice. These two specialties can help provide substantive educational underpinnings for areas in which obstetrics and gynecology residencies typically cannot provide adequate education. On the other hand, obstetrics and gynecology may continue its leadership role in providing necessary education for family physicians in obstetrics and to internists for gynecologic ambulatory health care services. Departmental faculties in the future will probably contain, on a part-time basis, physicians and educators who are not strictly working within their own specialties. Academic faculties will contain physicians who are certified in more than one specialty, enabling them to provide more broad-based education and a widened perspective for their medical students and resident graduates.

Further speculation relates to how the board certification process may evolve to accommodate a larger cohort of physicians who can take on the expanded tasks of primary health care provision for women. Within the existing certification process, areas of ambulatory/primary care are receiving and will continue to receive a high priority. Whether separate board certification accommodations are made for the future trainee in obstetrics and gynecology remains to be seen.

The necessity of a new "subspecialty" of women's health care in internal medicine could become a moot point if appropriate broad-based education becomes well established within our own specialty. The educational leadership of our specialty should become more aware of the need for these training modifications to avoid conflicts with existing political groups that are serving as advocates for the development of yet another specialty in women's health.

Screening, Counseling, and Immunization

Screening can identify individuals who are free of evidence of or at low risk for the development of a disease or a condition. It also identifies individuals who are susceptible to the development of a disease or a condition or who have a precursor of a disease or condition. Finally, screening may identify an individual who has a disease or condition before it becomes clinically manifest, when it is more likely to be cured, or a person who has a disease or a condition that poses risk to others.

Tests for screening need to be evaluated in terms of accuracy, risks, and cost. These factors are usually expressed in terms of sensitivity:

$$\text{Sensitivity} = \frac{\text{No. of persons with disease correctly identified}}{\text{No. of persons actually having the disease}}$$

Also of importance is specificity, which is the number of persons correctly identified as not having the disease divided by the number of persons who do have the disease. The value of a test used in a population is affected by how many persons in that population have the disease or condition.

Because screening is generally considered to involve testing a person who does not have signs or symptoms of the disease or condition under consideration, there is a distinct contrast to the use of the same test for diagnosing a disease based on symptoms or findings. However, screening also applies to the use of tests in individuals or populations who do not have manifestations of the disease but are identified as being at high risk for the disorder because of a distinctive characteristic. Therefore, the presence of a high-risk factor may be the primary indication for screening, or it may determine the age at which screening is started or influence the frequency with which it is done.

Identification of high-risk factors by means of a medical, social, or behavioral history is becoming increasingly important, as is the physician's responsibility for detecting them. Self-administered histories offer one method by which more complete data can be obtained with an economy of physician time. A system by which risk factors are identified and displayed in the record for easy review at subsequent visits will enhance the quality of an office practice.

In addition to high-risk factors related to each age group, the physician should be aware of the leading causes of death and leading causes of morbidity of women by age group. This will assist in selective application of screening tests and efficient use of counseling time.

A new order of obstetrician-gynecologists is evolving. This is the most significant change in ambulatory care practice patterns in the history of the specialty. The emphasis is no longer placed on episodic, interventional, hospital-based medicine, but rather on an approach similar to that outlined here. This change in health care emphasis crosses many specialty lines and is underscored by a new direction in educational efforts beginning in medical school and progressing through postgraduate education. The paradigm shift is complete with attendant changes in health care economics, political influence, and interspecialty cooperation.

Domestic Violence

The problem of intimate partner (domestic) violence permeates all strata of society. It has no barrier based on age, race, and religious, educational, and

Table 1.6.   History and physical findings suggestive of abuse.

Inconsistent explanation of injuries or delay in seeking treatment
Somatic complaints
Psychiatric illness
Frequent visits to emergency department
Injuries, especially to the head and neck
Low birth weight

Source: Reprinted, with permission, from Punukollu M. *J Family Pract* 2003; 52:537–43.

socioeconomic status, etc. Unfortunately it can result in homelessness for the affected spouse and children. A definition of the problem includes "violence perpetrated against adolescent and adult females within the context of family or intimate relationships" (ACOG Educational Bulletin #257, December 1999). It is important to recognize that both males and females may be the victim, although the vast majority are women.

The National Center for Injury Prevention and Control was developed in 1993 and served to provide guidelines for evaluation and management of domestic violence. In 1994 the Violence Against Women Act (PL 103–322) was established by the federal government and provides legal protection for victims. Policies, protocols, and services are outlined in this document. Of note, women who are victims of domestic violence tend to use health care facilities more often than those who are not victims. All women should be screened, as advocated by the American Academy of Family Practice, the American College of Physicians, the American Medical Association, and the American College of Obstetricians and Gynecologists. Leaving information in a bathroom where a patient can take it without being seen is useful. A number of approaches to screening have been recommended (see Tables 1.6 and 1.7).

Table 1.7.   The HITS screen.

Hurt	How often does your partner physically hurt you?
Insult	How often does your partner insult or talk down to you?
Threaten	How often does your partner threaten you with physical harm?
Scream	How often does your partner scream or curse you?

Source: Reprinted, with permission, from Punukollu M. *J Family Pract* 2003; 52:537–43.

Domestic violence takes its toll on children. In infants, whose need for attachment tends to be disrupted, poor sleeping habits and eating habits are observed. The preschool child notes a lack of feeling safe in the home environment. In this age group separation anxiety, regressive behaviors, and insomnia are common. The school-aged child exhibits somatic complaints, self-blame, as well as both aggressive and regressive behaviors. Adolescents exhibit school truancy, delinquency, substance abuse, and early sexual activity.

When the diagnosis is suspected, the clinician should know the appropriate referral sources in the area. It is necessary to assess "immediate risk." Safety behaviors, i.e., self-protection, should be discussed and an escape plan should be part of the overall recommendation. Listening to the patient in a nonjudgmental manner is of paramount importance.

Contact resources:

National Domestic Violence Hotline: 800 799-SAFE (7233)
National Resource Center on Domestic Violence: 800 537-2238
Family Violence Prevention Fund: www.endabuse.org
Minnesota Center Against Violence and Abuse: www.mincava.edu

Substance Abuse

While we often equate the term substance abuse with illegal or "street" substances, the most common instances of substance abuse we are likely to encounter in the practice of obstetrics and gynecology involve alcohol and tobacco. Alcohol and tobacco use are ubiquitous in our society. Cigarette smoking has been labeled the largest preventable public health hazard in the United States, and nearly two-thirds of Americans over the age of 14 drink alcoholic beverages. It has been estimated that one-sixth of all deaths in the United States (almost 400,000 deaths per year) can be directly or indirectly attributed to cigarette and tobacco use. In 1990, $136 billion was spent on alcohol-related health problems. As primary care providers, we cannot ignore health risks of this magnitude.

Scope of the Problem

Alcohol

Consumption of alcoholic beverages in the United States is almost universal. Per capita annual consumption is equal to 9.7 gallons of whiskey, 89 gallons of beer, or 31 gallons of wine. Half of all the alcohol consumed is used by only 10% of drinkers (about 7% of the overall adult population). It is also this group of heavy or abusive drinkers that accounts for nearly all of the social and medical complications of alcohol use. It has been estimated that the prevalence of alcohol-related problems among hospitalized patients may be as high as 25%. In 1990, two-thirds of women of childbearing age reported being current drinkers. Of this group, 5–9% reported consuming two or more drinks per day with approximately one-third of all women continuing some level of alcohol consumption during pregnancy. It has been estimated that 7–10% of women seeking prenatal care are alcohol abusers.

Although we often presume that alcoholics are male, women are not immune; alcoholism occurs in 3.5% of all adult women. Alcohol even has different effects for women than for men: In women, serum alcohol concentrations rise faster and higher following a given dose of alcohol, even when adjusted for body weight. Women are more prone to alcohol-related medical complications than are men. Women also suffer from unique alcohol-related effects including reduced fertility, increased rates of complications of pregnancy, sexually transmitted diseases, and abuse.

Tobacco

Annual cigarette consumption has declined somewhat from its peak of 4336 cigarettes per capita in 1963 (the year before the Surgeon General's landmark report), but it still represents a dramatic increase from the 54 cigarettes per capita consumed in 1900. The rise in the popularity of smoking has been followed by an equally dramatic rise in the incidence of lung cancer deaths. Increased health awareness in general, a greater appreciation of the health risks of cigarettes specifically, and a growing social trend to restrict locations that permit smoking have resulted in a decline in cigarette use from the 1963 high. Despite this general trend, there are more than 50 million smokers in the United States. In 1990, 27% of white women between the ages of 18 and 44 still smoked and this number is up by 2% from just 5 years earlier. Roughly one million teenagers begin smoking each year. This number is important because about 90% of smokers begin smoking before the age of 20.

The onetime image of a macho-male smoker has given way to equality of the sexes, and with it, equality of health problems due to smoking. About 26% of all American women of reproductive age smoke, with about 35% of the women between the ages of 18 and 25. Somewhere between 19 and 30% of pregnant women continue to smoke during pregnancy.

Medical Impact

Alcohol

Alcohol is rapidly absorbed from the stomach and small intestines and circulated within the body. Because there is no blood–brain barrier for alcohol, neurologic symptoms appear rapidly and can persist for long periods. These symptoms can be found with blood levels of 50–150 mg/dl and are most noticeable when the levels are rising. Both short- and long-term tolerance develops rapidly, leading to progressively larger intakes of alcohol to obtain the same effects. Typical effects of alcohol are given in Table 1.8.

Alcohol has potentially deleterious effects on the entire body, ranging from nutritional deficiencies such as reduced folate and thiamine, to hepatic and cerebral damage. Women who abuse alcohol are prone to menstrual

Table 1.8.   Clinical impact and blood ethanol level.

mg/dl	Sporadic drinker	Chronic drinker
50–100	Euphoria Gregariousness Incoordination	Minimal or no effect
100–200	Slurred speech Ataxia Drowsiness Nausea	Sobriety or incoordination Euphoria
200–300	Lethargy Combative Stuporous Incoherent speech Vomiting	Mild emotional and motor changes
300–400	Coma	Drowsiness
>500	Death	Lethargy, coma

irregularities and amenorrhea, reduced fertility, and increased pregnancy losses. They also suffer the consequences of alcohol-associated problems such as depression, sexually transmitted diseases, abuse, and assault. Alcohol is both a morphologic and behavioral teratogen with an estimated 5000 newborns per year affected by fetal alcohol syndrome.

Tobacco

Tobacco has been used for almost 15 centuries, though the medical impact of its use has only been known for the past 30 years. Tobacco use began with religious ceremonies by the Mayans and spread north to the native Americans who greeted European explorers. Introduced into Europe by the returning voyagers, most of the known world was using tobacco by the mid-seventeenth century. Though the southern states found tobacco a major cash crop even in colonial times, it took the development of cigarette-making machines in the 1880s, American's involvement in two world wars, and aggressive marketing to change the popularity and image of cigarettes.

Tobacco smoke is made up of pyrolysis and distillation products in a particulate and gas phase that is composed of some 4000 compounds and constituents. The particulate matter (once water and nicotine have been removed) is what makes up "tar." The gas phase of smoke contains a high concentration of carbon monoxide as well as other irritating and ciliotoxic agents. The risks attributable to smoking are related to these chemicals, the person's smoking habits, environmental exposure, and other risk factors. Risk increases with the number of cigarettes smoked, depth of inhalation, and the duration of the smoking habit. There is evidence that these risks are magnified when smoking begins at an earlier age. Risks do return to roughly normal if a person can stop smoking for 10 years or longer.

It is well documented that smoking is associated with large increases in the risk for heart disease, lung cancer, and other cancers. Smoking contributes greatly to chronic lung disease, peptic ulcer, esophageal reflux, and bladder cancer. Smoking is associated with a less favorable course in patients with Crohn's disease. Paradoxically, smoking cessation is associated with the onset or worsening of ulcerative colitis.

Women who smoke have lower fertility rates, more frequent ovulatory dysfunction, and earlier menopause, and increased rates of tubal pregnancy and spontaneous abortion. Once pregnancy is established, smokers have higher rates of pregnancy complications including premature rupture of the membranes, prematurity, and low-birth-weight infants.

Establishing the Diagnosis

While it would seem easy to spot the patient who is abusing alcohol or tobacco, it is often well hidden because of the stigma that is increasingly placed on the use of these substances. When we realize that the greatest impact we can have will be with those patients who have not yet reached the extremes of use, some form of strategy for diagnosis is in order.

Alcohol

Establishing the presence of alcohol abuse or dependence is not as simple as determining the amount of alcohol consumed per day or month (e.g., greater than 45 drinks per month or 5 per day). While these may be indicators of problems, the diagnosis of alcohol abuse requires evidence of craving, tolerance, and physical dependence (see Table 1.9). Screening for alcohol-related problems may be based on either intake measures (such as the Single Screening Question or the Ten Question Drinking History) or outcome measures (such as the NET, TWEAK, CAGE, TACE, or SMAST questionnaires). Examples of these questionnaires are shown in Tables 1.10–1.15. For complete information on the application and scoring of these tools, please consult the relevant references provided.

Laboratory studies are of limited help in assessing alcohol use or abuse. Blood ethanol levels of greater than 0.1 mg% on a random sample, greater than 0.15 mg% without signs of intoxication, or a level of greater than 0.3 mg% at any time are indications of abuse. Suggestive of abuse are elevated liver enzymes, bilirubin, amylase, or prothrombin times. Similarly,

Table 1.9.   Criteria for alcohol abuse and dependence.

Abuse (at least 1)
  Use despite awareness of harm
  Recurrent hazardous use
  Symptoms of greater than 1 month or recurrence
Dependence (any three)
  Larger amounts or over a longer time than intended
  Persistent desire or failed attempts to quit
  Larger amount of time spent to obtain or recover from alcohol
  Intoxication or withdrawal that affects life obligations (school, work,
    family)
  Social changes to accommodate alcohol
  Continued use in face of adverse impact
  Tolerance leading to increased use
  Has experienced symptoms of withdrawal
  Use of alcohol to avoid withdrawal

Source: Reprinted from American Journal of Obstetrics and Gynecology, Mullen, PD,
"Identifying Pregnant Women", pg. 1429–1430, Copyright 1985, with permission
from Elsevier.

decreased blood urea nitrogen (BUN) or serum protein is suggestive, but
not diagnostic. Depression, anxiety, bipolar personality disorders, diabetes,
gastritis, and solar skin damage may all mimic alcohol abuse and must be
considered.

Table 1.10.   Intake based screening questionnaires for alcohol abuse.

Single screening question
  Which describes your use?
    1.   I drink regularly now (unchanged)
    2.   I drink regularly now, but less
    3.   I drink once in a while
    4.   I have quit drinking
    5.   I wasn't drinking (still not)
Ten question drinking history
  For beer, wine, and liquor:
    How often?
    How much?
    Ever more?
  Any change in the past year?

Source: Reprinted from American Journal of Obstetrics and Gynecology, Mullen, PD,
"Identifying Pregnant Women", pg. 1429–1430, Copyright 1985, with permission
from Elsevier.

Table 1.11. The NET questionnaire.

Do you consider yourself a **N**ormal drinker?
Do you ever have an **E**ye-opener?
How many drinks does it **T**ake to get high?

Source: Bottoms SF, Martier SS, Sokol RJ. Refinements in screening for risk drinking in reproductive-aged women: the "NET" results. Alcoholism 1989; 13: 339.

Table 1.12. The "TWEAK" test.

Tolerance: How many drinks does it take to feel the first effects?
Have friends or relatives **W**orried or complained about your drinking?
Eye-opener: Do you sometimes take a drink in the morning when you first get up?
Amnesia: Are there times when you drink and can't remember afterward what you said or did?
Do you sometimes feel the need to **K**(c)ut down on your drinking?

Source: Susan S Sokol, Russell M, Robert J. Mudar, Pamela Bottoms, Sidney Jacobsen, Joseph Jacobson (1994) Screening for Pregnancy Risk Drinking Alcoholism: Clinical and Experimental Research, 19(5): 1156–1161. Blackwell Publishing.

Table 1.13. The CAGE questionnaire.

Have you ever felt the need to **C**ut down on drinking? What was it like? Were you successful? Why did you decide to cut down?
Have you ever felt **A**nnoyed by criticism of your drinking? What caused the worry or concern? Do you ever get irritated by their worry? Have you ever limited what you drink to please someone?
Have you ever felt **G**uilty about your drinking, or about something you said or did while you were drinking? Have you ever been bothered by anything you said or did while you were drinking? Have you ever regretted anything that has happened while you were drinking?
Have you ever taken a morning "**E**ye-opener" drink? Have you ever felt shaky or tremulous after a night of heavy drinking? What did you do to relieve the shakiness? Have you ever had trouble getting back to sleep early in the morning after a night of heavy drinking?

Source: Ewing, JA (1984) Detecting Alcoholism: The CAGE Questionnaire. JAMA: Journal of the American Medical Association, 252, 1905–1907.

Table 1.14.   The TACE questionnaire.

How many drinks does it take to make you feel "high"? (Tolerance)
Have people Annoyed you by criticizing your drinking?
Have you ever felt you ought to Cut down on your drinking?
Have you ever had a drink first thing in the morning to steady your nerves
or to get rid of a hangover? (Eye-opener)

Source: Sokol RJ, Martier SS, Ager JW. The T-ACE questions: Practical prenatal detection of risk-drinking. Am J Obstet Gynecol. 1989 Apr; 160(4): 863–870.

Cigarettes

Unlike alcohol abuse, cigarette use and abuse are more likely to be accurately reported by the patient when questioned. To assess the risk of tobacco use, the amount and duration of use are established. For cigarettes, this is expressed as the number of "pack-years" (packs per day times years of use). The depth of inhalation, the age at which smoking began, and the presence of other risk factors all play a part in the medical impact of the smoking habit. Potentially just as dangerous is environmental exposure to cigarette smoke. It has been

Table 1.15.   The SMAST questionnaire.

Do you feel you are a normal drinker—that is, do you drink less than or as much as most other people?
Does your partner, a parent, or other close relative ever worry or complain about your drinking?
Do you ever feel guilty about your drinking?
Do friends or relatives think you are a normal drinker?
Are you able to stop drinking when you want to?
Have you ever attended a meeting of Alcoholics Anonymous?
Has drinking ever created problems between you and your partner, a parent, or other close relative?
Have you ever gotten in trouble at work because of drinking?
Have you ever neglected your obligations, your family, or your work for 2 or more days in a row because you were drinking?
Have you ever gone to anyone for help about your drinking?
Have you ever been in a hospital because of drinking?
Have you ever been arrested for drunken driving, driving while intoxicated, or driving under the influence of alcohol?
Have you ever been arrested, even for a few hours, because of other drunken behavior?

Source: Adapted with permission from Selzer ML, et al. A Self-Administered Short Version of the Michigan Alcoholism Screening Test (SMAST). Journal of Studies on Alcohol, 36:117–126, 1975.

Table 1.16.   Indications of cigarette addiction.

1. Do you smoke your first cigarette within 30 minutes of waking up in the morning?
2. Do you smoke 20 cigarettes (one pack) or more each day?
3. At times when you can't smoke or haven't got any cigarettes, do you feel a craving for one?
4. Is it tough for you to keep from smoking for more than a few minutes?
5. When you are sick enough to stay in bed, do you still smoke?

Two or more "yes" answers may mean addiction

estimated that between 500 and 5000 cancer deaths a year are due to "second-hand" smoke exposure and wives of one pack-per-day smokers have a two-fold increase in their risk of developing lung cancer. Questions that can help assess the degree of cigarette dependence are listed in Table 1.16.

Medical Interventions

Clearly, intervention to decrease the risks caused by alcohol and tobacco is appropriate. Many studies indicate that interest, support, and counseling (with referral when needed) by a physician greatly increase the chances of a patient altering risky behaviors.

Alcohol Interventions

The cornerstone of intervention to decrease alcohol use is nonjudgmental support. Care must be taken to safeguard the medical condition of the patient during the process. This is done by providing nutritional support through multivitamins and thiamine (100 mg IM). Sedation and seizure precautions during acute withdrawal are necessary, though cross-tolerance to sedatives may require increased dosages (e.g., diazepam 5–10 mg every 4–6 hours). Seizures may develop in up to one-third of patients during the first 12–24 hours of withdrawal. Seizures may occur after as few as 5–7 days of binge drinking. Phenytoin will not prevent alcohol withdrawal seizures. Delirium tremens may occur abruptly after 2–4 days and end just as rapidly 1–3 days later. Death, generally due to injury or dehydration, may occur in up to 15% of cases. The best success rates for long-term alcohol withdrawal come through trained detoxification centers and will involve the help of the patient's friends and family.

Smoking Cessation

Forty-five percent of people who have ever smoked have quit. Despite this number, two-thirds of current smokers are not ready to take any action to quit. Because 65% of those who quit smoking will relapse within 3 months, continuing support is required. Often all that can realistically be accomplished in any one encounter is to move the patient gradually along toward eventual cessation. For those who have never considered quitting, we can get them to start considering it, for those who have thought about it, get them to try, and for those who have failed in the past, get them to try again. Modification of the patient's habits and environment will be required in addition to addressing nicotine withdrawal.

Nicotine withdrawal is characterized not only by a craving for tobacco, but also by irritability, anxiety, hostility, restlessness and difficulty concentrating, drowsiness with insomnia, headaches, and altered appetite. These symptoms will begin as soon as 24 hours into the withdrawal process. Women smokers generally report more withdrawal symptoms than men. To help combat these symptoms, transdermal nicotine has been useful in conjunction with smoking cessation programs. In one trial, success rates of 61%, and 48% were achieved with 21- and 14-mg transdermal patches, versus 27% for the placebo group (group counseling only). In general, nicotine replacement therapy is of greatest help to those who smoke more than 20 cigarettes a day.

Most smoking cessation plans advocate stopping smoking all at once ("cold turkey") rather than tapering the amount smoked or switching to lower tar cigarettes. Unlike other types of addiction, nicotine withdrawal is only prolonged and not eased by tapering the dose. Most smokers who switch to lower tar or nicotine cigarettes will, unconsciously, increase their use to deliver the same net doses of nicotine.

Any smoking cessation program must take into consideration the patient's fears of weight gain and oral cravings. These are best addressed early and in a positive way. Increasing fluid intake (not alcohol), the use of chewing gum, eating raw vegetables, and avoiding skipping of meals will all help to decrease these problems.

Suggested Reading

American College of Obstetricians and Gynecologists. Primary and preventive care; periodic assessments. ACOG Committee Opinion 246. Washington, DC: ACOG; 2000.

American College of Obstetricians and Gynecologists. *Guidelines for Women's Health Care,* 2nd ed. Washington, DC: American College of Obstetricians and Gynecologists; 2002.

Bartman BA, Weiss KB. Women's primary care in the United States: a study of practice variation among physician specialties. *J Women's Health* 1993; 2:261–8.

Laube DW. Precis: *Primary and Preventive Care,* 2nd ed. 1998.

Leader S, Percales PJ. Provision of primary-preventive health care services by obstetrician-gynecologists. *Obstet Gynecol* 1995;85(3):391–5.

2

Pediatric and Adolescent Patients

Mary Anne Jamieson and Joseph S. Sanfilippo

Introduction

The field of pediatric and adolescent gynecology (PAG) encompasses a host of clinical conditions spanning a variety of disciplines and specialties. Primary care providers including obstetricians and gynecologists are often called upon to diagnose and treat problems of the genitourinary system that occur in children and adolescents, especially when a subspecialist is not available. Even in centers where there is PAG expertise, a working knowledge and understanding of the common clinical problems can be very useful in determining if and when a referral is necessary. Table 2.1 lists those scenarios under the pediatric and adolescent gynecology umbrella and it will serve as a framework for this chapter.

Prepubertal Vulvovaginitis

Vulvovaginitis is a somewhat descriptive term used often to imply any combination of genital irritation or pruritis, vaginal discharge or odor, and vulvar erythema or inflammation. It is probably better to use the term vulvitis when there are complaints or findings isolated to the external genitalia and the term vaginitis when referring to vaginal discharge or odor and to reserve the term vulvovaginitis when there is a combination of both (Fig. 2.1).

Table 2.1.   Clinical scenarios in pediatric and adolescent gynecology.

Vulvovaginitis	The first gynecologic examination
Genital bleeding in childhood	Menstrual dysfunction
Abnormal/ambiguous genitalia	Amenorrhea
Childhood sexual abuse	Androgen disorders
Pubertal aberrancy	Pelvic pain
Müllerian anomalies	Adolescent sexuality
Breast abnormalities	Contraception
Pelvic masses	Adolescent pregnancy
	Sexually transmitted infections

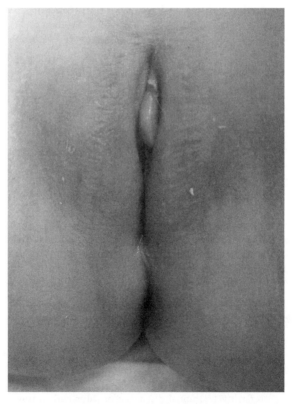

Fig. 2.1. Chronic vulvovaginitis.

Vulvitis

External genital irritation often accompanied by erythema or inflammation (vulvitis) is most often a consequence of irritants or allergens, but infection and dermopathy should also be considered. Identifying the underlying cause or contributor(s) is paramount to proper treatment and obtaining a meticulous history cannot be overstated. Once identified, irritants or allergens should be eliminated and plain water tub soaks (three times per day initially) should be reinforced. Some advocate bath products such as oatmeal colloidal "Aveeno®" to soothe, but plain water is often all that is necessary. Very rarely a mild corticosteroid ointment used sparingly will be necessary to facilitate resolution, but conservative strategies should be maintained to prevent recurrence.

There are very few organisms that cause vulvitis without vaginitis. Group A streptococcus would be one example. Often there is a history of coexisting or preceding strep throat or impetigo and a penicillin agent would be indicated. Finally, dermopathies such as lichen sclerosis and eczema can exist on the vulva necessitating mild to moderate potency corticosteroid ointments used sparingly. Conservative strategies such as plain water soaks and avoidance of irritants and allergens are paramount with these conditions too.

Vaginitis

Vaginitis is most often caused by colonization of the vagina with fecal or upper respiratory tract (URT) flora. The anatomy of the prepubertal child is such that there is easy access of bacteria into the vagina because of its close proximity to the anus. There is often a history of fecal soiling in undergarments from inadequate wiping or a history of wiping back to front. Similarly, chronic rhinitis or nose-picking would raise suspicion of colonization with upper respiratory infection (URI) flora. The discharge from vaginitis can create a secondary vulvitis (vulvovaginitis). If swabs are to be taken from the vagina, gentle labial traction allowing the hymen to gape open will facilitate passage of a calgiswab without contact with the hymenal edge. While a calgiswab is often used, some clinicians prefer a nasal dropper filled with saline to gently irrigate the vagina and collect a specimen. Using labial traction is the only acceptable way to perform vaginal sampling without causing pain or discomfort and every effort should be made to accomplish this assuming a culture is considered necessary even if it requires an assistant. Treatment involves increased attention to hygiene and toileting along with plain water tub soaks. Occasionally a broad-spectrum antibiotic such as clavulanate potassium/amoxicillin trihydrate is necessary for 7 days to clear up the current problem, but diligent soaks, good hand-washing, and wiping front to back should be encouraged to prevent recurrence. In the event that the discharge clears up while on antibiotics then recurs almost immediately or in the event that the discharge is bloody or particularly malodorous, consideration should be given to a vaginal foreign body (Fig. 2.2C) and vaginoscopy

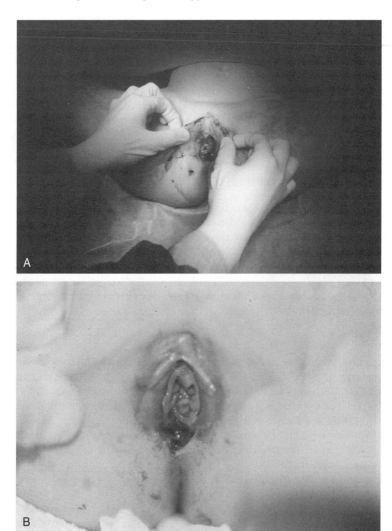

Fig. 2.2. (A) Straddle injury sparing hymen. (B) Deliberate penetrating genital injury (hymen transected).

Fig. 2.2. (C) Vaginal foreign body seen with labial separation. (D) Hemangioma (of scalp). (E) Diaper from 10-day-old female: neonatal estrogen-withdrawal bleed.

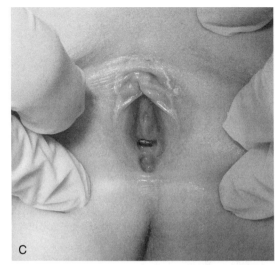

C

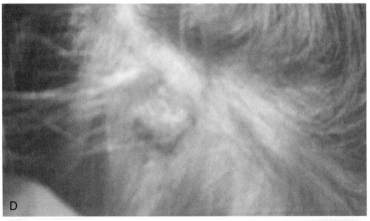

D

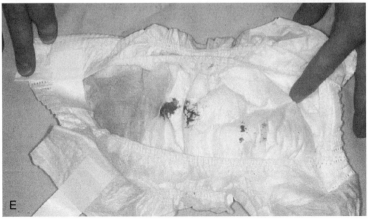

E

should be performed. Various techniques are used for vaginoscopy including pediatric speculums and hysteroscopes with warmed saline to visualize the vagina, but anesthetics may be necessary and these procedures should be performed by qualified providers.

Table 2.2 lists the most common underlying etiologies for vulvitis, vaginitis, and the combination vulvovaginitis. Of particular importance is the recognition that *Candida* is usually not the "culprit" unless the child is still in diapers, is diabetic, is immunocompromised, or has received recent antibiotics. Pinworms predominantly present with extreme pruritis that can awaken the child from sleep. Scratching can, in turn, cause genital soreness. Fortunately, while sexual child abuse must always be considered, sexually transmitted infections (STIs) account for very few cases of vulvitis, vaginitis, or vulvovaginitis. Table 2.3 can be used as a handout for children and their caregivers to address good genital care.

Table 2.2. Vulvitis in childhood.

Irritants/allergens
  Bath products
  Urine
  Chlorine
  Trapped moisture and heat (noncotton undergarments, leotards, sports equipment)
  Laundry product residue
  Topical products
  Trauma/friction
Infections
  Fecal flora
  Upper respiratory flora
  Group A streptococcus
  Pinworms
  Foreign body: toilet paper, small toys, etc.
  Candida[a]
  Sexually transmitted organisms[a]
Dermopathy
  Lichen sclerosis
  Eczema, psoriasis

[a] See text.

Table 2.3.   Genital care in childhood.

The following suggestions may be helpful in reducing or eliminating genital itch or irritation with or without a vaginal discharge in the female child:

1. Tub soaks with warm water (nothing added ____X per day including after each bowel movement. After tub soaks, air dry–blow dry
2. Cotton uderwear only
3. Avoid use of nylon tights, leotards or other tight clothing
4. Don't sleep in restrictive garments that cause sweating
5. Rinse underwear after washing/drying to remove any detergent or fabic softener residues
6. Hypoallergenic soap (if necessary), rinsed well
7. Eliminate any potential irritants or allergens such as bubble bath, lotions or creams, panty liners, colored or fragranced toilet paper
8. Don't stay long in wet bathing suits
9. In the context of urinary incontinence (wetting), change to dry underwear frequently
10. Improve urinary incontinence by encouraging regular voiding at least six times per day (including before bed and first thing in the morning)
11. Encourage thorough hand washing BEFORE and AFTER washroom use
12. Eliminate constipation by using fruits, vegetables, plenty of fluids, and fiber in the diet. Regular daily BMs must be encouraged
13. Continue these measures even after the problem has resolved

---

Genital Bleeding in Childhood

Any of the vulvovaginitis conditions discussed previously can cause inflammation and irritation that results in a minor amount of bleeding. Repeated scratching can cause small fissures and excoriation and in addition to the treatment strategies mentioned above, it may be necessary to add a medication such as hydroxyzine hydrochloride ("Atarax®"), especially at bedtime, if nighttime scratching is a problem. Unfortunately, drowsiness can often result from antihistamine-type medications limiting their use during the day. Other causes of genital bleeding in childhood include hymenal/vaginal polyps, inadvertent trauma (straddle injuries, rarely penetrating injuries), deliberate trauma (abuse), a vaginal foreign body, urethral prolapse, hemangiomas, premature menarche, and a neonatal estrogen withdrawal bleed (Fig. 2.2). Sinister malignancies such as rhabdomyosarcoma are fortunately very rare, but vaginoscopy with or without anesthetic would be indicated if unexplained vaginal bleeding occurs or recurs.

With estrogen exposure *in utero, hymenal/vaginal tags and polyps* may grow such that they protrude from the introitus in the neonate. While a genital examination should be performed with labial traction to determine the etiology and origin of any introital mass in a child, reassurance is often all that is needed once the diagnosis has been made. As the estrogen environment is withdrawn, the polyp regresses and seldom requires any intervention. Caregivers should be aware that occasionally the polyp will lose its smooth resilient surface (a consequence of estrogen) before it retracts to within the confines and shelter of the labia. This can lead to ulceration and bleeding, albeit scant.

Straddle injuries (Fig. 2.2A), involve a clear, consistent, and plausible history or mechanism of injury. The child need only be taken for EUA, etc., if the child cannot void, there is ongoing bleeding, there is an expanding or large hematoma that needs to be evacuated, anal sphincter integrity may have been compromised, or a penetrating injury is suspected and the upper vagina must be inspected. Soaks should be encouraged and the child may even need to void in water to avoid stinging. Intermittent ice packs to reduce swelling are useful, analgesics should be provided, and follow-up arranged. Inadvertent straddle-type injuries very rarely tear the hymen or lower vagina. If the hymen has been compromised (Fig. 2.2B), an assessment for abuse by experienced and skilled care provider(s) should be undertaken.

Urethral prolapse presents with either blood in the undergarments, dysuria, or hematuria. There will be a beefy red and somewhat friable ring of tissue around the urethral meatus. There is often a history of repeated valsalva either from constipation, urinary tract infection, or chronic cough. This condition occurs in hypoestrogenic females such as the prepubertal child or the postmenopausal woman. It is not a condition of the neonate because of maternal and placental estrogen exposure. Treatment involves resolving the repeated valsalva problem and using topical estrogen. The urethral mucosa will often then regress over a few days to a few weeks. Excision, may be necessary if conservative treatment fails or if the problem is recurrent.

Premature menarche can occur in isolation, but most often will coexist with thelarche as evidence of estrogen exposure. It is important to look for and stage other signs of puberty as discussed later in this chapter (pubertal aberrancy).

A *neonatal estrogen-withdrawal bleed* (Fig. 2.2E) presents as a small self-limited episode of vaginal bleeding that occurs between 1 and 3 weeks of life as the result of *in utero* exposure to maternal and placental estrogens. Reassurance is all that is needed.

Abnormal Genitalia

Hymenal Variations

There are a number of variants of hymenal shape. Most commonly, the hymenal shape is circular/annular, horseshoe/crescentic, or fimbriated (Fig. 2.3). These are considered normal variants, whereas other configurations such as sleeve-

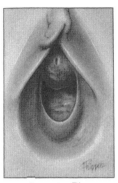
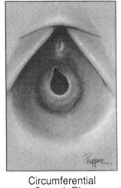
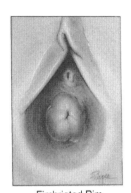

Posterior Rim

Circumferential
Smooth Rim

Fimbriated Rim

Fig. 2.3. Hymenal variants. (Reprinted from Pokorny SF: Configurations of the prepubertal hymen. *Am J Obstet Gynecol* 1987;157:950–56, Copyright 1987, with permission from Elsevier.)

like, septated, cribriform or fenestrated, microperforate, and imperforate may cause symptoms or sequelae. The cribriform, microperforate, and imperforate hymens must be surgically corrected (hymenotomy or modified hymenotomy) to allow adequate drainage of menstrual blood, prevent or treat hematocolpos, and allow for tampon insertion or intercourse. Essentially a square introitus is created and reabsorbable sutures are placed around the perimeter for hemostasis. This requires an anesthetic. The patient with a septate hymen may present with difficulty inserting or removing tampons, difficulty with intercourse, or even postcoital bleeding. The latter occurs when this band gets torn. Bleeding is often self-limited but occasionally will require a few reabsorbable sutures for hemostasis. The remnant can be removed, but a ligature/suture should be placed for hemostasis at the point(s) of attachment to the vaginal or hymenal mucosa. Often this type of procedure can be performed on a post-pubertal patient in the office setting with or without local anesthetic.

Hymenal/Vaginal Polyps or Tags

See the section on Genital Bleeding.

Labial Agglutination (Fig. 2.4)

Labial adhesions form between the labia minora of prepubertal girls when the labia are allowed to lie in apposition for extended periods of time. There may be an episode of inflammation that serves as a precipitant, but that is not a prerequisite. Urine may become trapped behind the wall of the labia causing postvoid dribbling after the child stands up from the toilet. Trapped secretions and urine can cause a secondary inflammation that leads to genital irritation. In the

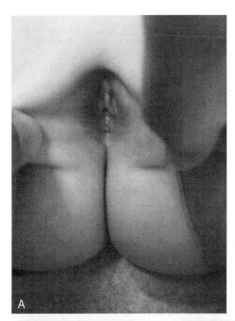

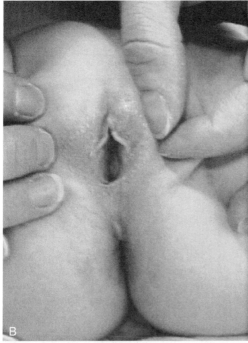

Fig. 2.4. (A) Labial agglutination. (B) Posttopical estrogen therapy with successful separation.

worst case scenario, the child may present with urinary retention or incomplete emptying with or without a urinary tract infection. The examination is diagnostic revealing a translucent or gray line running from somewhere under the clitoral hood posteriorly to the perineal body (Fig. 2.4A). Efforts at gentle labial traction fail to reveal the introitus/hymen or urethral meatus. There will be no scrotalization of the labia and no clitoromegaly in contrast to ambiguous genitalia with congenital labial fusion. The condition of labial adhesions is acquired as opposed to congenital, but often the caregiver assumes the child was born with the fusion, especially if genital care has not often involved labial separation. Treatment depends on the urgency of the situation. Unless there is concern over a coexisting urinary tract infection (UTI) or urinary retention, topical estrogen cream can be applied with gentle traction to the line of agglutination every night. The adhesions should separate within 3 weeks (Fig. 2.4). Follow-up is recommended. Occasionally, manual separation is required and this does necessitate some form of sedation, but can be accomplished with flavored midazolam in the clinic setting (Table 2.4) although some clinicians prefer more complete anaesthesia in the operating room. Recurrence is a problem with this condition unless the caregiver is educated and diligently inspects the introitus with labial separation at least twice per week. The principle is to avoid prolonged episodes in which the labia lie in apposition to one another and have the opportunity to reagglutinate. After puberty, the problem should not recur.

Ambiguous Genitalia (Fig. 2.5)

The birth of an infant with ambiguous genitalia can be a devastating experience for parents and a challenge to all caregivers. It is essential to have a logical approach to determining the underlying etiology and to gathering data in a timely

Table 2.4.   Sedation in clinic with midazolam.

Chocolate flavored mixture 3 mg/ml
0.75 mg/kg to maximum dose of 20 mg
If child weighs more than 27 kg, then results not optimal

Alternatively:
Acetaminophen elixir 80 mg/ml or 160 mg/5 ml
15–20 mg/kg
mixed with 0.5–1.0 mg/kg of injectable midazolam

Administer midazolam 30–45 minutes prior to procedure
Child should be supervised ± O_2 saturation monitor

Topical lidocaine/prilocaine (EMLA) cream 30 minutes prior to procedure when indicated

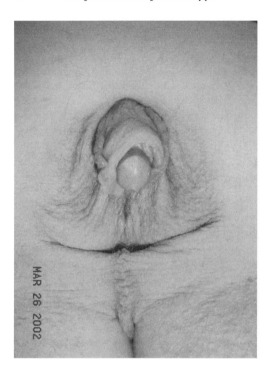

Fig. 2.5. Ambiguous genitalia.

fashion so as to manage the child medically and/or surgically and counsel the family insightfully. Fortunately the birth of a child with ambiguous genitalia is rare. The workup and management of the newborn with ambiguous genitalia should be performed by a multidisciplinary team and should involve specialists in neonatology, genetics, pediatric gynecology and/or pediatric urology, social work, and nursing. Ethicists may even be necessary when sex of rearing is being addressed. Any primary care physician who encounters this clinical scenario should be supportive toward the parents but refrain from speculating about the gender of the infant until all facts have been gathered. It is often helpful to emphasize to the parents that they have a "beautiful (and healthy) baby but that the genitals have not properly formed which is making it difficult at this time to tell whether the child is male or female." The infant may be an overvirilized female (female pseudohermaphrodite), an undervirilized male (male pseudohermaphrodite), a true hermaphrodite or have more complex gonadal dysgenesis. Salt-wasting 21-hydroxylase deficiency congenital adrenal hyperplasia is one of the most important diagnoses to be considered and is the diagnosis that accounts for the largest number of ambiguous genitalia cases. These newborns can be lacking in both glucocorticoids and mineralocorticoids, which can lead to sodium and potassium imbalance and life-threatening cortisol deficiency. In this context the child will be an overvirilized female with internal female organs but can present with a spectrum of labial fusion, clitoromegaly, and urethral/vaginal malformations.

Vaginal Agenesis (Fig. 2.6)

Patients born without a vagina are most often going to have a condition known as Mayer–Rokitansky Kuster Hauser (MRKH) syndrome. In this condition, the patient has a normal 46,XX karyotype, normal ovaries, and normal pubertal development but presents with primary amenorrhea. A Müllerian remnant may be present and it may contain endometrium. If there is a trapped nidus of endometrium, the patient may complain of intermittent lower abdominal cramps very similar in character to dysmenorrhea but without coexisting flow. This is termed cryptomenorrhea, "hidden menses," and if the patient is ovulating regularly, there will be a monthly pattern to her complaints. Even when the uterus has a focus of endometrium within its cavity, there is often cervical hypoplasia and it is extremely rare to be able to surgically create anatomy capable of reproduction. Specialist involvement is essential in the care of these patients. Having said that, surgical vaginoplasty has become second-line and the preferred method of creating a vagina, if only for sexual function, is through

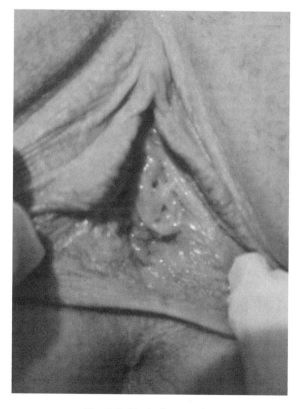

Fig. 2.6. Vaginal agenesis.

patient-centered dilators. These patients need their renal anatomy and their spine imaged for well-recognized coexisting anomalies.

When a patient is found to have a blind-ended or absent vagina, the two other conditions to be considered are imperforate hymen and an androgen action disorder such as androgen insensitivity syndrome (AIS) (testicular feminization). An imperforate hymen may be recognized by a conscientious care provider who includes a mini-genital examination with childhood visits. Most often, however, the peripubertal young woman presents with pain or urinary retention approximately 1–2 years after thelarche when menstrual blood has accumulated within the vagina. Genital inspection reveals a bulging introitus and rectal examination confirms a mass anteriorly (hematocolpos). Assuming an imperforate hymen has been ruled out, a physical examination showing normal axillary and pubic hair usually discriminates MRKH syndrome from AIS. In contrast to patients with Mayer–Rokitansky syndrome who have normal pubic and axillary hair, patients with AIS do not (although they may have some). Other distinguishing features include male level serum testosterone and male karyotype found in AIS patients. AIS patients need to have their gonads removed after puberty because of the risk of malignancy. Patients with partial AIS can present with ambiguous genitalia (see above) but patients with complete AIS appear phenotypically female. Both acquire breasts at puberty and experience primary amenorrhea because they do not have a uterus.

Labial Hypertrophy

Labia minora are seldom the exact same size and shape. Patients who present with concerns over the appearance of the labia often only need reassurance. Patients in whom the labia minora are significantly redundant can present with problematic genital irritation, problems with athletic activities, and/or problems with intercourse. In the former, secretions accumulate in the redundant genital folds and cause irritation or pruritis. Bathtub soaks daily may be all that is required. Some patients find the hypertrophied labia particularly bothersome as it/they get(s) caught in the elastic of undergarments or get(s) drawn up into the vagina with intercourse or tampon insertion. In these patients, surgical resection of the hypertrophied labia whether unilateral or bilateral is effective but is best performed under anesthetic and with appropriate pre-surgical discussion of risks and benefits.

Pubertal Aberrancy

Puberty is now considered delayed in a girl if there has been no sign of secondary sexual characteristics by the age of 14 years. Similarly, any secondary sexual characteristics before the age of 8 is still considered precocious, but we now recognize that up to 15% of "normal" African-American girls will have breast development and/or early pubic hair at age 7–8. Specifically, based on odds ratios, menarche occurs earlier in Mexican-American girls than in white or African-American girls. However, African-American girls experienced menarche on average 3 months earlier than white girls, i.e., 12.3 versus 12.6 years of age respectively. These findings were part of the Bogalusa, Louisiana Heart Study, which evaluated a semirural community. Furthermore, less than 10% of American girls reach menarche before 11 years of age and 90% menstruate by 13.75 years, with a median age of 12.43. Figure 2.7 is a useful tool in guiding

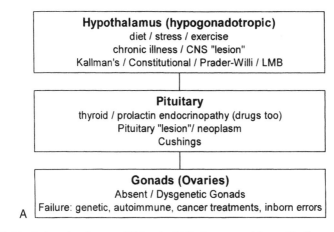

Fig. 2.7A. Delayed puberty—HPO axis. LMB, Laurence–Moon–Biedl.

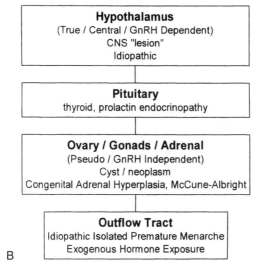

Fig. 2.7B. Precocious puberty—HPO axis.

Table 2.5.   Basic Workup.[a]

For delayed puberty
CBC, FSH, LH, TSH, estradiol
Ultrasound pelvis
Bone age
When indicated: CT or MRI head, karyotype, bone density, autoimmune
   workup, MRI pelvis

For precocious puberty
CBC, FSH, LH (+/− GnRH stimulation test), TSH, prolactin, estradiol
Ultrasound pelvis
Bone age
When indicated: CT or MRI head, imaging adrenals, serum androgens

---

[a] CBC, complete blood count; FSH, follicle-stimulating hormone; LH, luteinizing hormone; TSH, thyroid-stimulating hormone; GnRH, gonadotropin-releasing hormone.

the history and physical examination (H&P) and laboratory investigations when trying to sort out the patient with delayed or precocious puberty. Note that there are several underlying etiologies and conditions that are common to both. Table 2.5 provides a basic set of guidelines for investigating delayed and precocious puberty. Accessory testing will depend on the findings of the H&P and laboratory investigations and might include a computed tomography (CT) scan or magnetic resonance imaging (MRI) of the brain, imaging of the adrenals, karyotype, bone density, and serum androgens. The basic principles of therapy include identifying and treating the underlying cause, searching for and treating comorbidities, normalizing the pubertal stage and progress, preserving the final stature/height, optimizing bone density, and educating the patient and her family.

Menstrual Dysfunction

The most common menstrual disturbance in an adolescent is menometrorrhagia (heavy and irregular menses) occurring as a consequence of hypothalamic/pituitary/ovarian (HPO) axis immaturity. The average female takes 1–2 years after menarche to establish regular ovulatory cycles. Some remain anovulatory or oligoovulatory and this may be idiopathic or due to a variant of polycystic ovarian syndrome (PCOS). Often care providers need only provide reassurance and communicate expectations, especially if the young woman has just begun to menstruate within the past few years. If, however, the young woman is finding unpredictable or heavy flow to be dysfunctional, then intervention is warranted, if only temporarily, until the physiologic maturation process is complete. Combined oral contraceptives (OCPs) are an excellent and safe medical option to regulate cycles and decrease flow. Alternatives include progestins, nonsteroidal antiinflammatory drugs (NSAIDs), and even antifibrinolytics. When the primary complaint is menorrhagia (heavy but regular flow), and it is severe enough to cause anemia, then coagulopathy should be ruled out. Von Willebrand's disease, idiopathic or immune thrombocytopenia, and even medications/drugs can cause a bleeding disorder. Even in the context of coagulopathy, however, OCPs are often effective at reducing flow.

Dysmenorrhea can be problematic for the adolescent causing her to miss school or activities. NSAIDs and OCPs are very useful in the treatment of primary/physiologic dysmenorrhea. If the combination of OCPs and aggressively administered NSAIDs fails to treat dysmenorrhea, consideration should be given to the possibility of endometriosis, Müllerian anomalies, or even chronic pelvic adhesions. In fact, it is estimated that 50% of adolescents with dysmenorrhea or chronic pelvic pain failing to respond to conventional therapy will have endometriosis. Table 2.6 lists a complete differential diagnosis for dysmenorrhea and pelvic pain in adolescent females.

Figure 2.8 represents a revised hypothalamic/pituitary/ovary/outflow tract (HPOO) axis to assist in the assessment of an adolescent with menstrual dysfunction. Very few of the etiologies listed in Fig. 2.8 will present the same way in all patients and in fact many of the items listed also appear in Fig. 2.7. The spectrum of clinical presentation will depend on when the disorder is acquired and how severe it becomes. For example, an anorexic patient early in the course of her disordered eating may present with irregular menses only if the onset is postmenarche, or she may present with delayed puberty and primary amenorrhea if she begins the eating disorder behavior prior to puberty. The exceptions include Female Kallman's syndrome and ovarian agenesis or dysgenesis, which will, with very rare exception, always present with delayed puberty and primary amenorrhea. Similarly, vaginal agenesis and androgen insensitivity will always present as primary amenorrhea. Recall that the first menses is expected within 4 years of thelarche or by the age of 16, and when these criteria are not met, the patient should be considered to have *primary amenorrhea* and assessed as appropriate.

The key to diagnosing and treating menstrual dysfunction in teens is a focused history and physical examination taking into consideration the HPOO axis schematic in Fig. 2.8. Key features are outlined in Table 2.7.

Table 2.6. Causes of recurrent pelvic pain and dysmenorrhea in adolescence.

Genitourinary
Primary dysmenorrhea
Mittelschmerz
Ovarian cyst/neoplasm: torsion/hemorrhage/rupture/infection
Endometriosis
Pelvic inflammatory disease/chronic pelvic adhesions
Müllerian anomalies and outflow obstruction
Pregnancy-related complications
Urinary tract infection or calculus
Pelvic kidney
Interstitial cystitis

Gastrointestinal
Constipation
Inflammatory bowel disease
Irritable bowel syndrome, lactose intolerance
Meckel's diverticulum, volvulus, intestinal obstruction
Infectious diarrhea disorder or gastroenteritis
Appendicitis
Mesenteric adenitis
Hernia

Musculoskeletal system
Myofascial pain syndromes
Pelvic, hip, and low back: strain/malalignment/fracture/inflammation/
   infection

Miscellaneous
Psychosomatic/stress/drug seeking
"Migraine-equivalent"
Sickle crisis
Porphyria
Lupus

Fig. 2.8. Menstrual disorders/amenorrhea—HPOO axis. AI, androgen insensitivity; PCOS, polycystic ovarian syndrome; FB, foreign body.

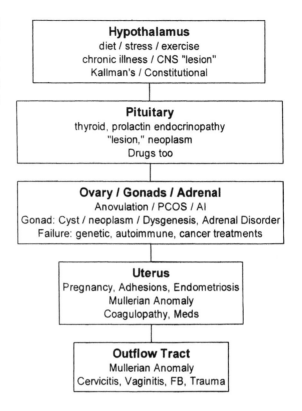

Table 2.7.   Basic principles for menstrual dysfunction and amenorrhea.[a]

History	Physical Examination
Specific complaint	Stature and Tanner staging
Age of menarche	Stigmata—use HPO(O)
PMS molimina?	Abdominal examination
Puberty/growth/development	Individualize re: gynecologic examination
PMH and medications	Evidence for Estrogenization of the vagina
Sexual hx and risk-taking	
R of S—use HPO(O)	

[a] PMS, premenstrual syndrome; PMH, past medical history; R of S, review of systems; HPO(O), hypothalamic/pituitary/ovary (outflow).

Contraception

Approximately 1 in 10 American teens conceive per year and this translates into about 800,000 adolescent pregnancies. Twenty-five to fifty percent of these pregnancies will be terminated and certainly parenthood during adolescence costs society billions of dollars per year. While some adolescents actually desire pregnancy, most conceive because contraception failed or was omitted, forgotten, or used incorrectly. While barriers such as condoms should always be reinforced to protect the adolescent from sexually transmitted infections (STIs), the fact remains that adolescents oftentimes do not use condoms properly and consistently. Ongoing reliable family planning must be accessible and acceptable for it to be used. The oral contraceptive pill, the contraceptive patch, and the vaginal ring have many noncontraceptive benefits that can be exploited to increase compliance in teens. These include cycle control, decreased flow, decreased acne, and decreased cramps. Obviously with pills, the teen must adhere to the daily regimen to achieve efficacy. Reminder beepers, stickers, Web and phone hotlines, and 28-day packaging are all intended to increase compliance. If daily pill-taking is too demanding or not acceptable, the weekly contraceptive patch is a useful option and the vaginal ring should also be explored. Similarly, in the adolescent who either cannot or will not take a pill daily but who wishes reliable birth control, depomedroxyprogesterone acetate (DMPA) given as an IM injection every 3 months is often a solution. The side-effect profile is not quite as consistent as with OCPs, causing irregular nuisance bleeding in approximately one-third of patients, but the 60–70% chance of amenorrhea can be an asset if the patient is properly forewarned. Weight gain, while not a problem in all patients using DMPA, is still more likely than with the OCP and bone density issues certainly need to be explained. Proper diet and exercise must be reinforced. Even intrautine contraceptive devices can be considered in properly selected and counseled adolescents. Finally, while not optimal as a reliable ongoing method of family planning, emergency contraception can prove to be a useful "back-up" method for the adolescent with a "mishap." Teens need to know that this type of resource exists and can be administered up to 72 hours after an act of unprotected intercourse.

Case Studies

Case 1: A 6-year-old female presents with genital irritation and pruritis. She is toilet trained but her panties have a faint odor of urine each evening. She is frustrated because she seems to dribble as she leaves the bathroom. She loves swimming and is a healthy child.

   Guidelines for management: Take a good history trying to identify irritants/allergens, any associated vaginal discharge, bleeding, or odor and eliciting genital care routine. Include routine one on one private time to inquire about the possibility of abuse.

   Case 1 (cont.): The child showers daily and swims three times per week. There is no history of vaginal discharge or bleeding. She has "sensitive skin" and the family is very conscientious about laundry products, bath products, and soaps. The child denies any abuse.

Guidelines for management (cont.): Examine the child using the frog-leg position with gentle bilateral labial traction to expose the introitus. Look for inflammation, excoriation, discharge, labial agglutination, dermopathy, and the size and shape of the hymen. If discharge is present and using proper technique, swab the lower vaginal canal and be sure that the laboratory knows that this is a vaginal specimen on a prepubertal child.

Case 1 (cont.): There is a thin translucent line where the labia minora are fused in the midline. With labial traction, you can see an opening anteriorly just under the clitoral hood. The external labia are mildly erythematous.

Guidelines for management (cont.): The diagnosis is labial agglutination. The child is probably irritated by postvoid dribbling and urine exposure. Tub soaks daily and estrogen cream applied nightly; along the line of agglutination with gentle traction will usually allow the labia to separate within 3 weeks. The parent must be encouraged to inspect and gently separate the labia minora at least two times per week until puberty to prevent recurrence. This child, because of her "sensitive skin," should probably be encouraged to include tub soaks in her genital care routine indefinitely and everyone should recognize that chlorine should be rinsed thoroughly after swimming as it is a common irritant.

Case 2: A 12-year-old child presents with severe menstrual cramps that began with menarche 6 months ago. She has regular cycles, has never been sexually active, and has tried (unsuccessfully) prescription NSAIDs taken proactively.

Guidelines for management: It is unusual for primary prostaglandin-mediated dysmenorrhea to occur with menarche as first menses are not usually ovulatory. Having said that, this is still the most likely etiology for her complaint. It is necessary to take a good history exploring the nature of the pain, the treatments tried thus far, and a past medical, surgical, and family history focusing on genitourinary or pelvic problems. Often adolescents are not able to take NSAIDs in a timely fashion while at school and this can lead to treatment failure.

Case 2 (cont.): The girl complains that her pain is predominantly left-sided and occurs despite taking naproxen regularly beginning the day prior to expected menses/pain. She has had a left ectopic ureter reimplanted at the age of 6 years but otherwise has been well.

Guidelines for management (cont.): Unilateral dysmenorrhea occurring immediately with menarche and a previous history of genitourinary anomaly suggests the possibility of Müllerian anomaly. Other considerations include ovarian cyst, endometriosis, pelvic adhesions, and constipation. An examination that focuses on the abdomen, the introitus, and a single-digit vaginal or rectal examination may prove helpful. In this type of scenario, there is a low threshold for imaging the pelvis with an ultrasound (3-D) because the gynecologic examination may be limited or not tolerated. If the examination and ultrasound assessment are negative, then an OCP would/should be tried in combination with an NSAID. If still suboptimal or ineffective then MRI (or 3-D ultrasound if not yet done) of the pelvis or laparoscopy can be considered depending on the suspicion for Müllerian anomaly (noncommunicating uterine horn) or endometriosis/adhesions respectively.

Suggested Reading

Black A, et al. Canadian Contraception Consensus Parts 1–3. *J Soc Obstet Gynecol* Feb, Mar, and April 2004.

Black YA, Jamieson MA: Adolescent endometriosis. *Curr Opin Obstet Gynecol* 2003;14:467–74.

Carpenter SE, Rock JA. *Pediatric and Adolescent Gynecology*, 2nd ed. Philadelphia: Lippincott Williams & Wilkins; 2000.

Davis AJ. Adolescent contraception and the clinician: an emphasis on counseling and communication. *Clin Obstet Gynecol* 2001;44(1):114–21.

Emans SJ, Laufer MR, Goldstein DP. *Pediatric and Adolescent Gynecology*, 4th ed. Philadelphia: Lippincott Williams & Wilkins; 1998.

Gidens-Herman ME, Slora EJ, Wasserman RC, Bourdony CJ, Bhapkar MV, Koch, GG, Hasemeier CM. Secondary sexual characteristics and menses in young girls seen in office practice: a study from the Pediatric Research in Office Settings Network. *Pediatrics* 1997;99(4):505–12.

Jamieson MA, Ashbury T. Letter to the Editor: Flavoured midazolam elixir in the office. *J Pediatr Adolesc Gynecol* 1999;12(2):106–7.

Laufer MR, Sanfilippo J, Rose G. Adolescent endometriosis: diagnosis and treatment approaches. *J Pediatr Adolesc Gynecol* 2003;16(3 suppl): S3–11.

Sanfilippo JS, Jamieson MA. Physiology of puberty. In *Gynecology and Obstetrics*, Vol. 5. JJ Sciarra (ed). Philadelphia: Lippincott Williams & Wilkins; 2003. (Book on CD-ROM.)

Sanfilippo J, Muram D, Dewhurst J, Lee P (eds). *Pediatric and Adolescent Gynecology*, 2nd ed. Philadelphia: Saunders; 2001.

Spence JEH. Vaginal and uterine anomalies in the pediatric and adolescent patient. *J Pediatr Adolesc Gynecol* 1998;11:3–11.

3

Elderly Patients

Hugh R.K. Barber[†] and Roger P. Smith

Background Information

Geriatric gynecology includes the prevention, diagnosis, care, and treatment of illnesses and disabilities in women aged 65 years and older. It is a subdivision of the overall emerging specialty of geriatric medicine. Gerontology, on the other hand, is the study of normal aging and assists us in knowing what to expect as the patient grows old. It is obvious that there is an overlap between geriatric gynecology and gerontology.

For the geriatric patient, time seems to race, cognitive thinking increases, insomnia and sleep disorders are common, and the sleep/wake rhythm becomes diverse. Eating patterns become more varied and there is great variation in the sense of taste. Perhaps it is better for the geriatric patient to have five small meals rather than three large ones.

American literature during the first half of the twentieth century reflects little improvement in the status of the aging. This may be explained by the fact that at the turn of the century, the average age expectancy in the United States was 40 years. The first significant attention given to the aging patient occurred with the passage of the SOSA (Security Act of the Federal Old Age Insurance Law) in 1935, which provided some financial security for the aging woman.

[†]Deceased.

The aging process causes a decrease in body mass (primarily muscle and bone) as opposed to fat and total body weight. In calculating food replacement and the dosage of drugs, this must be taken into consideration; otherwise, the patient may be overtreated to the point of toxicity. As aging occurs, the muscles lose elasticity and the blood pressure tends to increase. The ability to metabolize sugar tends to decrease and it is not uncommon to hear that a mother, father, or aunt had developed Type II diabetes.

Demography

There has been a change in the age of the population in the United States. In the 1990s, there were more than 50 million people over the age of 50. The fastest growing segment of the population is aged 85 years and there are more than a million Americans over 100 years of age, with most being women. The epidemiologists and statisticians have calculated that American women at the age of 50 can expect to live another 32 years, and, therefore, will live one-third of their lives after ovarian failure and will exist in an estrogen-deprived environment. Knowing the changes that occur in the cardiovascular and skeletal systems, the gynecologist must direct attention to providing a healthy life-style for those patients, with hormone replacement as needed when there is no contraindication. Since coronary heart disease and osteoporosis account for a great deal of morbidity and mortality, management of the hormonal system in the aged 65 years and older group is cost effective.

Alternatives to Hormone Therapy

As women continue to seek alternatives to traditional hormone therapy (HT), gynecologists must be prepared for questions about unconventional methods.

Designer estrogens, also called selective estrogen receptor modulators (SERM), have evolved from laboratory curiosity into drugs that hold promise for preventing several major disorders in women.

Estrogen's effects on a woman can be good or bad. Research scientists in the pharmaceutical companies hope that SERMs will mimic estrogen's effects on the liver, heart, and bone, but will combat its harmful effects on the breast and uterus. The aim is to protect the health of postmenopausal women who manufacture low levels of estrogen of their own.

SERMs bind estrogen receptors, producing estrogen-like (agonistic) effects on some tissues and estrogen blocking effects on others (antagonistic).

Studies have shown that SERMs have beneficial effects on the breasts, skeleton, and some markers of cardiovascular risk on postmenopausal women. These benefits can be obtained without some of the disadvantages of HT, potentially enhancing acceptance and long-term compliance.

The National Surgical Adjuvant Breast and Bowel Projects (STAR) and the raloxifene use for the heart (RUTH) supply detailed information on designer estrogens.

The star study noted raloxifene to have fewer side effects than tamoxifen. The study population included 19,747 patients.

Complementary and Alternative Medicine

Disenchantment with and the rising cost of conventional medicines are driving people to reach out to alternative methods of health care.

Transmission of an herbal therapy to a Food and Drug Administration (FDA)-approved medication has occurred in approximately half of currently prescribed medications in traditional medicine. Digitalis, aspirin, narcotics, and hormonal contraceptives and several anticancer therapies have their origin in plants.

Herbs are often referred to as natural. Natural does not necessarily mean healthful or beneficial. Hemlock and poison ivy are natural, but cannot be listed as healthful or beneficial. Women often refer to estrogen purchased at a health store as natural, but there is no natural estrogen.

Herbal remedies are becoming increasingly popular among patients receiving treatment for such varied medical problems as arthritis, back problems, allergies, insomnia, spasms, headaches, digestive problems, anxiety, and depression.

United States law currently does not provide control and supervision of herbal remedies and dietary supplements and much work is being done to improve regulation of these products. Currently the United States is following the Dietary Supplement Health and Education Act of 1994. Senator Orrin Hatch of the state of Utah (which has an active herbal product industry) introduced this law. It permits the marketing of dietary supplements with no required approval of any government agency as long as there is a label on the product stating (1) no FDA evaluation of that product has occurred, and (2) the product is not intended to diagnose or prevent illness. The FDA may choose to try to prove that a product is unsafe, but this is their limitation. The manufacturers can suggest doses on the labels but these products are not standardized.

The most common herbs used by American women are evening primrose, black cohosh, horse chestnut, grape seed extract, and saw palmetto. Black cohosh, a native plant of North America, was called squaw root because it was a favorite herb of Native American women. It was the chief ingredient of Lady Pinkham tonic medicine, which was a favorite medicine for women for a variety of ailments.

Herbal remedies need more regulation, quality control, and standardization. They often contain toxic ingredients, including pesticides, nondeclared drugs, added chemicals, arsenic, mercury, lead, and cadmium, as well as prescription drugs such as phenylbutazone, aminopyrine, prednisone, testosterone, and diazepam.

The public is demanding to know more about herbs. Doctors will be forced to answer questions and the government will need to set up an agency to establish more regulations, quality control, and standardization.

On July 1, 1983, for the first time in the history of the United States, there were more elderly people than there were teenagers, and never again will teenagers outnumber senior citizens, at least not for the next several decades. The percentage of the population that reaches age 85 years and beyond is growing faster than the percentage that reaches age 65–84. As the phenomenon accelerates, the advantage in female survivorship will become more pronounced. Dr. R. Butler, who was the first director of the National Institute on Aging, is calling the next century "The Century of the Older Woman." The trend will continue and our greatgranddaughters, who will be born in the year 2030, may expect to live for 84 years, adding more than 5 years to their life expectancy. By then, women will be outliving men by 8.5 years. Because of this tremendous increase in the older population, the U.S. government should project a plan to meet the tremendous cost and the burden that it will put on the current younger generation, who will be paying taxes. There are many ways to prepare for this and obviously one would be a fund into which everyone would pay. The hope would be that this fund would yield enough interest to ease the burden for the young Americans who will be paying taxes to support the aging population, which will be predominantly women.

Morbidity and Mortality

Women's advantage in mortality and life expectancy does not extend to morbidity. Women have more illnesses and disabilities than men. They visit doctors more often and are hospitalized at a much higher rate. Women also have a higher incidence of respiratory (except pneumonia) disorders, digestive disorders, and infectious disease than men. It has been stated that the problems of old age in America are largely the problems of women. Chronic disease is the major health problem among the elderly and in the population group aged around 45–65 approximately 72% have one or more chronic illnesses and the percentage increases to over 86% for a person 65 years of age or older (see Tables 3.1 and 3.2). In addition, the incidence of multiple chronic conditions increases as does the incidence of arthritis and hypertension.

It is known that a woman's chance of having a heart attack or stroke rises to that of a man within 10 years after menopause unless there has been

Table 3.1.   The most common chronic diseases.

Arthritis	38%
Hearing impairment	29%
Vision impairment	20%
Hypertension	20%
Heart condition	20%

Table 3.2. The most serious potential consequences of aging.

Cardiovascular disease
Osteoporosis
Cancer

active therapy and improvement in the life-style of the patient. This may be due to the decreased level of estrogen or the elevated testosterone in the level in the blood. Currently, the thought is that replacement therapy with a conjugated estrogen will protect the cardiovascular system.

Establishing a Diagnosis

Most geriatric women have two to four specific medical complaints and the vast majority are on four to eight medications. Many medications are not taken correctly and, since most of these patients do not have a principal or primary physician, the medications are not well-regulated. Each specialist provides a medication without thought to the interaction with drugs prescribed by other specialists. A gynecologist is in a unique position to serve as the principal physician for the elderly woman. It is important to inquire not only about prescription drugs but also over-the-counter medications as well as those given to them by a friend or alternative practitioner. The best way to judge the medication and the possible adverse interaction of the drugs is to have the patient bring in everything that she is taking. Often she may enter with a bag filled with drugs, some of which are not compatible. As an example, drugs for depression often adversely interact with pain medication, causing high temperatures and confusion. Some of the medications are incompatible with a glass of wine, producing confusion and making the patient unsteady on her feet, which often results in a fall with danger of a fracture.

Adjustment to Temperature Changes

The aging woman has difficulty adjusting to long exposure to heat or cold. During cold weather she may develop an accidental drop in internal body temperature. This can be fatal if not detected and treated proportionately. On the other hand, hot and humid weather can result in a body heat buildup that may lead to heat stroke or heat exhaustion. This is especially true for those with heart and circulatory disease, stroke, and diabetes.

Hypothermia

This is a condition in which the body temperature drops to 95°F (35°C) or under, but may occur in anyone who is exposed to severe cold without enough protection. On the other hand, there are some aging women who can develop accidental hypothermia after exposure to relatively mild cold.

The chronically ill and the poor, who are unable to afford enough heating fuel and also do not take steps to keep warm, are the most likely to develop hypothermia. If there is an impairment of temperature regulation the dangers are greater for the elderly woman. Though it is yet undetermined why, patients with an imbalance of temperature regulation apparently do not feel the cold nor do they shiver.

When patients shiver, they produce body heat, but these elderly women have lost the ability to do this. Actually, there are aging women who have felt cold for much of their life and, in observation, these aging women have a lower risk of hypothermia.

Since it is almost impossible to clinically detect hypothermia, it is important to take the temperature with a special low-reading thermometer, which is available in most hospitals. A regular thermometer must be shaken down very well and, if the temperature is below 95°F (35°C) and does not register, it is important to give emergency medical help. Although clinical signs are not as accurate as the thermometer reading, it is important to note unusual changes in appearance or behavior during cold weather, such as slow and altered heart rate, slurred speech, very slow breathing, sluggishness, and confusion. The treatment consists of slowly rewarming the patient and this is best done under a doctor's supervision while the patient is hospitalized.

Prevention

No specific room temperatures for the elderly woman have been established. However, setting the heat at 65°F (18.3°C) in living and sleeping areas is adequate for most cases, but some sick people may need more heat. The following steps can be taken to prevent accidental hypothermia: dress warmly enough when indoors, eat enough food, and stay as active as possible. Since hypothermia may start during sleep, it is important to keep warm in bed by wearing enough clothing and blankets. Heating blankets can be set at the desired temperature. The elderly woman who is being treated for anxiety, depression, nervousness, or nausea must consult a physician about the effects medication can have on the control of body temperature. It is wise to ask friends and neighbors to look in and check on the elderly woman twice a day, particularly during a cold spell. Most communities have a telephone check-in and personnel as a service for the elderly or homebound and this number should be kept easily available.

Hyperthermia

A medical emergency referred to as heat stroke requires immediate attention and treatment, preferably by a physician. Among the symptoms are dizziness, fainting, headache, nausea, loss of consciousness, and a body temperature of 104°F (40°C) or higher, measured rectally. There is also a rapid pulse and flushed skin.

As opposed to heat stroke, which may be sudden, heat exhaustion takes longer to develop. It is directly due to loss of body water and salt. Symptoms include weakness, heavy sweating, nausea, and giddiness. It is best treated by resting in a bed away from the heat and drinking cool fluids with salts added such as is found in Gatorade.

The best program is prevention against heat-related illnesses. The aging woman is advised to remain indoors in an air-conditioned room during hot spells. Some homes have no air-conditioning and the elderly woman is advised to go to a cool place like a library, movie theater, or store during the hottest hours. The health department in many cities directs patients to a shelter where they can stay cool. If none of these is available, the aging woman should take cool baths or showers, place ice bags on the back of her neck, and use electric fans.

It is advisable to stay out of direct sunlight and avoid strenuous activity and it is advisable to wear lightweight, light-colored, loose fitting clothing that permits sweat to evaporate. The aging woman should drink plenty of fluids, such as water, fruit and vegetable juices, and iced tea to replace fluids lost by sweating. It is best not to drink alcoholic beverages or fluid that contains too much salt, since salt can complicate existing medical problems such as high blood pressure. Salt tablets should be used cautiously and under medical supervision.

The aging woman should take heat seriously and must not ignore danger signs like nausea, dizziness, and fatigue. It is important to make sure that a family member or friend or neighbor checks on the condition of the elderly woman two or three times a day.

It is important for the elderly woman to accept the fact that the extremes of temperature are not usually adjusted to and therefore the key is prevention. Hypothermia is a condition of below-normal body temperature, typically 95°F (35°C) or below. Heat stroke may occur at a body temperature of 104°F (40°C) or higher, measured rectally. It is usually accompanied by faintness, dizziness, headache, nausea, loss of consciousness, rapid pulse, or flushed skin.

Osteoporosis

Morbidity and mortality from fractured hips is very high, especially among women, and prophylactic and preventive treatment ideally must be started during the premenopausal years. Osteoporosis, the silent epidemic, affects 25 million people in the United States and most of these are women. There are about 1.5 million fractures annually, including 500,000 vertebral crush fractures, more than 250,000 hip fractures, and 200,000 distal radius fractures. The three areas of the skeleton most commonly fractured in osteoporosis are the spine, hip, and forearm. Sites containing substantial amounts of cancellous bone tend to fracture at earlier ages. Each fracture has different characteristics and effects (Table 3.3). Vertebral fractures result in height loss and kyphosis, back pain, significant morbidity, especially when there are multiple fractures,

Table 3.3.   Complications associated with hip fractures.

Excessive mortality due to peri- and postoperative complications such as deep vein thrombosis, pulmonary embolism, pneumonia	5–20%
Long-term morbidity, loss of some function	60%
Long-term care	30%
Complete return in function	20%

anterior rib pain, a protuberant abdomen and abdominal discomfort (due to the reduced lumbar vertebral height), negative body image, and difficulty fitting into clothes. Hip fractures occur twice as frequently in women, particularly after age 75 years.

The incidence of distal radial fractures (Colles' fractures) increases with age, causing short-term morbidity and significant loss to the work force because they generally occur in the younger portion of the population. Other common fracture sites are the proximal humerus, pelvis, tibial plateau, and ribs. It is obvious that osteoporosis is primarily a women's issue and is painful, disfiguring, and debilitating. Osteoporosis may result in marked changes in the thoracic skeleton. Thoracic changes may result in an increase in the dead space, decrease in alveolar ventilation, reduction in oxygen uptake, and decrease in partial oxygen pressure (PO_2) and ventilatory reserve. Changes that predispose a patient to respiratory infection are particularly important when the patient is being evaluated for preoperative anesthesia.

Measurement of bone mass confirms the existence of osteoporosis and determines the extent of osteoporotic changes. Dual-energy photon absorptiometry and dual-energy X-ray absorptiometry are primarily used. These can measure what is present, but they do not indicate what the rate of bone loss is. Biochemical markers identify how much bone is being destroyed or, following treatment, how much bone has been restored or whether the condition has plateaued (Table 3.4).

Table 3.4.   Biochemical markers that allow a determination or rate of bone turnover.

Serum osteocalcin
Urine hydroxyproline
Osteocalcin acid
Calcium
Phosphatase
Deoxypyridinoline

Table 3.5. The most common cancers in women (arranged by incidence—most to least frequency.

Lung
Breast
Colon and rectum
Uterus
Ovary and cervix
Urinary bladder (due to increase in smoking)
Pancreatic cancer

Cancer

The risk of cancer in all organs increases with age, particularly with each decade during the aging period (Table 3.5). When cancers are detected early, they are more likely to be treated successfully. Chances of surviving cancer today are better than ever before. Because many cancers occur more often in people in the aging and geriatric age group, it is in this group that screening can make a significant contribution to the welfare of the aging and geriatric patient.

Blood Transfusion

The older population receives the highest rate of blood transfusions during routine medical care. As a result, the second most common cause of acquired immunodeficiency syndrome (AIDS) in people aged 60 years and over (after homosexual and bisexual activity) has been exposure to contaminated blood transfusions received before 1985, when the public blood supply was not being screened carefully for the virus. Currently, blood banks now offer assurance of cleaner blood products; however, the number of older persons who receive contaminated blood and may now be unintentionally infecting spouses or other sexual partners remains unknown. A further complication is that older patients have a decline in their immune system functions, making them more susceptible to a variety of illnesses, such as infections and cancer. Since early symptoms of age (such as fatigue, loss of appetite, and swollen glands) are similar to those of the common illnesses, many people, including health professionals, may dismiss these symptoms as a minor ailment. The point to emphasize is that a careful history should be taken to determine whether these patients ever received blood or any blood products and to assess their exposure to environmental and occupational conditions.

Screening: Preventive Medicine

Screening is the clinical backbone of preventive medicine. Screening is not a diagnostic measure but does identify patients who need additional testing.

Screening tests have the greatest value when they are carefully employed, all steps are followed, and the responsible physician communicates with the laboratory or is familiar with the laboratory and how it works.

Colon and rectal cancers are on the increase among women. The aging and geriatric patient should undergo a digital rectal examination and have a fecal occult blood test annually. Since there is a high rate of colorectal cancer in the American population, endoscopic screening of the colon and rectum has become commonplace. Patients should be encouraged to have this screening test. Urinary bladder cancer is on the increase and one of the contributing factors seems to be heavy smoking.

The Cancer Information Service (CIS), a program of the National Cancer Institute, is available to answer cancer-related questions. The number to call is 1-800-4-CANCER. The CIS staff answers questions confidentially and mails free booklets about cancer concerns, including places where help is available in a particular region.

White lesions and vulvar dystrophies are commonly seen in the elderly patient. Pruritus is common and is often difficult to treat in elderly patients. It is associated with knobby skin lesions and, if accurately diagnosed, treatment is usually prompt and effective. However, pruritus associated with an ill-defined, variable change in vulvar skin, for which no specific cause is apparent, is much more difficult to manage.

A temporary but effective treatment to stop itching is to place two Kleenex side by side in the freezer. Coat them with plain yogurt and leave them there until itching is intolerable. Then take one out and place it over the pruritic area. The relief is almost instant. The yogurt holds the coolness and also supplies lactobacillus to the area, which helps control bacteria and fungal contamination. It can be used often since there are minimal side effects.

Sexuality and Sense of Well-Being

The notion that sex does not matter in old age is a cultural fallacy prevalent in our youth-oriented society. Since women remain sexually active through their eighth decade, it is important to explore this with the patient and be prepared to offer advice and any help that is needed.

A careful sexual history and gynecologic examination are very important in treating the elderly patient. This approach often establishes a close patient–physician relationship and facilitates the care of the geriatric patient. There is minimal evidence to support the view that hormonal deprivation is the primary cause of a reduction in sexual activity. It has been adequately demonstrated that sexual decline is a matter of circumstance, not potential.

There is a hierarchy of human needs: after food, water, and safety comes the need to belong, to feel loved. Aging does not alter this. There is a great myth that sexuality is no longer a major concern for a person when he or she become old, and this must be dispelled. In obtaining the history, it is important to explore sexuality as a matter of fact and not be judgmental. Sexuality has often been limited to responsiveness for men and to reproduction and youthful beauty for women. Elderly women see themselves as asexual too often. They describe sex much more broadly, namely as touching, hugging, comfort, warmth, and joy. Masturbation may become more common, since women may have lost control of their sex lives, usually due to loss of partners. Pleasure may include self-pleasure and fantasy, but women also feel guilty. In addition, women often lack privacy for masturbation and fear that somebody may see them.

There have been three major studies of sexuality—one in 1920, Kinsey's report (1951), and, subsequently, Masters and Johnson. The 1926 report showed that 4% of males aged 70–79 years had intercourse every third day and 9% had weekly intercourse. The 1951 report showed that 65% of males between the ages of 56 and 70 years had intercourse and 40% of males over the age of 80 years still had intercourse 10 times per year, and this has been borne out by the Kinsey study and the Masters and Johnson report. This information suggests that sexual activity decreases with age, but does not cease, and that women are capable of and better prepared for intercourse than men.

For those women who have no partner and who are embarrassed to talk about masturbation, the subject should be explored and an attempt made to dispel their sense of guilt and the feeling that it may be harmful to them. They must realize that intercourse and masturbation are physiologic functions and are not detrimental to their health. It can be stated that both serve the same purpose as aerobics and are probably more satisfying and pleasurable. It should be carefully explained to women that the female response cycle is the same as it was when they were younger but that the duration is probably shorter, with the exception of the excitement stage; however, they still go through the excitement plateau, orgasm, and resolution stages. Elderly women should be told that having multiple orgasms is not harmful, either physically or psychologically.

Urinary Incontinence

Urinary incontinence (UI) denotes a sign, a symptom, or a specific condition. Clinically significant, incontinence is defined as a condition in which involuntary loss of urine is a social or hygiene problem and is objectively demonstrable. There are several types of UI and the most important for the gynecologist includes stress, urgency, and mixed and overflow incontinence. Genuine stress incontinence is the immediate and involuntary loss of urine when the intravesicle pressure exceeds the maximum urethral pressure in the absence of detrusor contraction. Urge incontinence (bladder unstable) is subdivided into two categories. The first category, motor urge incontinence (unstable bladder), is associated with uninhibited detrusor contractions; the second, sensory urgent incontinence (irritable bladder syndrome), is not due to inhibited detrusor contraction, but to the result of strong sensory input from the bladder and urethral sensory receptors. It is caused by inflammation, mechanical irritation, neoplastic epithelia changes, or epithelia changes due to hormone deficiency or irradiation. Patients with sensory incontinence are able to inhibit detrusor contraction, but often have a smaller bladder capacity and experience discomfort with bladder filling.

Patients complaining of UI should be thoroughly evaluated (Table 3.6). The physician should take a basic evaluative history with a focused medical, neurologic, and genitourinary history and medication review, including nonprescription medications, and a detailed exploration of the UI-associated symptoms and factors, such as duration and characteristics of the incontinence, as well as the frequency, timing, and amount of continent and incontinent voids. It is important to determine what precipitates the incontinence, such as situational antecedents, abdominal pressure, surgery, trauma, and disease. The role that dementia plays in incontinence must be carefully evaluated, particularly when planning treatment.

The general examination should detect comorbid conditions, such as edema, and assess cognition and manual dexterity when functional urinary stress incontinence is suspected (Table 3.7). The preliminary workup should be fairly straightforward with a urine analysis to clarify symptoms and identify abnormalities directed to guide therapy. The patient should have a voiding diary explained to her and she should return with this. At the initial examination, a postvoiding residual should be evaluated; greater or equal to 200 ml is considered abnormal, 50–199 ml requires clinical judgment, and less than 50 ml is normal.

Involuntary voiding of small amounts of urine is very common in women. It is known, perhaps incorrectly, as stress incontinence and its treatment calls for an understanding of bladder and urethral physiology. The bladder displays the phenomenon of adaptation to increased urinary volume.

Table 3.6.   Elements of basic evaluative history.

Lower urinary tract symptoms
    Nocturia
    Hesitancy
    Straining
    Interrupted stream
    Hematuria
    Pain
    Frequency
    Urgency or increased leakage
Establish
    Careful fluid intake pattern?
    Any alteration in bowel habit or sexual function?

Table 3.7.   **Elements of the physical examination.**

Abdominal	Pelvic	Rectal	Bimanual
Detect masses	Evaluate atrophy, prolapse	Test for rectal sensation	Test for postvoid residual
Detect fullness	Evaluate skin conditions, tenderness	Test for rectal tone	Estimate any fullness in pelvis
Detect tenderness	Evaluate muscle tone, hypermobility	Test for fecal impaction, masses	Palpate urethra

The pressure remains below 10 cm H_2O until over 500 ml of urine is contained. Urethral pressure is maintained by the internal sphincter composed of longitudinal and circular plain muscles and elastic tissue in an external sphincter, which contributes striated muscle. The urethral pressure profile shows the changes in pressure along the length of the urethra. This is normally much greater than intravesicle pressure, thus incurring continence. There is an intercommunicating sympathetic, parasympathetic, and somatic supply. The parasympathetic stimulates detrusor contraction and the sympathetic fibers (chiefly through the α receptors) stimulate contraction of the bladder neck and urethra. There is some degree of reciprocal activity, but the precise function of each type of nerve and the exact control of the mechanism of the bladder neck are not completely understood. The striated muscle has been shown to have a dual autonomic/somatic supply via the pelvic plexus and the long-held concept of pudendal innervation is debatable. The normal urethral closure and the components of the sphincter mechanism must function together, the striated muscle has more to do than merely contract voluntarily, and the desire to micturate must be resisted.

Cystometry recording demonstrates the timing of events. The intraabdominal pressure increases (measured per rectum), the detrusor contracts (intravesicle pressure increases), the sphincter relaxes (electromyelogram of anal sphincter), and urine flow begins. The urethra and bladder neck are maintained in the closed state of the trigonal condensation of muscle (the base plate) and the urethral sphincter (plain and striated muscle). When cortical inhibition is withdrawn, the detrusor contracts and the bladder neck relaxes (funneling). The sphincter also relaxes and urine is voided. As the flow continues, the bladder neck moves downward and backward and the urethral vesicle (UV) is obliterated.

The patient experiences an irresistible desire to micturate. Detrusor instability, or unstable bladder, is the most common cause. It may also be due to inflammatory disease of the bladder without detrusor contraction. All forms of bladder pathology must be considered, including calculus and carcinoma. There is usually an associated complaint of frequency.

A very common cause of incontinence of urine in the elderly is detrusor instability or an unstable bladder. This is defined as a contraction exceeding 15 cm H_2O and pressure, occurring during the filling of the bladder or while standing erect, coughing, or straining. This may also cause involuntary incontinence, but the mechanism is altogether different from that of genuine stress incontinence. In the elderly, the cortical inhibition is decreased and there is an unstable bladder, spontaneous detrusor contraction, and incontinence.

The urethral syndrome includes complaints of frequency, dysuria, urgency, and a sensation of incomplete emptying in a patient whose urine is clear and with no evidence of infection. The cause is not known and there are several explanations. Urinary infection is strictly defined as being present only when 10 or more typical urinary pathogens are grown per milliliter of freshly voided midstream urine and it may be that the urethral syndrome is simply a condition caused by fewer than the usual number of organisms or by organisms that cannot be cultured in the medium used for conventional organisms. Clinically, these patients must be regarded as suffering from a urinary tract infection and investigation must be pursued. Even if no evidence of infection is obtained, some empirical treatment will need to be prescribed. These patients can be helped with an estrogen cream "rubbed in" from the UV angle down to the external meatus. This should be applied daily for 1 week, then every other day for another week, and then once weekly. This will address the atrophic urethritis and provide comfort to the patient.

There are several diagnostic procedures that can be carried out without any elaborate equipment. Uroflowmetry is a noninvasive procedure providing an evaluation of micturation. The volume of urine voided, as well as the length of time voiding, should be noted. The average flow has been found by dividing the volume of urine voided by time. The normal female completes voiding in less than 20 seconds and voids at a flow rate of greater than 20 ml/second. A flow rate of less than 15 ml/second indicates abnormal voiding. Residual urine is measured after this test is performed.

A simple neurologic test is the pinprick of the saddle area of the perineum; the appropriate response is contraction of the external sphincter and sphincter muscle. If sensory or motor defects are noted in the area supplied by the sacral nerves 2, 3, and 4, further neurologic evaluation is indicated.

Clinical Intervention

Osteoporosis

Prophylaxis and prevention are important and must start in the premenopausal years with an increased attention to life-style, limiting smoking and alcohol and providing enough exercise and a well-balanced diet. Treatment includes calcium supplementation, which should be a total of 1500 mg a day; if the patient is taking estrogen, this can be lowered to 100 mg a day. The regimen should be outlined for patients who have no contraindication to estrogen replacement therapy and who are symptomatic. If the patient has a uterus, estrogen therapy must be supplemented by progestin.

Exercise is an important physical activity for protecting bone mass. Exercise must be antigravity, which includes a brisk walk for 20–30 minutes, bicycle riding, and walking on a treadmill three times a week. Although swimming is excellent for toning up muscle, it is not helpful in maintaining or improving bone mass. The point to emphasize is that too much exercise can contribute to osteoporosis, so there must be a balance between too little and too much. Too much would include marathon running and too little would be continually sitting with no weight-bearing activity.

Calcitonin is currently available as an alternative to estrogen replacement treatment for therapy of established osteoporosis. It inhibits osteoclasts from functioning and diminishes their number over a prolonged period, thus inhibiting bone resorption. The disadvantage is that it must be given subcutaneously and must be very carefully controlled by a physician. Etidronate has been used in the past but lacks potency and selectivity for antiresorptive surfaces. Alendronate, a nonhormonal therapy, can be taken orally, has great potency, and is able to increase bone mass. Currently it is being used for those with marked symptoms and has not replaced estrogen as a long-term preventative against bone mass loss. Alendronate, 70 mg per week, is gaining great favor. Boniva, a once a month pill, is on the market.

Fluoride is a bone-seeking ion that can reduce bone resorption and increase bone formation. In addition to some of the side effects such as nausea and dyspepsia, there is a decrease in cortical bone mineral density and increased peripheral skeleton fragility. Currently, sodium fluoride treatment is not recommended for clinical use outside of research studies. Vitamin D, 400 IU/day, must be included in all regimens.

Vulvar Irritation

The vulvar area in elderly patients is thin and can easily be irritated by tight clothing and improper hygiene. It is important to explain to patients that many soaps, including Ivory and detergent soaps, are very alkaline and dry out the area, resulting in irritation and particularly pruritus. It is very important to tell elderly patients to take their own soap when traveling, preferably a mild (baby) soap, because the soaps provided by most hotels are often very irritating to the vulva.

It is important to teach elderly women to be cautious about having nylon touch the vulva because many become sensitive to nylon and will develop vulvitis. Colored and perfumed toilet tissue should not be used and commonly used perineal sprays are often very irritating. When the elderly develop discomfort in the vulvar area, they often get immediate relief by use of one of the local anesthetic agents. However, these may sensitize the area and give rise to a delayed hypersensitivity reaction, which is often difficult to treat. Women who have repeated vulvar discomfort may receive relief during the night by a simple process (Table 3.8).

When patients have itching, very often application of a 0.5–1% hydrocortisone cream will give them relief, but the effect is usually only temporary, lasting for 2 or 3 days. If the patient has not responded by that time, it is better to give her a prescription for crotamiton (Eurax) (one-third) and hydrocortisone 1% (two-thirds), made up to 60 g, which are applied to the vulva on a per-need basis.

It is assumed that diabetic changes that might account for vulvar irritation have been ruled out because it is obvious that these patients very often have a resistant monilia. If the lesion does not respond to local antifungal treatment, fluconazole may provide relief; however, it does have side effects, particularly gastrointestinal upset. If there is an allergic response superimposed on the fungal infection, a preparation such as Mycostatin (Nystatin/triamcinolone acetonide) may be of benefit. Preparations such as Flagyl (metronidazole) instilled into the vagina usually successfully treat bacterial vaginosis, restore the lactobacillus to the vagina, and do not increase the incidence of fungus infection secondary to the treatment.

There are some patients who complain of burning and for whom most treatments are not effective. Cancer should be ruled out and the patient told that there is a change in the metabolism of the tissue. Two percent testosterone propionate in a petrolatum base is usually very helpful. Excessive use of this results in enlargement of the clitoris and an unpleasant increase in libido, so it is important over the first few weeks to use the treatment two or three times a day and then, after that, increase the interval between treatments. Not only does it give relief, but it has also been shown to have a therapeutic effect on restoring healthy tissue to the area. For those unable to tolerate testosterone, a similar preparation can be made up using progesterone in oil. Although not quite as successful as the testosterone, it usually works

Table 3.8. Treatments of vulvar irritation.

Symptom	Treatment	Method	Effects
Burning	Plain yogurt	Placed on gauze or paper towel, chilled in freezer, applied directly	Quick relief—temporary
Burning	Ice bag (never place next to bare skin)	Place in cloth on area	Quick relief—temporary

successfully in most patients with burning. The use of estrogen combined with androgen provides help in increasing the libido. An estrogenic cream applied locally decreases the discomfort of atrophic vaginitis. The secret is to rub the cream into the area, starting just above the anus and going about 1 cm into the vagina and around the introitus. It is important to rub the cream into this area, otherwise when the penis touches the area there is great discomfort and it sends the levator muscle into spasm, which adds to the discomfort.

Incontinence and Urethritis

For patients with urethritis, even if no evidence of infection is obtained, some empirical treatment will have to be given. These patients can be helped by applying an estrogen cream from the UV angle down to the meatus. The cream should be rubbed in daily for 1 week and then every other day for 1 additional week, decreasing to once weekly. This will change the atrophic urethritis and provide comfort to the patient.

There are pharmacologic treatments for incontinence due to detrusor overactivity. Anticholinergic/antispasmodic agents serve to relax the bladder and increase bladder capacity. All anticholinergic agents are contraindicated in patients with narrow angle but not wide angle glaucoma. Oxybutynin is recommended at a dose of 2.5–5 mg orally 3 times a day. Tricyclic agents such as imipramine and oxepine are often helpful at 10–100 mg orally per day, initially on divided doses. α-Adrenergic agents increase urethral resistance by stimulation of the urethral smooth muscle acting on α-adrenergic receptors in the urethra. Phenylpropanolamine (PPA) is recommended in a dose of 25–75 mg every 12 hours. These drugs should be used with caution in patients with hypertension, hyperthyroidism, cardiac arrhythmias, and angina. Calcium channel blockers can reduce smooth muscle contractility in the bladder and occasionally can cause urinary retention and overflow incontinence. Benzodiazepines, such as flurazepam and diazepam, are especially long-acting agents and accumulate in elderly patients causing confusion and secondary incontinence. Alcohol, frequently used as a sedative, can cloud the sensorium, impair mobility, and induce a diuresis, resulting in incontinence. It is very important to take a very careful history of all drugs, prescription and over-the-counter, to determine whether they are causing retention or incontinence.

Special Considerations

Preoperative Evaluation

The preoperative evaluation of the elderly patient is very important (Table 3.9). There have been important therapeutic advances relating to anesthesia, water and electrolyte balance, methods of measuring impaired function to determine the individual's capacity to withstand surgical procedure, and the expanded use of monitoring devices, such as the Swann-Ganz catheter.

Table 3.9.   The most important systems and changes to be evaluated preoperatively.

Cardiovascular	Pulmonary	Renal
More prominent arteries in head, neck, extremities	Weaker respiratory muscles; 50% increase in residual capacity	Decreased size of kidneys
Decreased cardiac output up to 40%	Alveoli fewer in number and larger in size	Loss of nephrons
Blood pressure increased to compensate for increased peripheral resistance	Thoracic muscles more rigid; maximum breathing capacity reduced	Decrease of renal blood flow
Loss of elasticity in vessels	Decrease in ciliary action	Decrease in glomerular filtration rate
Less efficient oxygen utilization	Lungs appear larger due to loss of elasticity	Weaker bladder muscles with loss of inhibition from central nervous system
Valves become thicker and more rigid	PO_2 reduced as much as 15%	Decreased bladder capacity and tubular function

PO_2, partial oxygen pressure.

The usual evaluation is carried out with standard testing, but it is important to consider the diminished reserve that the elderly patient has and compensation should be made for such. If not, medication may be administered to decrease toxicity and increase oxygen delivery, which, if not supplied early enough and with the right flow, results in pulmonary changes that may lead to early pneumonia.

Summary

A variety of preventive and detective programs have been established that focus on health care in the elderly. There are a great number of common problems that arise among the elderly and the gynecologist must be prepared to evaluate and treat these common conditions.

There comes a time when "death is the best life has to offer." The responsible physician must prolong life, but not prolong dying. This raises many ethical and moral questions that are currently being addressed as geriatric gynecology is being established as a subspecialty.

Suggested Reading

Barber HRK. *Perimenopausal and Geriatric Gynecology.* New York: Macmillan; 1988.

Bygny RL, Speroff L, eds. *A Clinical Guide for the Care of Older Women.* Baltimore: Williams & Wilkins; 1990.

Dempster DW, Lindsay R. Pathogenesis of osteoporosis. *Lancet* 1993; 341:797.

Eliopoulous C. *Gerontological Nursing,* 2nd ed. Philadelphia: Lippincott; 1987.

Hyblick L. *How and Why We Age.* New York: Ballantine Books; 1994.

Lebow MA. A look at older Americans. In *The Gynecologist and the Older Patient.* Breen JL (ed). Rockville, MD: Aspen; 1988.

Rowe JW, Grossman E, Bond E, et al. Special report: academic geriatrics for the year 2000. *N Engl J Med* 1987;316:1425–87.

4

Lesbian Patients

Joseph S. Sanfilippo and Ruth Schwarz[†]

Background Information

Attitudes of health care professionals affect the quality of care we provide to both heterosexual and lesbian populations. Many lesbians feel health care providers are "homophobic" and have negative attitudes toward lesbians. Homophobia is defined as antipathy or disdain for gay men and lesbians. Theories regarding how and why homosexuality occurs abound and reflect genetic, embryologic, hormonal, and personal experiences with and without associated sociopathology as possible contributing factors. The psychiatric literature conveys that gay and lesbian individuals are an integral part of normal expression of the natural diversity of human sexuality. Homosexuality was included in the 1981 edition of the *Diagnostic and Statistical Manual*, but the *Manual* has since been revised to exclude homosexuality as a psychiatric

[†]Deceased.

disorder. While there are no solid data it is quoted that 10% of the female population is homosexual, yet many health care providers assume everyone is heterosexual. Most often "negative" experiences are with male practitioners. Fear of a provider's response to the gay patient "disclosing" or "coming out" remains paramount in the mind of lesbians. One report from Oregon noted it was easier for lesbians to be open with "alternative practitioners" than with allopathic health care providers. Several studies indicate that lesbians delay or totally avoid seeking medical care because of the insensitivity of health care providers and poor prior experiences with the system.

Homosexuality is believed to begin in adolescence when gays and lesbians are in reality no different from their peers. But there is a distinction; it is the emotional, psychological, and physical trauma that may result from the homophobia they experience in their daily lives. Furthermore, some sources note a higher incidence of sexually transmitted diseases, suicide, and substance use among this population. The reality is that most homosexual youth grow up to be healthy, happy contributors to society.

Data indicate that this population of women accesses preventive health screening less frequently, delays treatment, and more commonly does not have a primary level health care provider when compared to heterosexual women. Lesbians are less likely to obtain Pap smears and screening mammograms than heterosexuals but at the same time have the same incidence of cervical cytologic abnormalities. Health care providers must keep in mind the challenges, unique problems, and risks that this population faces.

There is a need for better understanding of health issues related to sexual orientation. Sexual orientation is in essence a woman's self-perception of being lesbian, bisexual, or heterosexual. Sexual behavior and orientation may vary over time, with different characteristics: desire, identity, and behavior. There are definitions of sexual differences. The word *homosexuality* indicates a sexual orientation involving an attraction for a person of the same sex with affection, fantasy, or erotic desire. A homosexual is one who prefers an erotic, sexual, and usually genital relationship with an individual who has the same genital morphology. Homosexuals can be celibate, promiscuous, or have moderate sexual activities. A lesbian is a woman with an exclusive sexual preference for females. Bisexuals are persons with both homosexual and heterosexual attractions. A transvestite is an individual who attempts to adopt the behavior and mannerisms of the opposite gender. The female tends to prefer male-oriented clothing and jewelry. Transsexuals are individuals who feel a discordance or incongruity (gender dysphoria) between their own anatomic sex and their psychological orientation (they feel "trapped in the wrong body"). Ego-deptonic homosexuality is characterized by internal conflict and disturbance and a strong desire to change sexual orientation (Table 4.1).

The overall concern is missed treatment and lack of early diagnosis of medical conditions. Carroll has summarized it succinctly: "lesbians, like other marginalized groups of women, underutilize health care services. Lesbians also present later for health care (related problems) than heterosexual

Table 4.1.   Terminology.

Term	Definition
Homosexuality	Attraction for a person of the same sex
Lesbian	Woman with a preference for females and if sexually active—exclusively with females
Bisexual	Both homosexual and heterosexual attractions
Transvestite	Attempts to adopt the behavior and mannerisms of the opposite gender
Transsexual	Incongruity between your own anatomic sex and psychological orientation ("trapped in wrong body")
Homophobia	Negative feelings toward homosexuals
Homophilia	Positive, accepting response to homosexuality

women. Lack of awareness of health issues of lesbians by some health care professionals has produced lesbians' abstention from health services."

How Common Is Female Homosexuality?

Both heterosexual and homosexual women became more sexually active during the second half of the twentieth century, and life-styles have changed significantly since the 1950s. The "coming out process"—the discovery of gay networks and organizations, bars, and other gathering places—is usually delayed until lesbians are in their mid-20s or older.

Some reports have estimated that there are about 10 million lesbians in the United States; various studies show that 1.3–4% (and one study 12%) of women are homosexual or bisexual, which suggests that homosexuality is not uncommon. This sexual orientation is much more common than the general society and physicians recognize, discuss, or accept.

Most lesbians sustain relationships with their partners for a year or more, which differs from gay males, among whom only 60% of relationships last a year or more. Homosexual affairs occur in 50–70% of women in prison, although most were not homosexuals before imprisonment. Unlike male prisoners, female prisoners rarely face sexual coercion and assaults.

Neuroendocrinology of Homosexuals

There is no evidence that inherited organic or nonpsychogenic factors have an effect on homosexuality. The levels of sex hormones, estradiol, progesterone, testosterone, and androstenedione in lesbians and heterosexual women are not different. One study showed elevated testosterone in lesbians, but not above the normal female level. Another study of a small group of women who had diethylstilbestrol (DES) exposure *in utero* showed a higher incidence of homosexuality. However, my own experience over many years with a large number of DES-exposed women has shown no apparent increase in this incidence.

Most females with congenital adrenal hyperplasia who received endocrine therapy were heterosexual. Also there was no increase in incidence of homosexuality in children with 5α-reductase deficiency, even though they were raised as girls and converted to the male gender at puberty, although there are obvious stressful impacts of this unusual change.

Family Relationships and Other Factors

There is a distinct difference in parental–child relationships for gay men and lesbians. Some lesbians show more indifference to parents, or consider the father to be weak, inadequate, or rejecting. Others have close bonds with their fathers, while mothers are considered dominant and independent. Many lesbians tend to feel rejected by their parents.

About two-thirds of lesbians have a childhood history of "tomboyishness," avoiding household activities and games seen as feminine. This behavior does not elicit a negative response by parents as often as does "sissiness" in boys.

Almost 50% of lesbians had a romantic attachment to a man at some time; for two-thirds, this occurred during adolescence. During adolescence, heterosexual arousal occurred in 70% of lesbians, and homosexual arousal was noted in only 5% of heterosexual women.

Families whose child has "come out" may benefit from PFLAG (Parents, Families and Friends of Lesbians and Gays).

Sexuality and Safe Sex

In one sense reduction in the risk for contracting sexually transmitted diseases should focus on in-depth knowledge of the complex sociocultural patterns of sexuality in specific communities and specific subgroups. Lowering the risk for human immunodeficiency virus (HIV) requires specific recommendations for behaviors and educating patients regarding safe sex. One retrospective study from Sydney, Australia, reported a higher prevalence of bacterial vaginosis, hepatitis C, and HIV risk behaviors among women having sex with women compared with controls, i.e., heterosexuals. Overall, 17% of self-identified lesbians in the United States have had a documented sexually transmitted infection (STI). There is a direct correlation between frequency of STI and number of lifetime partners. Cervical cytology was not different between groups. Genital herpetic and wart lesions were lower among the homosexual group.

Diagnostic Considerations
Sexually Transmitted Diseases

Women who have sex only with women are at less risk for contracting *Trichomonas*, syphilis, gonorrhea, or *Chlamydia*. However, if there are signs or symptoms of sexually transmitted diseases (STDs), appropriate testing should be undertaken because some women might not completely explain their sexual behavior. The risk of virus infection, especially with human papilloma virus (HPV), is lower for lesbians than for heterosexual women. HIV is rare in lesbians except for those using drugs intravenously or engaging in bisexual relations, especially with bisexual men. Herpes has been reported as more common because of direct contact.

Bacterial Vaginosis

This may be more common. It is unknown if orogenital or direct genital contact can transmit this disease. Candidiasis rates are lower. In work reported from London, evaluating the effect of nonheterosexual factors on vaginal flora, bacterial vaginosis (BV) was identified in 51.6% of the 91 lesbians studied. The study population was composed of women who had not had sex with a male for a minimum of 12 months.

Human Papilloma Virus Infection

The epidemiology of HPV among homosexuals is an area of discussion and research. The prevalence of HPV determined by DNA amplification assays has been reported to be 19–21% among female populations who never had sexual contact with men. The Australian National Cervical Screening Program identified the need to encourage lesbians to have Pap smears at the same frequency as heterosexuals. Their campaign, titled "Lesbians need pap smears too," continues to identify lesbians as a target group for HPV.

Cystitis

This occurs in about 15% of women in the general population but is less common in lesbians.

Endometriosis

Abnormal menses, dysmenorrhea, pelvic pain, and the existence of endometriosis are the same in all women.

Cancer

Lesbians tend to assume that they are not at risk for gynecologic disease, such as breast or ovarian cancer. Studies comparing cancer rates of lesbians with those of heterosexual women are not available. However, breast cancer may be more common in those who have not given birth, and nulliparity may be a risk factor for ovarian cancer. Lesbians tend not to use oral contraceptives, which decrease the risk of ovarian and uterine cancer. They have a lower risk of cervical cancer because of a lower incidence of HPV; bisexual women have the same risk as heterosexual women because of exposure to HPV.

Pregnancy

Lesbians seem to have more of an interest in becoming parents than male homosexuals do. In middle-class homosexual women, 12% of whites and 34%

of blacks have had children. Some lesbians marry to have children; others have sex with men to become pregnant, but do not continue the relationship once pregnancy occurs; some have artificial insemination. Adoption is attempted, but is more difficult for lesbians due to discrimination.

Mental Health Issues

A high rate of mental illness has been reported among lesbian women compared to the general population. Homophobia in society is the primary source of stress and sickness in the homosexual population. Many situations create stress for these patients, including policies that exclude, segregate, or demean a person; homosexuals face ostracism and discrimination from many sources, including some health professionals. In the past, discrimination based on ethnic origin, race, sex, age, or socioeconomic status was accepted, but it is now illegal in business and social organizations. These pressures often lead to psychiatric complications such as depression in adult and adolescent homosexuals. The emotional disturbance related to their sexual identity is due to a sense of alienation, but they can be helped to become more comfortable with their status. The incidence of depression, anxiety disorders, and suicidal ideation is two to three times higher than in the general population. Furthermore, the incidence among bisexuals appears to be greater than among lesbians. They are more likely to be victims of childhood sexual abuse as well as of parental mistreatment. Domestic violence occurs with a frequency similar to that of the heterosexual population.

Substance Abuse

Homosexual women have a higher rate of alcohol and drug abuse than heterosexual women. This is related to psychological variables such as stress and the cultural importance of alcohol in bar settings, where lesbians tend to congregate for socializing. It declines substantially with age. Predisposing factors include increased risk-taking behaviors, higher levels of depression, and a social subculture that appears to incorporate substance use. The data are not clear-cut in that one study from New Zealand noted a lower level of alcohol intake among lesbians than heterosexual controls. On the other hand, a study from the United States reported just the opposite. Lesbians appear to have a higher rate of being in alcohol recovery and/or drug rehabilitation than their counterparts.

Physical Abuse

There is a very low rate of domestic abuse among lesbians. However, outside violence against homosexuals increased in the 1990s by 15%, with 80% of attackers being adolescents. Victims are unwilling to report the cause to police because police abuse of homosexuals has increased (a report from 1991 indicates a 29% increase). They may also be afraid to tell physicians how the episode occurred because of fear of rejection.

Intimate Partner Violence

The incidence of partner violence among lesbians is similar to that of heterosexual women. In a survey of 100 lesbians who reported that they were victims of intimate partner violence, mutual dependency was most strongly associated with abuse. In a survey from San Francisco, one in three lesbians reported emotional abuse in a current or recent lesbian relationship.

Preventive Health

Cancer screening among the lesbian population noted a perception among lesbians that cervical and breast mammography are not as necessary as among heterosexual women. In one study only 43% of lesbians had obtained a Pap smear within the past year. On average the interval is 32 months. With regard to breast self-examination (BSE), this practice is reportedly low among lesbians. Two national surveys noted that only 21% of lesbians do monthly BSEs.

Body Image and Eating Disorders

There appears to be a lower incidence of eating disorders and less body image dissatisfaction among lesbians. The theory is that lesbians reject the socially conveyed ideal thin body image and studies indicate generally higher weights among lesbians than among heterosexuals.

Reproductive Health

The National Lesbian Health Care Survey (NLHCS) reported that 30% of lesbians have been pregnant and 16% delivered a child. Work from a large Minnesota survey noted that adolescents who are lesbian are no more likely to have had heterosexual intercourse but are more likely to become pregnant than heterosexual teens.

Those desirous of pregnancy achieve it via self-insemination with a known donor's sperm or thorough a physician office-based donor insemination program. The legal aspects, i.e., paternal rights, vary to some degree from state to state and country to country. The American Academy of Pediatrics supports coparent adoption by same-sex parents and advocates that primary care (pediatricians) be knowledgeable with regard to gay and lesbian families.

Adolescent Health

The problems young girls are faced with include familial and societal condemnation for revealing their homosexuality. They experience problems with development of a new identity in association with the process of "coming out." Perhaps the greatest challenge they experience is frequent confrontation with societal "homophobia" and the ramifications of such. Religious institutions often view homosexuality as immoral and convey a "guilt trip" for each individual. The American Academy of Pediatrics, Committee on Adolescence, notes that while homosexual youth are making an effort to reconcile their feelings with negative societal connotations, there is a clear lack of knowledge and scarcity of positive role models, complemented by minimal opportunity for open discussion. All of this commonly results in rejection, isolation, runaway behavior, domestic violence, depression, suicide, and substance use, not to mention poor performance in academic endeavors.

Gynecologic Care

Most gynecologists provide care for lesbian patients, including some pregnant patients. However, they have a general lack of awareness of women's sexual orientation, and many do not know that their patient may be lesbian. Identification of lesbianism is generally based solely on clinical judgment and observation of the patient and not on patient disclosure.

One study in a medical society indicated that 37% of physicians were homophilic (favorable attitudes), 40% neutral, and 23% homophobic (unfavorable attitudes). Female physicians were more homophobic than male physicians, who tended to be more neutral. About one-third of obstetricians-gynecologists, family practitioners, surgeons, and orthopedists were homophobic. This implies personal prejudice in patient care, although many physicians may be unaware of their own biases.

The social stigma related to homosexuality compromises the willingness of patients to cooperate in verifying their life-style. Most bisexual women will not provide information about their sexual orientation because they have concerns about the response of the gynecologist. Black women are more reluctant than white women to disclose a homosexual experience, although the majority of black women have had heterosexual activity. Surveys have shown that only 49% of lesbians were specifically open about their sexual activity. One-third felt that their health care providers were unsupportive or hostile, and 25% had a "poor experience" with their gynecologists, 50% had a "neutral experience," and only 25% had an "adequate experience." Other studies have shown that the majority of physicians thought that very few or none of their patients were homosexuals; however, the percentage in their community was significantly higher than they realized.

How to Approach the Patient

The ability to diagnose and treat is dependent on awareness of accurate information about life-style, including smoking, use of alcohol, substance abuse, physical abuse, exercise, eating habits, and sexual orientation. Trust, confidence, and rapport need to be established between the physician and the lesbian patient. To obtain adequate information about the patient, there must be understanding and acceptance by the physician, to maintain her trust (Table 4.2).

Table 4.2. Approach to the patient.

1. Be aware of your own feelings, concerns, and attitudes toward homosexuality.
2. Obtain an appropriate sexual history.
3. Record sexual orientation in medical history with the patient's permission.
4. Recognize that a partner is as important to a lesbian as to a heterosexual.
5. Use gender-neutral pronouns (*lover* or *partner*).
6. Avoid the words *gay*, *lesbian*, or *homosexual*.
7. Most lesbians are primarily or exclusively homosexual; some are bisexual.
8. Do not assume all sexually active women are heterosexual.
9. Birth control should not be prescribed routinely for all sexually active women.
10. Avoid the question "Do you have intercourse?" Instead say "Tell me about your sexual activity."
11. Lesbianism per se does not require endocrinologic assessment to determine cause.
12. Confidentiality regarding sexual orientation is most important.

Categories and suggestions for how to establish a good doctor–patient relationship and provide appropriate care for *all* women include the following:

1.   The physician should be aware of his or her own feelings, concerns, and attitudes about homosexuality. Be nonjudgmental. Avoid assumptions of heterosexuality. Personal bias should be set aside so that the physician can relate to and coordinate with the patient.

2.   Taking a routine sexual history may alleviate difficulties for the physician and the patient and will encourage a more meaningful and mutually satisfactory relationship. The history should begin with routine, generalized questions. If the patient is in the office for sexually related concerns, then the physician should proceed into more specific areas.

3.   A place to record partnership status should be included on the medical history form. Options include *married*, *divorced*, *separated*, *widowed*, *single*, or *living with*. The name requested for a patient's partner may include her lesbian partner. The history sheet should include information about pregnancies, miscarriages, the patient's sexual activity, support

system, existence of a significant other, and previous disorders and diseases.

4.   Recognition of a partner is as important with a lesbian patient as it is with other patients.

5.   Gender-neutral language, e.g., "partner," should be used with new patients. For example, when inquiring about sexual activity, use *lover* or *partners*, rather than *he*, *husband*, or *boyfriend*. Be aware of disclosure or of the "coming out" process.

6.   It is preferable not to use the words *gay*, *lesbian*, or *homosexual*; many consider the use of these words offensive. Appropriate tones and language will convey the physician's openness to lesbian patients so as to better understand their life-styles and assist them with any problems.

7.   A physician should recognize that most lesbians are primarily or exclusively homosexual.

8.   It cannot be assumed that all sexually active women are heterosexual or that women who are not heterosexually active are celibate.

9.   Many physicians promote birth control to all sexually active women; it is *inappropriate* for those who are exclusively homosexual.

10.   The routine question "Do you have intercourse?" may discourage further communication. Instead say, "Tell me about your sexual activity," in the same tone as you say "Tell me about your menstrual period"; this will enhance communication with the patient.

11.   Lesbians are not more likely to have biological or endocrine abnormalities than other women. They should be investigated only for the same indications as heterosexual women who have some abnormality.

12.   If a patient has psychological problems and needs a referral for therapy, do not assume that all therapists are unbiased. Psychiatrists and psychologists vary in their adherence to the American Psychological Association (APA) standards of unbiased practice. Check out the attitudes of the psychiatrist or psychotherapist on homosexuality before the patient is referred.

13.   The confidentiality of the patient's sexual orientation should be maintained, regardless of whether a patient is homosexual, bisexual, or heterosexual.

14.   Do not share information of bisexuality or other affairs of the patient with her partner unless you have been given specific permission by the patient to do so. You should also obtain her approval before recording her sexual orientation in her record.

15.   Train your staff accordingly, i.e., have a written policy.

Summary

The practicing obstetrician-gynecologist is very likely to provide care for homosexual women. Therefore, it is imperative that the physician is knowledgeable about homosexuals and is accepting of and sensitive to the dialogue with the homosexual patient, including the fact that she might want to have a child. Appropriate history, psychological and societal data, and gynecological issues should be addressed and treated so that the woman's care is appropriate.

Case Studies

Case 1. A 29-year-old woman recently graduated from college. Her complaint is that of mild vulvar pain with pruritis for the past week. It hurts when she inserts a tampon. You ask her if she is sexually active and her reply is "no." She has been reluctant to see health care providers in the past. Her concern is that "they just don't understand me." Further inquiry on the physician's part reveals that the patient is a lesbian. It has been her assumption up to this point that there is no need for annual Pap smears and a pelvic examination because of her sexual orientation. She wants to know what her vulvovaginal problem is and seeks a consultation.

You tell her that the most likely diagnosis is that of vulvovaginitis. A discussion is then carried out in which you inform her that the incidence of bacterial vaginosis in lesbians is equal to or, based on several reports, higher than in heterosexual women. Hepatitis C and HIV are also reported and again, based on data, occur at an incidence equal to or even slightly higher than the incidence in heterosexual women. On the other hand, the incidence of *Chlamydia*, gonorrhea, syphilis, and *Trichomonas* is lower in a lesbian than in the heterosexual population. In this case a vaginal swab or a wet probe is most appropriate and likely to yield the correct diagnosis.

Case 2. A 17-year-old girl is brought in by her mother who feels that "something is wrong" with her daughter. She seems to avoid family member contact, doesn't go out on dates like her peers, and recently has had some change in appetite as well as hypersomnia, fatigue, and an inability to concentrate. These signs and symptoms are more common now than in the past. The teen states that every time she tries to talk to a family member she "gets the cold shoulder." She feels her interest in boys is "just not there." The mother seeks a consultation to determine "what is wrong with my daughter?".

Adolescence is often a time of increased stress. In this case there are clear manifestations of a major depressive episode. According to the American Psychiatric Association's *Diagnostic and Statistical Manual of Mental Disorders,* 4th ed. (1994), the presence of at least five of the following nine symptoms, present for 2 or more weeks, qualifies for a diagnosis of major depression: (1) depressed mood daily, (2) markedly decreased interest in pleasure (anhydonia), (3) significant weight or appetite change, (4) insomnia or hypersomnia, (5) psychomotor retardation or agitation daily, (6) fatigue, (7) feelings of worthlessness, (8) diminished ability to think and concentrate, and (9) recurrent thoughts of suicide or death. In this case the patient has developed a major depression based upon her attempt to "come out" and convey to her family her sexual orientation. The American Academy of Pediatrics, Committee on Adolescence, has brought particular attention to the evaluation and management of homosexuality in teens, as they attempt to provide open discussion. The problem can lead to depression, substance use, and runaway behavior.

Suggested Reading

American Medical Association. Policy 160:991: health care needs of the homosexual population. *AMA Policy Compendium.* Chicago, IL: AMA; 1994.

Bernhard L. Lesbian health and health care. *Annu Rev Nurs Res* 2001;19: 145–77.

Bevier PJ, Chiasson MA, et al. Women at a sexually transmitted disease clinic who reported same-sex behaviors. *Am J Public Health* 1995;85:1366–71.

Carroll N. Optimal gynecologic and obstetric care for lesbians. *Obstet Gynecol* 1999;93:611–13.

Denenberg R. Report on lesbian health. *Womens Health Issues* 1995;5: 81–93.

Falco KL. *Psychotherapy with Lesbian Clients: Therapy into Practice.* New York: Brunner/Malex; 1991.

Hall JM. Alcoholism in lesbians: developmental, symbolic interactions and critical perspective. *Health Care Women Int* 1990;11:89–107.

Lauman EO, Gagnon JH, Michaels RT, Michaels S. *The Social Organization of Sexuality: Sexual Practices in the United States.* Chicago: University of Chicago Press; 1994.

O'Hanlon KA. Lesbian health and homophobic perspectives for the training obstetrician/gynecologist. *Curr Probl Obstet Gynecol Fertil* 1995;18: 93–136.

Robertson P. Offering high-quality ob/gyn care to lesbian patients. *Contemp OB/GYN* September 2003;49–56.

Simkin RJ. Creating openness and receptiveness with your patients: overcoming heterosexual assumptions. *Can J Obstet Gynecol Women's Health Care* 1993;5:485–9.

Smith EM, Johnson SR, Guenther SM. Health care attitudes and experiences during gynecologic care among lesbians and bisexuals. *Am J Public Health* 1985;75:1085–7.

Spinks V, Andrews J, Boyle J. Providing health care for lesbian clients. *J Transcult Nurs* 2000;11:137–43.

Stein TS, Chen CJ. *Contemporary Perspectives on Psychotherapy with Lesbians and Gay Men.* New York: Plenum Publishing; 1986.

Stern PN, ed. *Lesbian Health: What Are the Issues?* Washington, DC: Taylor & Francis; 1993.

Web Sites

http://www.lesbian healthinfo.org Human information from the Lesbian Health Research Center at UCSF.

http://www.nclrights.org Legal information (power of attorney, parental rights).

http://www.pflag.org Information for parents of gay and lesbian children.

http://www.lesbianstd.com Sexually transmitted diseases in lesbians.

5

The Role of Genomic and Applied Molecular Biology

Randall S. Hines

Introduction

The world of genetics and molecular biology has exploded in the past 10 years. With the completion of the first phase of the human genome project, the genetic code has been deciphered. In addition, the rapid expansion of techniques, such as automated sequencing and analysis of gene arrays on microchips, has revolutionized research and will soon create a revolution in clinical medicine as well. The combination of understanding our own genetic sequence and the use of automated high-throughput technology will transform our world. In the near future, the understanding of organisms at a functional level, via proteomics, will expand our knowledge base by another order of magnitude. We start with a description of the fundamentals of genetics and move forward.

Background Information

DNA, or *d*eoxyribo*n*ucleic *a*cid, was first isolated in the 1940s by Oswald Avery. In 1952, James Watson and Francis Crick proposed their model for the structure of DNA, the now famous double helix. Essentially, DNA serves as the keeper of our genetic information within each cell. As such, it is equivalent to the operating system for a computer. In human cells, DNA is found in the nucleus as well as in the mitochondria.

A Quick Review of Molecular Biology

Basic Concepts about DNA

Despite the complex message that it carries, DNA has a rather simple structure consisting of three major components. Nitrogenous bases, or nucleotides, form the core and are divided into two major subgroups: the purines (adenine and thymine) and the pyrimidines (cytosine and guanine). The other two components are five carbon sugars and phosphate molecules. These three-component units are arranged in a linear fashion and are matched by a complementary chain. Adenine (A) and cytosine (C) form one complementary pair, while guanine (G) and thymine (T) form the other (Table 5.1). In this fashion, knowledge of the sequence of one chain provides the exact sequence for the matching chain.

DNA is composed of two chains that are coiled to form a regular helix, with about 10 nucleotide pairs per turn. Stretched, the total DNA of a human cell extends to about 2 m. Obviously, DNA is tightly packed to fit into the nucleus. This complex arrangement varies between cells and contributes to the different functions of the cells throughout the body.

Clusters of sequences along these strands of DNA form the building blocks for the key unit of genetic transmission, the gene. A strand of DNA therefore represents a string of different genes. Interspersed along this strand are sequences of DNA that are thought to have minimal function, often referred to as junk DNA, although this idea is currently in question. One string of DNA and its matching pair make up what has long been identified as a chromosome, a package of genetic material. There are approximately 30–35,000 genes in a human cell. Each gene behaves as a single

Table 5.1.   Nitrogenous bases.

Purines	Pyrimidines
Adenine	Thymine
Guanine	Cytosine

functional unit that provides a template for the ultimate formation of a polypeptide chain and a protein. This gave rise to the concept of one gene = one protein. We now know that through alternate splicing of genes, one gene can code for several different proteins, thus approximately 100,000 proteins are encoded by the 30–35,000 genes. Genes also segregate autonomously during meiosis according to the classic principles of Mendelian inheritance.

As stated above, it has been assumed that much of the DNA has limited function. To distinguish between those areas that behave as a gene or as part of a gene-functional unit and those that have no known function, terminology has been adopted. The DNA that contributes to genes is named genomic DNA, and the whole of the DNA is referred to as the genome.

Mutations represent alterations in the sequence of DNA. They are generally divided into three major categories. Point mutations refer to changes that involve only a single base pair in the gene. Sickle cell disease is a classic example of such a mutation. The difference between the normal gene and the sickle gene is a change from a single adenine to a thymine (A to T). This small change causes a change in the amino acid composition of the hemoglobin molecule by substituting a valine for a glutamic acid and alters the resulting protein enough to deform the red cell membrane. There are other types of point mutations, such as missense mutations, that lead to a change in the three-base sequence (codon = codes for one amino acid) causing a different amino acid to be inserted into the chain. Nonsense mutations, another type of point mutation, also cause a change in the codon. This can create a stop codon, truncating the formation of the protein. A second category of mutations, insertional mutations, refers to the situation where extra material is inserted into a gene. The extra material can be a single base pair or a whole string of DNA. An insertion may cause a disorder referred to as a trinucleotide repeat or expansion. A specific example of this type of disorder is Fragile X syndrome, the most common cause of mental retardation. The affected individual inherits an increasing number of repeated segments leading to an abnormal function of the gene. A third category is deletion mutation. As its name suggests, genetic material, consisting of one or many base pairs, is deleted from the DNA strand. In Duchenne's muscular dystrophy, 75% of the mutations involve large segments of gene deletions. Mutations can occur in DNA that is part of genomic DNA or in other areas of DNA. Certain regions of the genome are particularly prone to mutations. Such areas have been given the name of "hotspots."

The term *mutation*, or *mutant*, has often been associated with a negative connotation. Actually, the result of mutations can range from a total loss to greatly enhanced function. Loss-of-function mutations lead to decreased activity or absent activity of an enzyme, for example. Gain-of-function mutations also occur, such as when a protein takes on a toxic activity. Mutations that do not modify the function of a gene are said to be neutral. When an alteration in the base sequence does not result in a functional difference, the mutation is referred to as a polymorphism. Certain types of polymorphisms are used to detect genetic differences and are referred to as single nucleotide polymorphisms (SNPs). Because of these benign differences, any gene can have several variants. These alternate forms of the gene are called alleles.

One final basic concept is that of linkage. It has now well established that specific alleles not only are made up of their specific DNA sequence but are usually associated with specific sequences of DNA in their neighboring area. That neighboring DNA is said to be linked. The more likely a specific sequence of that adjacent DNA is to be associated with the specific variant of a gene, the closer the linkage is said to be. Analysis of linked sequences is called linkage analysis.

Summary Points

DNA is the basis of the genetic code.

Alterations in DNA sequences can lead to mutations, depending on their location, and this can lead to changes in gene function and potentially disease.

Where to Find DNA

Use of the term DNA most commonly refers to nuclear DNA. In actual fact, DNA is found not only in the nucleus but also in mitochondria. The potential of investigating mitochondrial DNA has just started to be realized. It holds great promise for understanding neurologic disorders but may also be extremely relevant to the reproductive process. It is generally accepted that the embryo has only maternal mitochondrial DNA, as the paternal complement of mito-chondria is retained within the sperm and does not participate in fertilization. Thus, maternal mitochondrial DNA will be transmitted vertically from genera-tion to generation, without the recombination seen in nuclear DNA. This will be a growing area of research in the coming years.

Principles of DNA Diagnosis

It should be obvious by now that the target of DNA diagnosis is the detection of problems at the level of a given gene or cluster of genes. This can be the search for the complete absence of a gene (a complete deletion), the lack of a portion of a gene (partial gene deletion), expansion of a repeating segment within a gene, or a mutation within a gene. Most genes contain between a few and several thousand base pairs (bp). To find a small sequence among the millions of base pairs that constitute the total DNA complement of a cell is literally like looking for a needle in a haystack. In other terms, DNA analysis aims at finding the equivalent of a microorganism on a strand spanning almost 2 m. To do this, several practical approaches have been developed which can be categorized simply into three groups.

Cutting Up DNA: Restriction Digest and Southern Blotting

If the total cellular DNA is cut into many tiny fragments, these then become more amenable to study (Fig. 5.1). This process is made possible by specific enzymes principally used by bacteria to lyse the DNA of invading organisms. Such enzymes are called restriction enzymes or restriction endonucleases. These restriction enzymes are identified by the bacteria that gives rise to them. For example, *Eco*RI refers to a restriction enzyme derived from *Escherichia coli*.

More importantly, restriction enzymes always cut at a specific site, determined by a specific sequence of DNA that is usually 4–6 bp in length. Thus, it is possible to reliably predict where restriction enzymes will cut. The resulting blend of DNA is referred to as a restriction digest, emphasizing the digested nature of the DNA cut at specific sites by the selected enzyme.

The digested fragments of DNA form charged particles. These can be electrophoresed on an agarose gel. The large heavy fragments will travel slowly down the gel and remain near the origin while the smaller fragments will distribute further down the gel, according to their size. The first scientist to describe this technique for DNA analysis was Dr. E.M. Southern, of the United Kingdom. In his honor, the resulting analysis blots are referred to as Southern blots.

Once the fragments have been spread out on the gel and transferred to a nylon membrane for ease of manipulation, a fragment of DNA that is complementary to the DNA of interest is used to pair up with it on the gel. This fragment of DNA is called a probe and is labeled for purposes of detection, with either a radioactive material or a fluorescent material.

Zooming in on a Segment of DNA: Polymerase Chain Reaction

In its natural state, DNA replicates itself short sequences at a time and is then assembled in its complex final form (Fig. 5.2). This process involves an enzyme known as DNA polymerase (DNA pol). It is now possible to replicate this process experimentally. In this fashion, it is possible to use the entire cellular DNA and target a specific area of interest. DNA replication of the specific area can then be performed. The process is repeated numerous times and follows exponential principles, giving rise to thousands of copies of a specific area of the genome. This process is referred to as polymerase chain reaction (PCR). PCR depends on two components. The first is a set of primers, usually about 20 bases long. One primer binds to the complementary strand upstream from the segment in question while the other primer binds to a complementary segment downstream. The second component is DNA polymerase that adds nucleotides to a growing strand. This enzyme can withstand dramatic temperature changes and facilitates replication of the growing strand at one temperature while remaining stable as the strands bind together or reanneal at a lower temperature. This has allowed PCR to be automated and performed quickly in a device called a thermocycler.

Genomic DNA

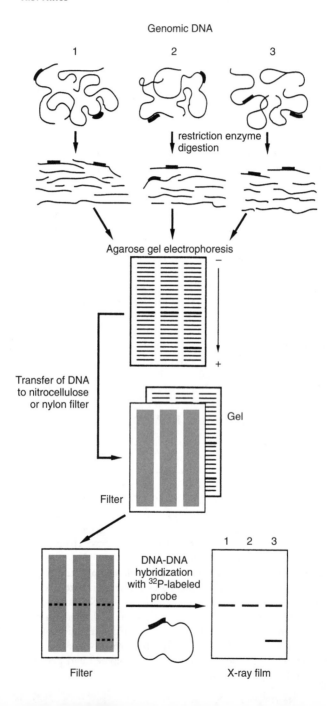

Fig. 5.1. Steps involved in the production of a Southern blot. (Reprinted from Thompson MW, McInnes RR, Willard HF. *Genetics in Medicine,* 5th ed. Copyright 1991, with permission, from Elsevier.)

Because PCR generates a very large number of copies of a specific segment of DNA, the DNA can be visualized directly under ultraviolet (UV) light, avoiding the need for molecular probes, as outlined for Southern blots. It is also possible to further cut up DNA obtained through PCR with

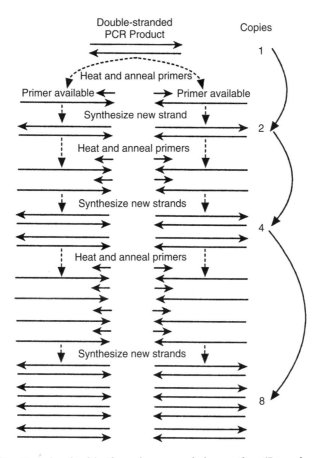

Fig. 5.2. Steps involved in the polymerase chain reaction. (Reproduced from Cogan JD, Phillips JA III. Polymerase chain reaction and DNA sequencing. *Infertil Reprod Med Clin N Am* 1991;5:143–56. Copyright 1994, with permission, from Elsevier.)

restriction enzymes. More recently, techniques have been developed to perform genetic diagnosis on a single cell, a remarkable undertaking considering that only two copies of a given gene may be located in a single cell.

Probing the DNA Within the Cell: Fluorescent *in situ* Hybridization

Chromosomes have been accessible for decades for cytogenetic analysis. Chromosome banding represents chemical labeling of the DNA sequences. In an analogous fashion, it is now possible to label specific regions of the DNA in the cell by using complementary DNA sequences known as DNA probes. These are tagged with a fluorescent label that lights up the specific chromosome location where the DNA probe has bound. This is the technique known as fluorescence *in situ* hybridization, or more commonly fluorescent *in situ* hybridization (FISH). FISH can be used to augment conventional cytogenetics, or karyotype analysis. Utilizing FISH, a large number of interphase nuclei can be examined, increasing the accuracy and eliminating a prolonged culture. This aspect of FISH can be helpful in prenatal diagnosis where time becomes important. FISH has also been used at the single cell level for preimplantation genetic diagnosis (PGD) of embryos.

Further Refinements

The three general approaches to DNA analysis are associated with further refinements that constitute the essentials of DNA diagnostic techniques.

Restriction Fragment Length Polymorphism Analysis

Restriction digests of DNA yields fragments of predictable length. If there is a mutation at an identified cut site for a specific enzyme, the result will be either the creation or the elimination of a predicted cut site. The former will yield shorter fragments than expected while the latter will give rise to larger fragments. If this mutation is associated with an abnormal allele, the difference in fragment length will be diagnostic (Fig. 5.3). The technique obviously involves Southern blotting to separate the different fragment lengths.

A key point to remember about restriction fragment length polymorphism (RFLP) analysis is that the mutation detected is frequently in DNA outside of the gene of interest, but closely linked to the allele of interest.

Oligonucleotide Probing

Another way of identifying a fragment of DNA of interest is by finding a complementary sequence of DNA that will bind specifically with the targeted DNA (Fig. 5.4). This can be accomplished by producing a short fragment of DNA, of between 20 and 100 bp, which is referred to as an oligonucleotide. This fragment will bind to the abnormal allele but not to the normal or wild type. This technique is therefore referred to as allele-specific oligonucleotide

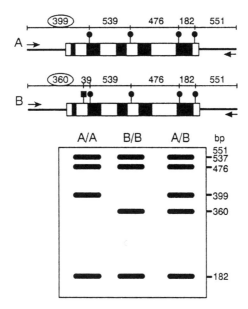

Fig. 5.3. Example of a diagnosis by RFLP technology. (Reproduced from Cogan JD, Phillips JA III. Polymerase chain reaction and DNA sequencing. *Infertil Reprod Med Clin N Am* 1991;5:143–56. Copyright 1994, with permission, from Elsevier.)

(ASO) probing. An attractive feature of this approach to diagnosis is that the probe used will bind only to the specific DNA sequence of interest. Instead of running the DNA on a gel to separate fragments, it becomes possible to put the entire digested DNA in a well and expose it to the probe. If the sequence that is sought is found, that spot of DNA will be highlighted relative to the other wells. This technique is called dot blotting or slot blotting, depending on the shape of the well.

Denaturing Gradient Gel Electrophoresis

Southern blotting separates fragments of DNA based on the molecular length. Another technique of separation is to use the principle that double-stranded DNA will denature differentially in gradients of chemical or thermal denaturants based on the unique sequence within the DNA strand. A gel is prepared that represents a gradient of denaturants. As the fragments travel down the gel, the double strands dissociate at different points and can therefore be identified on the gel by their different migratory properties.

Single-Stranded Conformation Polymorphism

Single-stranded conformation polymorphism (SSCP) uses PCR to first produce multiple copies of a gene of interest. The PCR product is separated

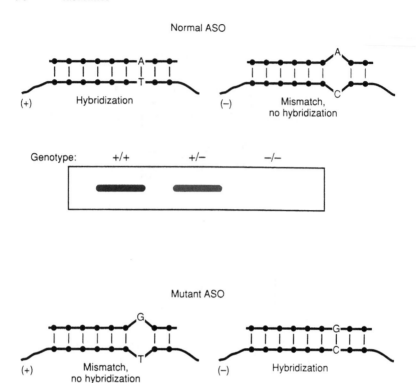

Fig. 5.4. Example of a diagnosis by oligonucleotide analysis. (Reprinted from Thompson MW, McInnes RR, Willard HF: *Genetics in Medicine,* 5th ed. Copyright 1991, with permission, from Elsevier.)

into single strands of DNA. Both a normal gene and an abnormal gene are electrophoresed in a polyacrylamide gel that allows for the detection of small differences between the genes as small as one base pair.

DNA Sequencing

The above-mentioned techniques are often used as screening techniques to rapidly determine if a given sample contains an abnormality. Subsequently, further identification of the mutation may be necessary. In this case, the specific sequence of the DNA will be determined often by utilizing a PCR-based method that incorporates radioactive material into increasing lengths of synthesized DNA strands. By arresting the lengthening strands at varying points using a method known as dideoxy chain termination, a step-by-step arrangement of the bases is determined. In this method, the radioactive label locates the arrested strand at various points and the base sequence is determined.

DNA sequencing can now be performed utilizing high-throughput technology and fluorescent-labeled oligonucleotides that are read by a scanning device as the sequence is electrophoresed on a gel. This innovation has remarkably shortened the time necessary for determining the genetic code in a segment of DNA.

DNA Arrays = The Chip

A rapid mechanism for screening multiple genes at one time is cDNA array analysis. These arrays are often used not for DNA, but for the ribonucleic acid or RNA for which the DNA codes. In analyzing RNA, the expressed genes can be examined. The arrays initially functioned in much the same way as the dot blots described above. Two tissues could be compared, a tumor and similar nontumor tissue, for example, determining for differences in gene expression between the two. The process would begin with extraction of the RNA from the two samples. RNA is converted to complementary, or cDNA, and labeled as if it were a probe. The labeled cDNA from each sample is hybridized to a membrane that contains large numbers of gene sequences of interest. This part of the process is similar to the Southern blot hybridization described above. Only a portion of the sequence is needed to allow correct hybridization and duplicate sequences placed on the membrane to provide controls. By comparing two identical membranes, each hybridized to one of the two samples, differences in gene expression are detected. Genes with greater intensity are suspected to be up-regulated relative to the normal or control tissue while other genes will appear down-regulated. A typical membrane might contain duplicated copies of some 600 genes, providing rapid analysis of all the genes at once.

From simple membranes containing fragments of gene sequences, this idea has now grown in sophistication with the creation of microarrays. Thousands of gene sequences are embedded on a glass slide. The cDNA of interest is labeled with a colored fluorochrome and a scanning device is used to detect differences in the two samples. This technique has had the greatest impact on research involving factors that change the gene expression of a tissue, but multiple clinical applications are possible. The use of large databases makes it possible to study how entire cascades of genes are related. Further, this volume of data has placed greater emphasis on the computational sciences or informatics.

Clinical Applications

All of the above techniques have been broadly utilized both in a research and in a clinical context. A gene becomes amenable to DNA diagnostics when the sequence has been identified or its location is known.

There are multiple areas where molecular techniques have important uses. A well-proven role for these techniques is in the area of prenatal diagnosis, such as identifying a sickle cell mutation in the fetus of carrier parents. Prenatal diagnosis can now be performed even before the creation of the fetus, by performing *in vitro* fertilization and testing day 3 embryos using single cell diagnostic techniques or PGD. PGD may use PCR-based technology for the identification of specific mutations or FISH for the identification of chromosomal abnormalities in the embryo. Single cell analysis allows the transfer of unaffected embryos to the patient, avoiding the need for pregnancy termination.

Another area that will have significant clinical impact is in the diagnosis of families at risk for cancer. The fundamental step, just as in prenatal diagnosis, is in first obtaining a good pedigree. This is a technique that even the busy practitioner can accomplish in a few minutes. While most cancer syndromes have yet to move from the research mode to practical application, risk analysis for family members is available for a small percentage of patients affected with breast and ovarian cancers due to mutations in *BRCA1* and *BRCA2* genes. Patients with BRCA1 mutations may have up to a 50% risk of ovarian cancer and may elect prophylactic surgery. The best treatment strategy has yet to be resolved. While inherited forms of cancer remain a minority of all cancers, they may represent the most important areas for prevention.

An additional use for molecular techniques is in the identification of infections. Currently PCR-based techniques are utilized for detection of bacterial infections like *Chlamydia* and viral infections like human immunodeficiency virus (HIV). Molecular-based studies decrease the time for detection relative to traditional culture approaches.

The analysis of tumor versus nontumor gene expression with cDNA arrays may lead to changes in cancer treatment. Rapid analysis of the whole genome from an individual, using a combination of arrays and automated sequencing, could reveal patients at risk for a number of disorders. A great deal of discussion will have to occur regarding issues of insurance coverage, the best use of risk assessment for a currently healthy individual, and the impact that detection of a disease risk could have on family members.

Keeping Up with the Developments in the Field

One of the greatest challenges for the clinician is keeping up with the rapid development in molecular biology. In addition to selected textbooks, it is necessary to be familiar with several resources. Journals such as *Science, Nature,* and *Molecular Endocrinology* have frequent comprehensive reviews about recent developments in molecular biology.

A tremendous source of information is the "On Line Mendelian Inheritance in Man" catalog, the computerized version of the outstanding reference catalog assembled by Dr. McKusick. This offers an exhaustive and constantly updated review on all disorders with a Mendelian pattern of inheritance. Much emphasis is placed on recent developments in molecular diagnosis. Most of these resources are now available through the Internet. The Human Genome Project will continue to have implications for years to come. In addition to deciphering our own genetic code, other organisms will yield important information as the code for each species is identified. We have explored the planet, space, and, now, the internal universe of our own DNA.

Case Studies

A male patient presents for an infertility evaluation and is found to have azospermia secondary to congenital absence of the vas deferens. What genetic test is indicated?

This patient may suffer from the same genetic mutation that is seen in cystic fibrosis (CF), despite the fact that he does not exhibit any pulmonary symptoms. This male may still be able to father a child, but he will require testicular biopsy to identify sperm, and his wife will have to undergo *in vitro* fertilization (IVF). Single sperm injection can then be performed on the retrieved oocytes, leading to pregnancy. The appropriate genetic test would be to test the husband and wife for the known CF mutations. The husband is almost certainly at least a heterozygote for one of these mutations and the critical aspect of this case is to determine if the wife is a carrier. If she is white of Northern European extraction, she has a 1/25 risk of being a carrier. If she is a carrier, then their child would have a 25% risk of having CF, a risk that some would find unacceptable. This could lead to an alternate decision to use donor sperm, or if desired, PGD on the embryos resulting from IVF.

A female patient reports a family history of a sister who was diagnosed at age 45 with breast cancer and a mother who died at 40 from the same disease. What is the appropriate genetic test to obtain?

Approximately 5% of breast cancer is inherited and the finding of two affected first-degree relatives would lead to testing for BRCA-1 and BRCA-2. This testing is best done on the affected individual or proband first, but may also be performed on archival material. The testing can be done only if the patient has been counseled appropriately and consideration given to a course of action if the testing is positive. Current options include prophylactic mastectomy and oophorectomy, although this approach remains controversial.

Glossary

Allele: Alternative forms of a gene.

CDNA: Complementary DNA or copy DNA, synthetic DNA obtained by transcription from an RNA fragment.

Codon: A trio of nucleotides specifying an amino acid.

Endonuclease: An enzyme that cleaves bonds with DNA or RNA.

Eukaryote: Organisms in which the cell has a well-developed nucleus and linear DNA. Human beings are thought to be the most famous eukaryotes.

Exon: That part of DNA that will ultimately be transcribed to mRNA to code for a polypeptide.

Gene: A segment of a DNA molecule involved in the synthesis of a polypeptide chain. The typical gene is composed of exons, the coding regions, and introns, the intervening noncoding regions.

Genome: The full complement of DNA in a cell.

Homeobox: One of many genes preserved in the phylogenetic scale and thought to play a role in cellular development.

Locus: The position of a gene on a chromosome.

Microarray: Contains sequences of different genes, potentially thousands, to which a cDNA population is hybridized.

Mutation: Any permanent heritable change in the sequence of DNA.

Nucleotide: A molecule composed of a nitrogenous base, a pentose and a phosphate.

Oncogene: One of many normal genes that have been preserved during the course of evolution and that play a role in normal and abnormal cellular development.

Probe: A labeled DNA or RNA sequence used to detect the presence of a complementary sequence by hybridization.

Southern blot: The technique used to transfer fragments of DNA on a special membrane and study their sequence by using complementary probes.

Triplet codon: the triplet codon is therefore the assembly of three nucleotides that code for a specific amino acid to be included in a polypeptide.

Suggested Reading

Gelehrter TD, Collins FS. *Principles of Medical Genetics.* Baltimore: Williams & Wilkins; 1990.

Genetics in Obstetrics and Gynecology. The American College of Obstetricians and Gynecologists; 2002.

Guttmacher AE, Collins FS. Genomic medicine—a primer. *N Engl J Med* 2002;347(19):1512–20.

Isada NB, Blakemore KJ. Basic concepts in molecular (DNA) diagnosis. *Obstet Gynecol Clin North Am* 1993;20:413–20.

Plouffe L Jr. Basic concepts of molecular biology for the reproductive endocrinologist. *Sem Reprod Endocrin* 1991;9(1):1–13.

Plouffe L Jr, Hines RS. Genetic considerations in common gynecologic disorders. *Infertil Reprod Med Clin N Am* 1994;5:143–56.

Thompson MW, McInnes RR, Willard HF. *Genetics in Medicine,* 5th ed. Philadelphia: Saunders; 1991.

6

Emergencies in the Office Setting

Mary Nan Mallory

Background Information

Although not widely reported in the literature, emergencies do occur in the office. Types and incidence will vary depending on patient demographics and specific office procedures. Providing definitive care for all emergency situations is obviously impossible, but the prudent clinician prepares to initiate treatment for the most likely and the most rapidly lethal diagnoses. Syncope, perhaps the most common, has many etiologies, some of which are life-threatening. Initial office management of cardiopulmonary arrest, hypoglycemia, seizures, and shock states, including anaphylaxis, can successfully avert morbidity and mortality.

When faced with a deteriorating patient in the office, the first minutes of care are focused not on diagnostics but on emergency medical services (EMS) notification and cardiopulmonary stabilization. Optimally, all office personnel are certified in basic life support (BLS). Current advanced cardiac life support (ACLS) training for the physicians and nurses allows for comprehensive resuscitation review and skill maintenance. A portable "office code cart" can provide the medications and equipment needed (Table 6.1). The cost of placing a cardiac monitor/defibrillator in the office may be offset by insurance premium discounts. Intervention priorities are guided by the systematic assessment of the "ABCDs" (Airway, Breathing, Circulation, neurologic Deficits).

Table 6.1.   Office code cart.[a]

Airway equipment
  Bag-valve-mask
  ETT (5, 6, 7, 8)
  Laryngoscope and blade
  Nasal cannula
  Oxygen tank
  Partial rebreather mask
  PTLV system (see text)
  Suction
  Stylet
  Syringe (10 ml)
  Trach tape
  Yankauer suction tip
IV equipment
  Catheters (14, 16, 18 gauge)
  Fluids (LR, NS)
  Heparin lock
  Saline flush
  Syringes (5, 10 ml)
  Tubing (two sets)
Medications
  Adenosine
  Atropine
  50% Dextrose
  Diazepam
  Diphenhydramine
  Epinephrine 1:1000
  Epinephrine 1:10,000
  Lidocaine
  Methylprednisolone
  Naloxone
  Nitroglycerin tablets 1/150
Monitoring equipment
  Cardiac monitor/defibrillator
ACLS reference algorithms

---

[a] ETT, endotracheal tube; PTLV, percutaneous translaryngeal ventilation; LR, lactated Ringer's; NS, normal saline; ACLS, advanced cardiac life support.

Establishing the Diagnoses

When faced with a life-threatening emergency in any setting, stabilization of the patient is best accomplished by systematic treatment of problems as they are identified. Unlike other clinical situations, in an emergency, this series of evaluation and treatment proceeds before a diagnosis is necessarily established. In fact, several diagnostic entities may occur simultaneously or in sequence. For example, a seizure may be the outward manifestation of sudden hypotension from an arrythmia portending cardiac arrest. It may also be the manifestation of hypoglycemia or inadequate/ineffective medical management of epilepsy. Regardless of etiology, for a prolonged seizure, the initial strategy is the same. Attend to the ABCDs of resuscitation and after a review of the patient's history, the events preceding the emergency situation, and the patient's response to treatment the diagnosis often becomes evident.

Clinical Intervention
Airway, Breathing, Circulation

Ensure the airway is open, clear, maintainable, and protected. After assessing the rate and depth of respirations, administer supplemental oxygen and positive-pressure ventilation as indicated. Intubation is appropriate to prevent aspiration when the airway is unprotected, spontaneous ventilations or oxygenation are inadequate, profound shock is evident, or therapeutic hyperventilation is necessary to emergently reduce increased intracranial pressure from a space occupying lesion. Selecting a smaller endotracheal tube may facilitate passage through an edematous upper airway.

When intubation is unsuccessful, percutaneous translaryngeal ventilation (PTLV) is a rapid, simple technique that may preclude an office cricothyrotomy. Although not a substitute for airway control with a cuffed tube, PTLV can provide effective ventilation for prolonged periods of time. After puncturing the inferior aspect of the cricothyroid membrane at a caudal angle with a 14-gauge over the needle catheter, remove the needle and advance the catheter tip toward the carina (Fig. 6.1). A three-way stopcock is interposed between the catheter and oxygen extension tubing. A flush open wall source or an oxygen cylinder without a secondary regulator valve can provide the necessary 50 psi, high-pressure oxygen source. Initially ventilate at only 25 psi until the correct catheter position is verified by auscultation. Intermittently occluding a hole cut on one side of the extension tubing with a finger will allow the chest to rise and the patient to be oxygenated. Passive exhalation occurs with finger release. When complete upper airway obstruction is present, harmful intratracheal pressures may occur. As a temporizing measure until cricothyrotomy, a second 14-gauge catheter similarly placed may facilitate exhalation.

Check for a central pulse and measure blood pressure. Initiate cardiac monitoring as soon as available and secure intravenous (IV) access. Trendelenburg positioning and a 500-ml crystalloid bolus are effective for transient

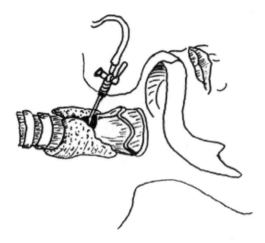

Fig. 6.1. Percutaneous translaryngeal ventilation. Oxygen tubing is attached by an interposed three-way stopcock to a catheter inserted through the cricothyroid membrane. (Mace, SE. Percutaneous translaryngeal ventilation. In Clinical Procedures in Emergency Medicine, 2nd ed. Roberts JR, Hedges JR (eds) Philadelphia: Lippincott Williams and Wilkins, 1991: 49–56.)

hypotension. When persistent, further therapy should be directed toward the underlying shock state.

Hypovolemic Shock

Gastroenteritis and hemorrhagic etiologies are the most likely causes. Hemorrhage should be controlled to the extent possible. Large-bore catheters allow rapid infusion of 1–2 liters or more of crystalloid until blood and definitive treatment are available.

Septic Shock

Suggested by a history of infection, fever, or warm, flushed skin, the persistent hypotension associated with sepsis results from capillary leakage and altered peripheral vascular resistance. Vital signs should dictate the need for repeat crystalloid boluses. Although not Food and Drug Administration (FDA) approved, naloxone may be helpful in reversing endotoxin-mediated hypotension. Begin with 0.8 mg IV, redose with 1.6 mg IV, and repeat every few minutes to a maximum of 4 mg. Consider empiric antibiotics when available.

Anaphylactic Shock

Anaphylaxis is an acute multiorgan system allergic response resulting in vasodilation, increased vascular permeability, and smooth muscle contractions. Any symptom that potentially represents a systemic reaction must be treated as rapid progression to circulatory collapse may occur (Table 6.2). Because the initiating agents are myriad, only a representative few are listed (Table 6.3). Parenteral penicillin accounts for about half of all anaphylactic fatalities annually. Early active airway management and crystalloid fluids are important, but epinephrine is the mainstay of treatment for all clinical manifestations and is dosed depending upon symptom severity (Table 6.4). If IV access is delayed, inject the intravenous dose into the sublingual venous plexus or instill endotracheally (Table 6.5). Transport will be indicated for all but completely asymptomatic patients observed for 3 hours after only a minor reaction.

Cardiogenic Shock

In addition to the pump dysfunction associated with myocardial infarction, arrythmias contribute to hypotension. Hemodynamic compromise from bradycardic rhythms and both wide and narrow complex tachycardias may be similarly manifest as ischemic chest pain, hypotension, altered mentation, hypoperfusion, or significant dyspnea. Judicious crystalloid boluses can be

Table 6.2. Clinical manifestations of anaphylaxis.

Organ system	Symptoms	Signs	Reaction
Respiratory tract	Nasal congestion	Mucosal edema	Rhinitis
	Itching, sneezing	Rhinorrhea	Laryngeal
	Throat tightening	Hoarseness,	edema
	Cough, dyspnea	stridor	
	Chest tightness	Tachypnea,	Bronchospasm
		cyanosis	
		Wheeze, rhonchi	
Cardiovascular system	Lightheadedness	Tachycardia	Circulatory
	Weakness, syncope	Hypotension	collapse
	Chest pain	Shock	
	Palpitations	Irregular pulse	Arrhythmia
		Pulseless	Asystole
Skin	Pruritis, flushing	Diffuse erythema	Urticaria
	Tingling, warmth	Hives	
	Swelling, numbness	Perioral	Angioedema
	Tongue thickening	Periorbital swelling	
Central nervous system	Apprehension	Anxiety	Seizures
	Impending doom	Tremor	(rarely)
Gastrointestinal tract	Dysphagia	Hyperactive bowel	Nausea
	Abdominal	sounds	Vomiting
	cramping		
Eye	Ocular pruritis	Edema and	Conjunctivitis
	Blurred vision	erythema	
		Lacrimation	

Table 6.3. Precipitating agents in anaphylaxis.[a]

Mechanism	Precipitant
Classic IgE antibody–antigen-mediated reaction	Antibiotics: penicillins, cephalosporins, sulfas
	Foods: nuts, shellfish, berries, eggs, milk, chocolate, grains, oils
	Foreign proteins: pollen, hymenoptera/snake venoms, hormones, vaccines
Immune complex mediated or complement mediated	Blood, fresh frozen plasma, immunoglobin
Direct, nonimmune mediated	Radiocontrast material
	Additives: food dyes, dextran
Anaphylactoid reaction	Drugs, aspirin, NSAIDs, opiates
	Exercise, physical agents

[a] IgE, immunoglobulin E; NSAIDs, nonsteroidal antiinflammatory drugs.

Table 6.4. Office management of anaphylaxis.

Remove inciting agent
Keep affected extremity dependent
Apply local ice for 15 minutes
ABCs/IV

First-line therapy is epinephrine[a]			
Reaction severity	Route	Concentration	Adult dose
Mild (urticaria, bronchospasm)	SQ	1:1000	0.3 ml
Moderate (respiratory distress, hypotension)	SQ or IM	1:1000	0.3–0.5 ml
Severe (laryngeal edema respiratory failure, blood pressure unresponsive to IM dose)	IV	1:10,000	Dilute 1 ml in 10 ml NS

Table 6.4.   *Continued.*

Second-line therapy		
Medication	Route	Adult dose
Mild		
Diphenhydramine	PO for 3–5 days	25–75 mg q6h
Prednisone	PO for 3–5 days	40–60 mg qd
Moderate		
Diphenhydramine	IM or IV	50–75 mg
Crystalloid	IV	1–2 liters prn
Cimetidine	PO or IV	300 mg
Methylprednisolone	IV	50–125 mg
Severe		
Repeat	IV	Repeat above dose every
Epinephrine		10 minutes

[a] Epinephrine may be aerosolized via an endotracheal tube. See Table 6.5.

temporizing. Atropine is reserved only for symptomatic bradycardias. For unstable tachycardiac arrhythmias with a ventricular rate of more than 150 beats/minutes, synchronized cardioversion (beginning at 100 J) is indicated after a brief trial of medication fails to restore sinus rhythm. Initial office resuscitation sequences can guide life-saving interventions for both unstable arrythmias and cardiopulmonary arrest in adults (Table 6.6).

Table 6.5.   Endotracheal drug administration.

Drug	Dosage
Atropine	1–2 mg
Diazepam	2–4 mg
Epinephrine	2–2.5 mg
Lidocaine	2–3 mg/kg
Naloxone	0.4–2.0 mg

Dilute drug volume to 10 ml with saline.
Suspend CPR. Rapidly push down the endotracheal tube.
Follow with three or four forceful ventilations. Resume CPR.

Table 6.6.   Initial office resuscitation sequences.

Ventricular fibrillation and pulseless ventricular tachycardia
ABCs/CPR
Defibrillate (200 J) → defibrillate (300 J) → defibrillate (360 J)
Reevaluate
CPR/intubate/IV
1 mg IV push epinephrine[a] repeated every 3–5 minutes
Defibrillate (360 J)
1.5 mg/kg bolus lidocaine[a] repeated once after 3–5 minutes
Defibrillate (360 J)

Pulseless electrical activity (PEA) and asystole
ABCs/CPR
Intubate/IV
Consider causes/(interventions)
Hypovolemia? (volume infusion)
Hypoxia? (oxygenation, ventilation)
Acidosis? (volume infusion, ventilation)
Drug overdose? (identification)
Massive, acute myocardial infarction? (fluid challenge)
Hyperkalemia/tension pneumothorax?
1 mg IV push epinephrine repeated every 3–5 minutes
For bradycardia, 1 mg IV atropine[a] repeated every 3–5 minutes (total
    0.04 mg/kg)

Narrow and wide complex tachycardias

Narrow QRS	Wide QRS
Vagal maneuvers	Lidocaine 1.5 mg/kg IV bolus
Adenosine 6 mg, rapid IV push	Lidocaine 1.5 mg/kg IV bolus
Adenosine 12 mg, rapid IV push	Consider adenosine trial
Consider lidocaine trial	

Synchronized cardioversion (100 J → 200 J → 300 J)
For ventricular rates >150 beats/minute
After a brief trial of medication fails and unstable cardiopulmonary
    symptoms are present

---

[a] Atropine, epinephrine, and lidocaine may be aerosolized via an endotracheal
tube; see Table 6.5.

Cardiac Arrest

For the unresponsive, apneic patient with absent pulses, begin cardiopulmonary resuscitation (CPR) and proceed with electrical and pharmacologic therapy as indicated by the cardiac rhythm. The immediate priority becomes the identification of pulseless ventricular tachycardia or ventricular fibrillation. Early, rapid defibrillation is the single most important intervention when these lethal rhythms are encountered. If the initial three defibrillation attempts are unsuccessful, proceed with intubation and a "drug/shock" sequence beginning with epinephrine. Early EMS notification with paramedic response should exclude the need for office administration of second-line antiarrythmics and sodium bicarbonate.

Pulseless electrical activity (PEA) and asystole are fatal unless reversible underlying causes such as hypoxia or hypovolemia are immediately identified and aggressively treated.

When cardiac arrest occurs in the pregnant woman, proceed with standard CPR. A wedge should be placed under the right flank and hip, displacing the gravid uterus leftward. Defibrillation and drug administration are performed without modification. With a fetus at a viable gestational age, the decision to perform a perimortem cesarean section must be made rapidly, with delivery effected within 4–5 minutes of maternal arrest to maximize both maternal and infant survival. When anticipated, the obstetrician may need to accompany the patient during transport to the hospital.

Neurologic Deficits/Disability

Perform a directed neurologic examination. Pupillary response and any gross lateralizing deficits should be noted. Naloxone will temporarily arouse most patients from opiate sedation. Dose titration and fetal monitoring for the addicted pregnant patient are important to prevent fetal narcotic withdrawal.

Syncope

Characterized by the sudden and temporary loss of postural vascular tone and a brief loss of consciousness with spontaneous, rapid recovery of full alertness, syncope is a symptom whose proximate cause is usually cerebral hypoperfusion. Underlying etiologies vary widely in clinical significance from a benign vasovagal faint to the portent of sudden death in cardiovascular disease (Table 6.7). As such, active medical intervention may not be indicated, but resources should be mobilized nonetheless to ensure adequate ventilation, perfusion, and cervical spine stabilization in the event the episode is not self-limiting or recurrent (Table 6.8).

Only those office patients who remain asymptomatic after vasovagal, hyperventilation, or reversed hypovolemic (hemorrhage excluded) syncope should be considered for discharge home. Hospitalization is indicated for monitoring and diagnostic testing in patients with frequent episodes, syncope while recumbent or associated with cardiac symptoms (palpitations, chest pain, dyspnea), or in elderly patients when the cause cannot be clearly explained as noncardiac. Emergency department screening evaluation for patients not clearly in a low- or high-risk group may further elucidate underlying pathology and guide disposition decisions.

Table 6.7. Causes of transient loss of consciousness.

Syncope
Vasomotor/circulatory
Vasovagal response
Hypovolemia, hemorrhage
Drug–induced
Autonomic insufficiency
Cough, micturition induced
Aortic dissection
Cardiac
Dysrhythmias
Valvular heart disease
Pulmonary embolus
Valsalva maneuver
Cardiomyopathy
Myocardial infarction
Metabolic
Hypoglycemia
Hypocapnia
Hypoxia
Central nervous system
Subarachnoid hemorrhage
Cerebral vascular insufficiency
Sleep disorders
Migraine
Subclavian steal syndrome
Psychogenic
Seizures
Drug induced
Head trauma

Table 6.8.   Initial office approach to syncope.

C-spine
Protect patient from further injury
Immobilize cervical spine after a fall
Airway
Open the airway with chin lift, jaw thrust
Clear the airway by finger sweep, suction
Prepare for (unlikely) intubation
Breathing
Apply supplemental oxygen
Assess rate and adequacy of effort
Positive-pressure ventilation if prolonged, poor effort
Circulation
Cardiac monitoring
Manage any symptomatic cardiac dysrhythmia
Pulse, blood pressure determinations
Identify and control hemorrhage
Establish intravenous access
Crystalloid replacement as indicated
Deficits (neurologic)
Rapid fingerstick glucose determination
If not available, empiric 50% dextrose for diabetics
Reevaluate
Obtain further history
Monitor vital signs
Evaluate for injuries secondary to fall
Transport unless etiology is clearly benign

Hypoglycemia

For an altered level of consciousness, routinely check a fingerstick glucose and treat for hypoglycemia with one 25-g ampule of 50% dextrose ($D_{50}W$) IV if measured less than 80 mg/dl. In the absence of IV access, the same dose administered rectally is effective. Empiric treatment is indicated when rapid glucose determination cannot be made. Once the patient becomes alert, a complex carbohydrate food should be eaten. Clinical judgment will determine the need for transport.

Seizure

When generalized seizure is noted, protect the patient from injury, immobilize the cervical spine if a fall has occurred, and provide oxygen by partial rebreather mask. Eclampsia is an obvious consideration. Check for and treat hypoglycemia. Most idiopathic generalized seizures are self-limiting, lasting less than 3–5 minutes followed by initial postictal combativeness and slowly resolving confusion. For prolonged or repeated seizure activity, intubate and administer diazepam 2 mg slow IV push or instill endotracheally. Repeat this every minute in 2 mg increments until the seizure ceases. Reassess the patient for adequacy of breathing and transport the patient to evaluate the underlying seizure etiology, most commonly a subtherapeutic anticonvulsant level.

Reevaluation

After all necessary and available resuscitation measures have been completed, reevaluate the airway interventions, the vital signs, and the patient's responsiveness. Obtain a further history and determine medications taken and known allergies. Copies of pertinent documentation should be provided to the transferring paramedic.

Once the patient is en route to the emergency department, phone communication with the receiving emergency physician will be appreciated.

Thought-Provoking Cases

Case 1. Fifteen minutes after an IM injection of ceftriaxone, a 23-year-old gynecology patient complains to your nurse's aide of lightheadedness and pruritus. The aide has placed the patient in an available room and reports that the blood pressure is 85/40 and the heart rate is 115. You note that the patient has stridorous breathing.

How do you proceed?

1. Identify one person to call EMS about a patient in respiratory distress who may be having a multisystem allergic reaction or anaphylaxis.
2. Prepare for airway management and call for the office code cart.
3. Assess the patient's breathing.
4. Because the patient's symptoms are characteristic of a *severe* reaction, treat the patient with epinephrine either SC or IV if rapid IV access is available.
5. Once an IV is established, bolus with crystalloid fluids.
6. Reassess and repeat epinephrine every 10 minutes as needed for hypotension or shortness of breath.
7. Treat with inhaled β-agonists, antihistamines, and steroids.
8. Prepare the patient for transport.
9. Call the receiving emergency physician to give a report of symptoms and treatment.

10. Debrief and review emergency procedures with the staff.
11. Pat yourself on the back for being prepared.

Case 2. The 64-year-old mother of one of your obstetric patients becomes distraught in your consultation room after hearing that an ultrasound of her next grandchild is abnormal. She complains suddenly of shortness of breath, chest tightness, and lightheadedness.
How do you proceed?

1. Position the patient in a supine position on the floor or in the examining room.
2. Identify one individual to notify EMS about an older woman with chest pains and breathing difficulty and call for an automated external defibrillator (AED) and office code cart.
3. Supply supplemental oxygen 2 liters/minute via nasal cannula.
4. Assess the patient's pulse rate.
5. Obtain vital signs, and a brief cardiopulmonary history, past history, and medications.
6. Obtain IV access.

As you assess the patient, she suddenly becomes diaphoretic, then unresponsive and pulseless. How do you proceed?

1. Initiate CPR and call for an AED and office code cart.
2. Identify one individual to renotify EMS that your patient is now in cardiac arrest.
3. Obtain IV access when possible.
4. As no AED or code cart arrives, continue CPR until EMS arrives 18 minutes after the first call.
5. Prepare the patient for transport.
6. Call the receiving emergency physician and give a report of the patient's status.
7. Debrief, review, and reconsider your office emergency procedures with the staff.

Summary

Initial resuscitative efforts for office emergencies such as syncope, hypoglycemia, seizure, anaphylaxis, hypotension, and cardiac arrest or a combination thereof can be accomplished in a rapid and organized manner by the prepared obstetrician/gynecologist and office staff.

When faced with an emergency in the office, proceed with simultaneous evaluation and treatment of the airway and breathing, the circulation, and any neurologic deficits.

Advanced preparation including a trained staff, dedicated equipment, and early notification of the local emergency medical services system will result in the best outcomes.

Suggested Reading

Danzl DF. Tracheal intubation and mechanical ventilation. In *Emergency Medicine: A Comprehensive Study Guide,* 5th ed. Tintinalli JE (ed). New York: McGraw-Hill; 2000:85–97.

De Lorenzo RA. Syncope. In: *Rosen's Emergency Medicine: Concepts and Clinical Practice,* 5th ed. Marx J, et al. (eds). St. Louis, MO: Mosby-Year Book; 2002:172–178.

Guidelines 2000 for Cardiopulmonary Resuscitation and Emergency Cardiovascular Care, American Heart Association. *Supplement to Circulation* 2000;102(8).

Mace SE. Percutaneous translaryngeal ventilation. In *Clinical Procedures in Emergency Medicine,* 2nd ed. Roberts JR, Hedges JR (eds). Philadelphia: Saunders, 1991:49–56.

Muelloman RL, Tran TP. Allergy, hypersensitivity, and anaphylaxis. In *Rosen's Emergency Medicine: Concepts and Clinical Practice,* 5th ed. Marx J, et al. (eds). St. Louis, MO: Mosby-Year Book; 2002:1619–1635.

Clinical Management Principles for the Office Setting

7

Abnormal Pap Smear: Gynecologic Pathology and Management

Richard S. Guido

Introduction

The introduction of the Papanicolaou (Pap) test as a routine screening test has resulted in a 70% reduction in the incidence of cervical cancer in the United States over the past five decades. In 2003 over 50 million women underwent cervical cancer screening, revealing close to 2.5 million abnormalities. Screening is offered by a variety of health care providers in various specialties.

In the past decade there has been a remarkable increase in knowledge concerning the natural history of cervical dysplasia, the role of human papiloma virus (HPV) in cervical cancer, and the development of new technologies for cervical cancer screening, specifically HPV testing and liquid-based cytology. The new information has prompted the American Cancer Society (ACS), the American Society for Colposcopy and Cervical Pathology (ASCCP), and the National Institutes of Health (NIH) to develop new guidelines pertaining to cervical cancer screening, cytologic terminology, and treatment of cytologic abnormalities. The objective of this chapter is to provide the most up-to-date recommendations on cervical cancer screening services for women.

Natural History of Human Papiloma Virus

Over 90% of all cervical cancer patients have evidence of HPV DNA present in the cancer cells, specifically high-risk HPV. The development of accurate tests for HPV, Hybrid Capture II and polymerase chain reaction (PCR), has drastically improved our understanding of the pathophysiology of cervical cancer and cervical dysplasia.

HPV is a group of common DNA viruses that infects squamous epithelium and is associated with a broad range of clinical manifestations. There are over 85 different types of HPV viruses. The genital tract represents one of the major sites of HPV infection. The majority of infections of the genital tract are asymptomatic in both men and women. Clinically apparent HPV is associated with genital warts, cervical intraepithelial neoplasia (CIN), vaginal intraepithelial neoplasia (VAIN), vulvar intraepithelial neoplasia (VIN), and squamous cell cancers of the cervix, vagina, and vulva.

The transmission of HPV is strongly associated with sexual activity. Natural history studies of HPV-negative adolescents with normal Pap tests who become sexually active clearly demonstrate the sexual acquisition of HPV. HPV is detectable in <2% of sexually inexperienced women yet is detectable in 45% of those who are sexually active. Studies that have followed a specific cohort of young sexually active women over time have demonstrated that over 50–60% of the population will be positive for HPV. The link between sexual activity and HPV infection is further strengthened by the identification of similar HPV types among sexual partners. Sexual transmission is the primary means of acquiring HPV but evidence of nonsexual transmission does exist. Although rare, there is some evidence for *in utero* infection, perinatal infection, auto- and heteroinoculation through close nonsexual contact, and possibly indirect transmission via fomites.

The majority of women infected with HPV will be asymptomatic. Those that are detected, either by an abnormal Pap test, HPV test, or the presence of clinically evident genital warts, will most likely resolve the infection without treatment. In natural history studies of adolescents with newly acquired HPV infection the average length of infection of detectable HPV is 13 months. The majority of patients with an intact immune system will resolve an HPV infection within 24 months. Further evidence for the resolution of HPV infection comes from the high resolution rate of CIN 1 and CIN 2, 70% and 50%, respectively. Unfortunately some individuals are susceptible to persistent HPV infection. In these individuals the HPV may be present for years, and may put them at high risk for the development of cervical cancer.

Cervical Cancer Screening Test

Cervical cancer screening programs based on the Pap smear have been highly effective in reducing the rate of cervical cancer in countries that have widespread screening programs. The system, however, is not without problems. The most common cause for a missed diagnosis of cervical cancer is the lack of screening. Despite the widespread availability of the Pap test in the United States, 50% of women diagnosed with cervical cancer have either never been screened or have not had a Pap test in the past 5 years.

Until the development of a reliable liquid-based Pap test the only available cervical cytology screening method was the conventional Pap smear. This test is an excellent screening test but it does have numerous limitations. The overall sensitivity of the Pap smear is believed to be 70%. The missed cases of cervical disease are more often due to the lack of transfer of the cells from the cervix to the smear rather than an oversight by the cytologist. Liquid-based cytology was in part developed to overcome the shortcomings of the traditional Pap smear. Presently two techniques have been approved by the Food and Drug Administration (FDA) for cervical cancer screening: ThinPrep (Cytyc, Boxborough, MA) and SurePath (TriPath, Burlington, NC).

ThinPrep requires sampling the cervix with either a broom-type device (e.g., Wallach Papette, Wallach Surgical Devices, Inc., Milford, CT) or a combination of a plastic spatula and a cytobrush (Medscand, Hollywood, FL). The spatula is then vigorously swirled in the collection medium and the cytobrush is rubbed against the side of the collection vial to remove as many cells as possible from the device. The broom is vigorously compressed against the base of the vial 10 times to separate the cells from the device.

The cervical cells are retrieved from the liquid medium via an automated device. The fluid is first agitated and then suctioned up through a filter that separates the cells from the liquid. The medium itself is both mucolytic and hemolytic and therefore the resulting monolayer sample is free of many of the obscuring problems that are present in a traditional Pap smear. This technology has demonstrated an increased sensitivity for low-grade as well as high-grade cervical abnormalities. ThinPrep prevents an air drying effect, has increased sensitivity for the detection of cervical abnormalities, and is FDA approved for the ancillary testing of residual fluid, specifically for HPV. Liquid-based cervical screening is now the most common method used in the United States. SurePath is FDA approved as an equivalent technique for cervical cancer screening and is in the process of seeking FDA approval for ancillary testing for HPV.

Bethesda 2001

The Bethesda system is designed to standardize the reporting of cervical cytology, improve quality assurance, and ultimately assist clinicians in the management of patients with abnormal Pap tests. Originally developed in 1988 the system has undergone its most recent changes in 2001. The entire classification is presented in Table 7.1. Bethesda 2001 has numerous changes, which not only make the system easier for the clinician to use but also reflect the importance of new technologies in the evaluation of cytologic abnormalities of the cervix.

Specimen adequacy is one of the most important components of the cytologic report. This aspect of the report has been simplified by eliminating

Table 7.1.   Bethesda 2001.

Specimen type: *Indicate conventional smear (Pap smear) vs. liquid based vs. other*

Specimen adequacy

- Satisfactory for evaluation (*describe the presence or absence of an endocervical/transformation zone component and any other quality indicators, e.g., partially obscuring blood, inflammation, etc.*)
- Unsatisfactory for evaluation (*specify reason*)
  - Specimen rejected/not processed (*specify reason*)
  - Specimen processed and examined, but unsatisfactory for evaluation of epithelial abnormality because of (*specify reason*)

General categorization (*optional*)

- Negative for intraepithelial lesion or malignancy
- Epithelial cell abnormality: see Interpretation/Result (*specify "squamous" or "glandular" as appropriate*)
- Other: see Interpretation/Result (*e.g., endometrial cells in a woman ≥40 years of age*)

Automated review

If case examined by automated device, specify device and result

Ancillary testing

Provide a brief description of the test methods and report the result so that it is easily understood by the clinician

Interpretation/Result

Negative for intraepithelial lesion or malignancy (*when there is no cellular evidence of neoplasia, state this in the General Categorization above and/or in the Interpretation/Result section of the report, whether or not there are organisms or other nonneoplastic findings*)

Organisms:

- *Trichomonas vaginalis*
- Fungal organisms morphologically consistent with *Candida* spp.
- Shift in flora suggestive of bacterial vaginosis
- Bacteria morphologically consistent with *Actinomyces* spp.
- Cellular changes consistent with Herpes simplex virus

Other nonneoplastic findings (*optional to report; list not inclusive*):

- Reactive cellular changes associated with
  - inflammation (includes typical repair)
  - radiation
  - intrauterine contraceptive device (IUD)
  - Glandular cells status posthysterectomy
  - Atrophy

Table 7.1. *Continued.*

Other
- Endometrial cells (*in a woman ≥40 years of age*) (*Specify if "negative for squamous intraepithelial lesion"*)

Epithelial cell abnormalities

Squamous cell
- Atypical squamous cells
  - Of undetermined significance (ASC-US)
  - Cannot exclude HSIL (ASC-H)
- Low-grade squamous intraepithelial lesion (LSIL) encompassing HPV/mild dysplasia/CIN 1
- High-grade squamous intraepithelial lesion (HSIL) encompassing moderate and severe dysplasia, CIS/CIN 2 and CIN 3
  - With features suspicious for invasion (*if invasion is suspected*)
- Squamous cell carcinoma

Glandular cell
- Atypical
  - Endocervical cells (NOS *or specify in comments*)
  - Endometrial cells (NOS *or specify in comments*)
  - Glandular cells (NOS *or specify in comments*)
- Atypical
  - Endocervical cells, favor neoplastic
  - Glandular cells, favor neoplastic
- Endocervical adenocarcinoma *in situ*
- Adenocarcinoma
  - Endocervical
  - Endometrial
  - Extrauterine
  - Not otherwise specified (NOS)

Other malignant neoplasms: (*specify*)

Educational notes and suggestions (*optional*)
   Suggestions should be concise and consistent with clinical follow-up guidelines published by professional organizations (references to relevant publications may be included).

Source: The 2001 Bethesda System JAMA, April 24, 2002; Vol. 287; 16.

the previously confusing category of "satisfactory but limited by." The specimen is now either "satisfactory for evaluation" or "unsatisfactory for evaluation." Minimum standards for the presence of endocervical and squamous cells have been established, and the cytology laboratory may comment with regards to the presence of obscuring inflammation. The presence of endocervical or metaplastic cells on a Pap test is considered evidence that the entire transformation zone has been sampled.

The presence of these cells is preferred, although their absence has not been shown to decrease the sensitivity for the detection of high-grade cytologic abnormalities.

The report includes a "general categorization" section, which is optional, but provides a one-sentence summary of the results of the cytology for easier triage. The sample is either "negative for intraepithelial lesions or malignancy" or an "epithelial cell abnormality" is present.

The "epithelial cell abnormality" interpretation has a number of important changes. The cytologic abnormality "atypical squamous cells of undetermined significance (ASC-US)" has been renamed and subdivided. The new abnormality is "atypical squamous cells (ASC)" and is subdivided into "of undetermined significance (ASC-US)" and "cannot exclude high-grade squamous intraepithelial lesions (HSIL)." This change mirrors the general understanding of cervical disease being subdivided into low- and high-grade abnormalities. The bulk of scientific data suggests that the majority of minor cytologic abnormalities [ASC-US and low-grade squamous intraepithelial lesions (LSIL)] represent clinical manifestations of various stages of HPV infection. The more dysplastic changes associated with HSIL represent a significant risk for the development of cervical cancer.

The ASC-H subcategory represents a small fraction (5%) of all ASC diagnoses and is characterized by a small number of moderate to severely dyplastic cells on the entire specimen. This group has been shown to harbor high-risk HPV in greater than 80% of samples and may be found to have moderate to severe dysplasia in 40% of cases within a 2-year period. As such this diagnosis requires more extensive evaluation and close follow-up.

The LSIL and the HSIL categories remain unchanged from the 1991 Bethesda system. These diagnoses are generally reproducible and in many ways reflect the dichotomous division in squamous intraepithelial lesions.

There have been numerous changes in the description of glandular cell abnormalities in the new Bethesda system. The previous system included the diagnosis atypical glandular cells of undetermined significance (AGUS), which was frequently confused with ASCUS, yet represented a more significant diagnosis. Glandular cell abnormalities are now separated into four separate categories: atypical glandular cells (AGC); atypical glandular cells, favor neoplastic; endocervical adenocarcinoma *in situ* (AIS); and adenocarcinoma. The first two groups should, when possible, characterize the cell of origin, endocervical or endometrial. The new system better describes the cellular abnormalities and is better suited for use by clinicians.

The final changes to the new Bethesda system are the addition of automated review and ancillary testing, and educational notes. This information gives the clinician information about the use of computerized cytologic anaylsis and ancillary tests (such as HPV testing), and provides the opportunity for the cytologist to comment about the validity and significance of an interpretation. Ultimately all these changes reflect the advancement in the technology used in the preparation and interpretation of cytologic specimens.

Screening Guidelines

The American College of Obstetricians and Gynecologists (ACOG) and the ACS have recently published evidence-based guidelines that cover a variety of issues relating to cervical cancer screening. In some cases these recommendations represent a significant departure from previous guidelines.

Onset of Screening

Traditionally cervical cancer screening has been initiated at age 18 years or at the onset of sexual activity. This time period corresponds to a period during which young women are very likely to become exposed to HPV infection. The majority of HPV infections in this population are transient yet they can produce cytologic abnormalities that prompt a colposcopic examination. Longitudinal studies of HPV-negative adolescents who acquire HPV demonstrate that 36 months is required to develop an HSIL Pap test. Finally, squamous cell cancer in women <21 years of age is exceedingly rare. Therefore the ACS and ACOG recommend the initiation of cervical cytology no later than age 21 years or 3 years after the onset of sexual activity.

Frequency of Screening

The optimal screening frequency for women is difficult to specify. Cytology, by its very nature, has a false-negative rate of 15–30%. Therefore its success in part depends on repeated tests that reduce the rate of false-negatives to an acceptable level. The ACOG and ACS recommend annual cytologic screening with traditional Pap smears and screening every 2 years if a liquid-based system is used. Both societies agree that screening intervals may be increased to every 2–3 years for women over the age of 30 who have three consecutive, technically satisfactory normal Pap smears. Women who are HIV positive, have a history of *in utero* exposure to diethylstilbestrol (DES), or are immunosuppressed should continue with annual examinations.

End of Screening

The absolute age at which cervical cancer screening may be discontinued is unclear. The ACS recommends women age 70 years and older with an intact cervix and who have three or more documented, consecutive, technically satisfactory normal/negative cervical cytology tests, and no abnormal/positive test within the 10 years prior to age 70, may discontinue cytologic screening. The U.S. Preventive Services Task Force has set 65 years of age as the upper limit of screening. Women for whom a complete history of cervical screening is unknown, those with a history of DES exposure, HIV-positive women, and those who may have multiple sexual partners warrant annual screening. It should be emphasized that continued gynecologic care is warranted even if a women does not have a Pap test performed.

Screening After Hysterectomy

There is no apparent benefit of performing cytologic screening of women who have undergone a total hysterectomy (removal of the cervix) for benign indications. Vaginal cancer is a rare event, occurring with an incidence rate of 1–2/100,000/year. There have been a number of large retrospective cytologic studies in patients with a history of total hysterectomy for benign indications demonstrating a low (<1%) rate of cytologic abnormalities and an even lower rate of biopsy-confirmed disease. The Pap test performed on a vaginal cuff is not cost effective. Women who have undergone a supracervical hysterectomy should continue annual screening as indicated above. Women who had a hysterectomy for CIN 2,3 should undergo continued screening until they have at least three consecutive negative smears. Before screening is discontinued it is important that the health care provider document the patient had a history of normal Pap tests. Women with a history of DES exposure should undergo annual screening due to a high rate of vaginal cancer.

Screening for Women Aged 30 or Older

The prevalence of HPV infection decreases with increasing age. There are behavioral and biologic reasons for this phenomenon. The process of metaplasia that is characteristic of the transformation zone gradually causes the squamocolumnar junction to move into the cervical canal. This reduces the chance of incorporation of HPV into the newly forming squamous cells. The number of sexual partners a women is exposed to and therefore the number of different types of possible HPV exposure decrease with advancing age. Recently the FDA approved the combination of HPV testing using Hybrid Capture II and cervical cytology for primary screening of women 30 years and older. Several large studies demonstrate that if a women is HPV negative and cytologically normal she is at very low risk for CIN 2,3 over the next 3–5 years. These patients should be screened no sooner than 3 years. These guidelines would change if the individual has a new sexual partner or develops a medical condition that interferes with her immune system. Patients who are screened using a combination of HPV testing and cytology and have an abnormal Pap test (≥ASC-US) require evaluation as per specific abnormality. Women who have a normal Pap smear and are HPV+ require closer evaluation with a Pap test and HPV testing every 6 months. The follow-up of any abnormality is summarized in Fig. 7.1.

Screening in HIV-Positive Women

HIV-positive women represent an at-risk population due to the impairment of their cellular immunity. With the advent of highly effective antiviral therapy this population may have a relatively normal immune response to HPV. All

Fig. 7.1. Algorithm for the management of women using a combination of cervical cytology and HPV DNA testing for primary cervical cancer screening. HPV, human Papillomavirus; ASCUS, atypical squamous cells of undetermined significance.

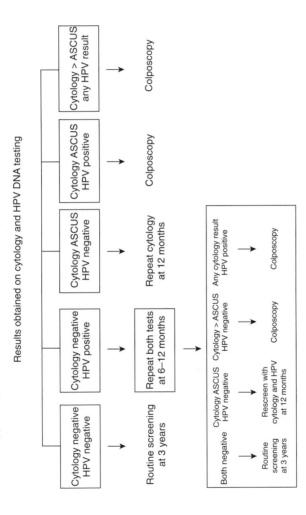

(Reprinted, with permission, from Wright TC: Algorithm for the management of women using a combination of cervical cytology and HPV DNA testing as adjunct to cytology. *Obstet Gynecol* 2004;103(2):307.)

women who are HIV positive should have two sequential Pap tests at 6 month intervals when initially diagnosed with HIV. If both tests are normal the patient should have regular cytologic screening at 12 month intervals. Women who have a low CD4 count (<200 cells/ml) are at increased risk for cervical disease and should have a Pap test every 6 months, especially if there is a history of an abnormal Pap test, HPV infections, or recent treatment for cervical dysplasia.

Triage for Cytologic Abnormalities
ASCCP Guidelines

The ASCCP held a consensus workshop in September 2001 to develop evidence-based guidelines for the management of both cytologic and histologic abnormalities of the cervix. The meeting included representation from 29 professional organizations, federal agencies, and national and international health organizations. The resulting clinical guidelines from this workshop are, when possible, evidence based. These guidelines represent the first well-organized, nationally accepted management strategies for treating cytologic and histologic abnormalities.

ALTS Trial and Its Role in the ASCCP Guidelines

The first Bethesda system included the new cytologic category AS-CUS. The net result was an increase in the number of colposcopies performed in the United States. In an effort to develop an effective method for the triage of low-grade cytologic abnormalities the National Cancer Institute funded a multicenter, randomized trial to determine if HPV testing could be used to separate those women at true risk for developing CIN 2,3 or cancer. The working hypothesis was that women who are positive for high-risk HPV using the Hybrid Capture II technique are at greater risk. The ASC-US/LSIL Triage Study (ALTS) provided critical information regarding the role of HPV testing in both the triage as well as follow-up of women with ASC-US and LSIL cytology. Table 7.2 summarizes the important findings of the ALTS trial. The following sections summarize the ASCCP consensus guidelines and highlight the key points for consideration.

Management of ASC-US (Fig. 7.2)

Highlight of management triage:

- Three separate triage methods exist, colposcopy, repeat cytology, and HPV testing.
- If liquid-based cytology is used, HPV triage (sent from the residual fluid) is the preferred management option.
- A negative HPV test allows a patient to return to routine annual screening.
- During serial cytologic follow-up any abnormality will warrant a repeat colposcopic examination.

Table 7.2.   ASCUS/LSIL triage study (ALTS).

---

1. Women with a diagnosis of LSIL are frequently positive for HPV (82.9%) and this technique is not useful in the triage of women with this diagnosis.
2. Triage of women with ASC-US using HPV testing is effective. The cytologic diagnosis harbors HPV in 50% of cases.
3. HPV testing is a very sensitive method for the initial detection of CIN 2, 3 (>90%).
4. HPV testing or repeat cytology using an ASC-US threshold (testing every 6 months) is similarly sensitive for the detection of CIN 2,3.
5. Women with ASC-US who are HPV positive and those with an LSIL cytology have very similar clinical outcomes.

- A single HPV test (without a Pap test) can be used for follow-up of women found to be histologically normal or without an obvious lesion on colposcopy.

  Management of ASC-US in special circumstances:

- **Postmenopausal patients:** An alternative acceptable option for post-menopausal women with a diagnosis of ASC-US who suffer from estrogen deficiency is treatment with vaginal estrogen for 1 month. If a repeat cytologic examination 1 week following the estrogen therapy is normal then the patient may be followed by Pap tests at 6-month intervals without a colposcopic examination.
- **Pregnancy:** Pregnant patients are to be managed in a fashion similar to patients who are not pregnant.
- **Immunosuppressed patients:** All immunosuppressed patients should be referred for colposcopy.

Management of ASC-H (Fig. 7.3)

Highlights of ASC-H:

- ASC-H are frequently >80% positive for HPV.
- ASC-H require immediate colposcopy and close follow-up.

Management of LSIL (Fig. 7.4)

Highlights of LSIL management:

- LSIL requires immediate colposcopy.
- Endocervical sampling is preferred in cases without a lesion or unsatisfactory colposcopy.

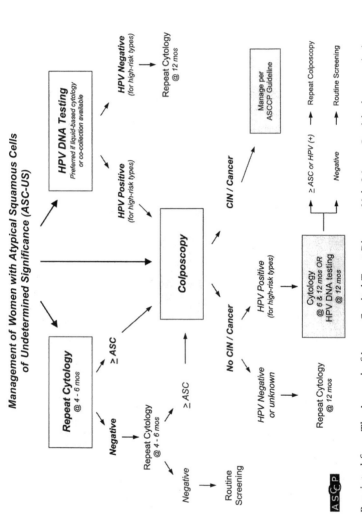

Fig. 7.2. Management of women with atypical squamous cells of undetermined significance (ASC-US).

Fig. 7.3. Management of women with atypical squamous cells: cannot exclude high-grade SIL (ASC-H).

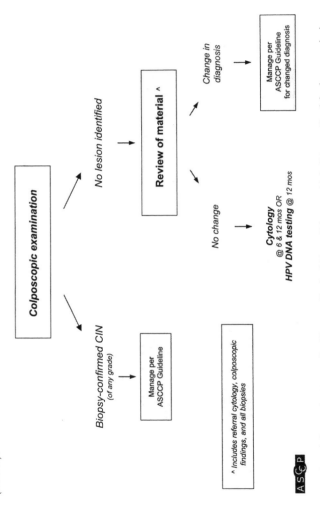

Colposcopic examination

Biopsy-confirmed CIN
(of any grade)

→ Manage per
ASCCP Guideline

No lesion identified

→ **Review of material** ^

No change → *Cytology*
@ 6 & 12 mos OR
HPV DNA testing @ 12 mos

Change in
diagnosis → Manage per
ASCCP Guideline
for changed diagnosis

^ *Includes referral cytology, colposcopic
findings, and all biopsies*

ASCCP

Reprinted from The Journal of Lower Genital Tract Disease, Vol. 6 Issue 2 with the permission of ASCCP © American Society for Colposcopy and Cervical Pathology 2002. No copies of the algorithms may be made without prior consent of ASCCP.

Fig. 7.4. Management of women with low-grade squamous intraepithelial lesions (LSIL).

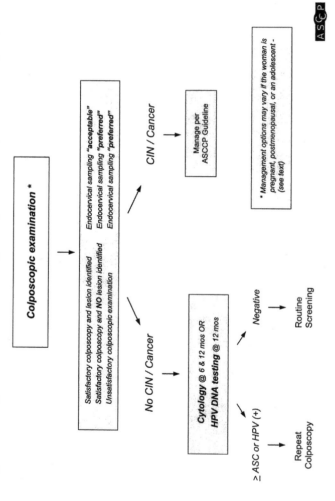

Colposcopic examination *

Satisfactory colposcopy and lesion identified
Satisfactory colposcopy and **NO lesion** identified
Unsatisfactory colposcopic examination

No CIN / Cancer

CIN / Cancer

Cytology @ 6 & 12 mos OR
HPV DNA testing @ 12 mos

Endocervical sampling *"acceptable"*
Endocervical sampling *"preferred"*
Endocervical sampling *"preferred"*

Manage per
ASCCP Guideline

≥ ASC or HPV (+)

Negative

Repeat
Colposcopy

Routine
Screening

* Management options may vary if the woman is
pregnant, postmenopausal, or an adolescent -
(see text)

ASCCP

Reprinted from The Journal of Lower Genital Tract Disease, Vol. 6 Issue 2 with the permission of ASCCP © American Society for Colposcopy and Cervical Pathology 2002. No copies of the algorithms may be made without the prior consent of ASCCP.

- Follow-up strategies reflect the high rate of HPV infection and risk for the detection of subsequent disease over a 2-year period.

  Management of LSIL in special circumstances (Fig. 7.5):

- **Adolescents:** Due to the high rate of HPV in this population and the lack of cervical cancer screening, colposcopy may be delayed.
- **Postmenopausal patients:** This population of patients suffers from vaginal atrophy and has a low rate of HPV infection. The available triage strategies reflect the unique nature of this population (Fig. 7.6).

Management of HSIL (Fig. 7.7)

Highlights of HSIL:

- Of patients with HSIL 70–75% will be found to have CIN 2,3.
- Endocervical sampling is preferred in all patients with HSIL.
- Diagnostic excisional procedures are frequently used when the source of the abnormal cytology is not identified.

  Management of HSIL in special circumstances:

- **Pregnancy:** Management should be conducted by individuals with considerable colposcopic experience. Treatment is reserved for invasive disease only.
- **Adolescents:** When biopsy-confirmed CIN 2,3 is not identified in an adolescent, repeat cytology every 4–6 months for a year is an acceptable option in a compliant patient.

Management of Glandular Abnormalities (Fig. 7.8)

Highlights of atypical glandular cells:

- This group of abnormalities carries a much higher rate of dysplasia, endocervical abnormalities, and endometrial abnormalities than atypical squamous cells.
- When an endometrial abnormality is suggested the initial evaluation involves an endometrial biopsy.
- When the abnormality favors dysplasia the responsibility lies with the clinician to rule out disease that quite frequently requires an excisional cone biopsy.
- Referral to an experienced clinician may be required for patients with this group of abnormalities.

Postcolposcopy Management

The ASCCP has published recommendations for the management of biopsy-proven CIN. These guidelines were developed during the 2001 workshop and represent in many cases evidence-based treatment guidelines.

The management of CIN 1 has changed drastically over the past 10 years. Treatment has evolved from all individuals being treated with ablative

Fig. 7.5. Management of adolescent women with low-grade squamous intraepithelial lesions in special circumstances.

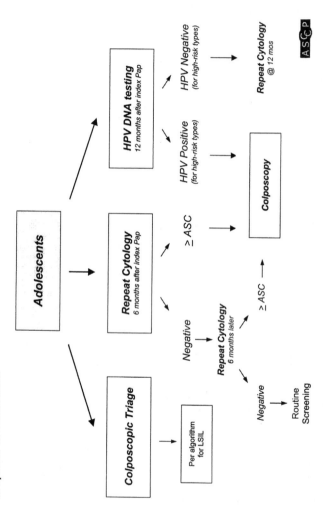

Fig. 7.6. Management of postmenopausal women with low-grade squamous intraepithelial lesions in special circumstances.

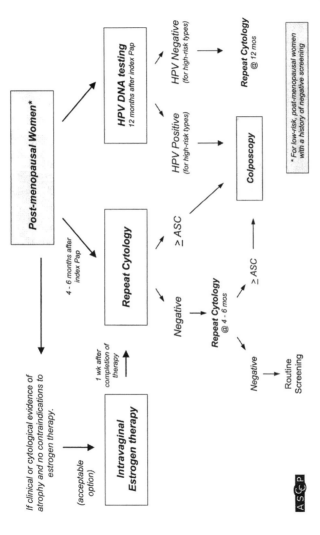

Reprinted from The Journal of Lower Genital Tract Disease, Vol. 6 Issue 2 with the permission of ASCCP © American Society for Colposcopy and Cervical Pathology 2002. No copies of the algorithms may be used without prior consent of ASCCP.

Fig. 7.7. Management of women with high-grade squamous intraepithelial lesions (HSIL).

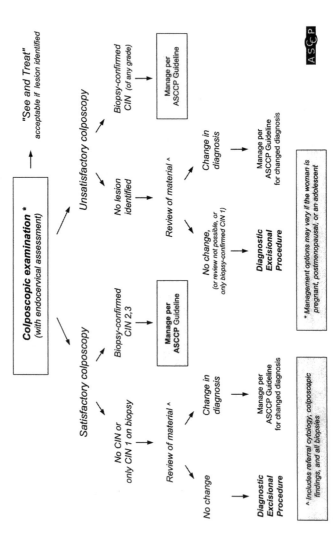

Reprinted from The Journal of Lower Genital Tract Disease, Vol. 7 Issue 3 with the permission of ASCCP © American Society for Colposcopy and Cervical Pathology 2003. No copies of the algorithms may be made without prior consent of ASCCP.

Fig. 7.8. Management of women with atypical glandular cells (AGC).

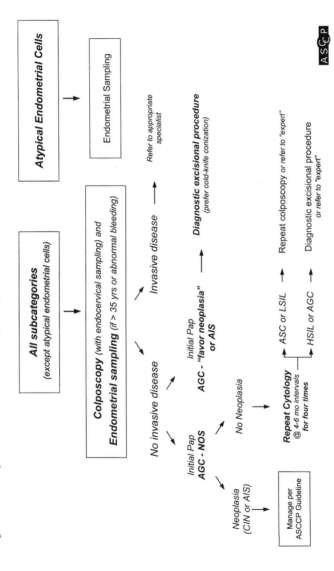

Reprinted from The Journal of Lower Genital Tract Disease, Vol. 6 Issue 2 with the permission of ASCCP. © American Society for Colposcopy and Cervical Pathology 2002. No copies of the algorithms may be made without the prior consent of ASCCP.

therapies to the majority of women being eligible for close follow-up. The rationale for the use of observation is the high rate of spontaneous resolution of CIN 1. In the adolescent population the rate of resolution approaches 90%, whereas in the older population the resolution is generally felt to be 70%.

Two methods are available when an individual is followed with observation, cytology every 6 months or HPV testing alone at 12 months. These recommendations were developed from the ALTS trial in which HPV testing and serial cytology where shown to have similar sensitivities for the detection of CIN 2,3 (93%) with a reasonable rate of referral for colposcopy. The addition of a repeat cytology to the HPV test at 12 months only marginally increases sensitivity with a significant increase in colposcopic referrals and is not recommended (Fig. 7.9).

Treatment of CIN 2 and CIN 3

CIN 2 and CIN 3 are generally accepted as cancer precursors and should be treated except in special circumstances. The treatments are divided into ablative therapies and excision therapies. The treatment methods available for ablation include cryotherapy, laser therapy, and loop electrosurgical excision procedure (LEEP). There are no significant differences in the success rates of the three therapies, and treatment decisions are at the discretion of the clinician. The following criteria must be met to use ablative therapy: (1) the lesion is on the outside of the cervix and does not extend significantly into the cervical canal, (2) there should be agreement between the cytology and the histology, (3) the endocervical sampling should be negative, and (4) ablative therapy is not acceptable for the treatment of adenocarcinoma *in situ*, adenocarcinoma, or squamous cell carcinoma.

Following treatment for CIN 2,3 the patient should undergo a series of cytologic examinations to confirm the appropriate treatment of the dysplasia. Following three normal cytologic examinations the patient may return to routine annual Pap tests. There is growing evidence that an HPV test done 6 months following therapy may replace serial cytologic examinations. A patient with a negative HPV test at 6 months can return to routine screening.

Adolescents are the only group for which the ASCCP offers observations for the treatment of CIN 2. The resolution rate of CIN 2 is 50%, and in this population, which is at low risk for the development of invasive cancer, CIN 2 can be observed without therapy in properly selected compliant patients.

During pregnancy CIN 2 and CIN 3 are not treated due to the high risk of an adverse outcome. Close observation with repeated colposcopic examinations during the pregnancy (each trimester) followed by postpartum colposcopy and appropriate treatment is recommended (Fig. 7.10).

Human Papiloma Virus Vaccines

The future for the prevention of cervical cancer lies in the reduction of the spread of HPV via vaccines. The most promising vaccines use the outer shell

Fig. 7.9. Management of women with biopsy-confirmed cervical intraepithelial neoplasia: grade 1 (CIN 1) and satisfactory colposcopy.

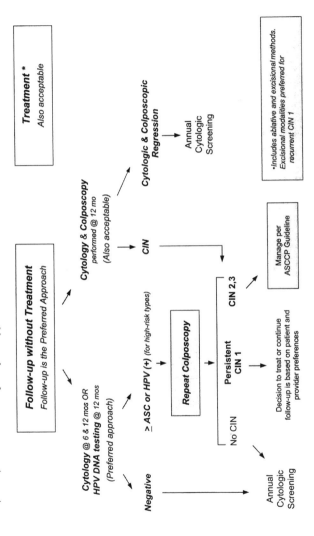

Fig. 7.10. Management of women with biopsy-confirmed cervical intraepithelial neoplasia: grades 2 and 3 (CIN 2,3).

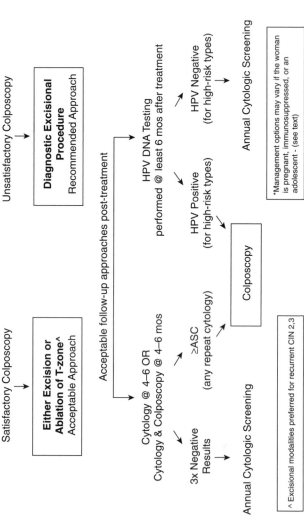

Reprinted from The Journal of Lower Genital Tract Disease, Vol. 7 Issue 3 with the permission of ASCCP © American Society for Colposcopy and Cervical Pathology 2003. No copies of the algorithms may be made without the prior consent of ASCCP.

of the HPV virus, the virus-like particle (VLP). The VLP presents an antigen to the host immune response that is specific to the particular type of HPV. The first large-scale randomized study of VLP for HPV 16 demonstrated complete protection against abnormal cytology and over 90% immunogenic response to the VLP. There are numerous efforts presently ongoing to develop a commercially available, multivalent, HPV vaccine. The widespread use of such a vaccine has the potential to reduce the rate of cervical cancer throughout the world.

Case Studies

Case 1. A 22-year-old G0 female presents for a routine yearly Pap test. She smokes 1 ppd, has no history of sexually transmitted diseases, has had five lifetime partners, and began sexual activity at age 16. The Pap returns as ASC and is HPV+. How should she be managed?

- The correct management would be a colposcopy based on the ASCCP guidelines.

Colposcopy is adequate, and the patient has a small acetowhite lesion that is biopsied and returns as CIN 1. The endocervical sampling is negative.

- The patient has various options at this point. She should be counseled extensively about HPV to improve her understanding of the disease and to incorporate her into the decision process for therapy. Although she could undergo an ablative therapy this patient would be best treated by expectant management. The high rate of resolution of the disease warrants a period of observation. The patient could have serial cytology or HPV testing. At this point either is acceptable. The patient can assist in the decision process.

Case 2. A 44-year-old obese G2 P2 female presents for annual screening. Her periods are irregular, but are not heavy. She is a borderline diabetic controlled with diet, is a nonsmoker, and has had one partner for 20 years. Her Pap returns as AGC, suggestive of endometrial type. How should she be managed?

- AGCs require a close evaluation due to the high rate of dysplasia. When endometrial cells are abnormal and specified the first evaluation should be an endometrial biopsy performed in the office.

The endometrial biopsy is normal proliferative endometrium.

- The patient should have close follow-up with cytologic examinations every 4 months until there are four negative examinations. In an individual with high risk for endometrial hyperplasia or cancer, hysteroscopy and dilation and curettage may be considered to further sample the endometrial lining.

If this individual had AGC, favor neoplastic, how would the evaluation differ?

- Colposcopy and endocervical sampling would be added to the evaluation. The results of the examination of the exocervix, endocervical canal, and endometrium will determine the next step in the treatment of this patient.

Suggested Reading

ASCUS-LSIL Triage Study (ALTS) Group. Results of a randomized trial on the management of cytology interpretations of atypical squamous cells of undetermined significance. *Am J Obstet Gynecol* 2003;188: 1383–92.

ASCUS-LSIL Triage Study (ALTS) Group. A randomized trial on the management of low-grade squamous intraepithelial lesion cytology interpretations. *Am J Obstet Gynecol* 2003;188:1393–1400.

ALTS Study et al. Human papillomavirus testing for triage of women with cytologic evidence of low-grade squamous intraepithelial lesions: baseline data from a randomized trial. *J Natl Cancer Inst* 2000;92: 397–402.

Cox JT, Schiffman M, Solomon D, for the ASCUS-LSIL Triage Study (ALTS) Group. Prospective follow-up suggests similar risk of subsequent cervical intraepithelial neoplasia grade 2 or 3 among women with cervical intraepithelial neoplasia grade 1 or negative colposcopy and directed biopsy. *Am J Obstet Gynecol* 2003;188:1406–12.

Fetters MD, Lieberman RW, Abrahamse PH, Sanghvi RV, Sonnad SS. Cost-effectiveness of Pap smear screening for vaginal cancer after total hysterectomy for benign disease. *J Lower Genital Tract Dis* 2003;7(3): 194–202.

Mao C. Do liquid-based Pap smears need a transformation zone component? *Cont Ob/Gyn* 2003;48(7):78–83.

McCance DJ. *Human Papilloma Viruses: Perspectives in Medical Virology*, Vol. 8. Amsterdam: Elsevier Science B.V.; 2002.

Monk BJ, Brewster WR. Does the ALTS trial apply to the community-based practitioner? *Am J Obstet Gynecol* 2003;188:1381–2.

Saslow D, Runowicz CD, Solomon D, Moscicki AB, Smith RA, Eyre HJ, Cohen C. American Cancer Society guideline for the early detection of cervical neoplasia and cancer. *CA Cancer J Clin* 2002;52:342–62.

Solomon D, Davey D, Kurman R, Moriarty A, O'Connor D, Prey M, Raab S, Sherman M, Wilbur D, Wright T Jr., Young N. The 2001 Bethesda System, terminology for reporting results of cervical cytology. *JAMA* 2002;287:2114–19.

Wright TC, Cox JT, Massad LS, Twiggs LB, Wilkinson EJ. 2001 concensus guidelines for the management of women with cervical cytological abnormalities. *JAMA* 2002;287:2120–9.

Wright TC, Schiffman M, Solomon D, Cox TJ, Garcia F, Goldie S, Hatch K, Noller K, Roach N, Runowicz C, Saslow D. Interim guidance for the use of human papillomavirus DNA testing as an adjunct to cervical cytology screening. Obstet Gynecol 2004;103:304–9.

8

Mood Disorders

G. Randolph Schrodt, Jr.

Major Depressive Disorder

Epidemiology and Clinical Course

The point prevalence for major depressive disorder has been established as 2.3–3.5% for men and 4.5–9.3% for women; the lifetime risk is 7–12% for men and 20–25% for women. This differential rate of affective disorders is primarily due to higher rates of depression between menarche and menopause. There is an increased incidence of the disorder in the primary care patient population; however, clinical depression has been both underdiagnosed and undertreated by primary care and other nonpsychiatrist physicians. Among "high utilizers" of medical services, there is an incidence of >40%. Risk factors include the following:

1. Female, especially during the postpartum period.
2. Family history of depression.
3. Prior history of depression or suicide attempts.
4. Stressful life events, particularly with first episode of depression.
5. Comorbid medical problems.
6. Lack of social supports.
7. Current alcohol or substance abuse.

The average age of onset for a major depressive disorder is the late 20s, but it may begin at any age. Untreated, about two-thirds of depressed patients will return to their premorbid level of functioning within 6–24 months; in addition, approximately 10% will have a persistent, chronic course, and 20–25% will have only partial recovery. At least 50% of depressed patients will subsequently have another episode (**recurrent depression**).

Diagnostic Criteria (*DSM-IV-TR*)

Five or more of the following symptoms have been present during the same 2-week period, most of the day, nearly every day. At least one of the symptoms is either criterion 1 or 2:

1. Depressed mood.
2. Markedly diminished interest (apathy) or pleasure (anhedonia) in activities.
3. Significant weight loss/gain.
4. Insomnia/hypersomnia.
5. Psychomotor agitation/retardation.
6. Fatigue/loss of energy.
7. Feelings of worthlessness/excessive or inappropriate guilt.
8. Impaired concentration/indecisiveness.
9. Recurrent thoughts of death or suicide/suicide attempt.

Symptoms are not due to substance abuse, medication, or a medical illness. In addition, symptoms are not a normal reaction to the death of a loved one (symptoms such as worthlessness, suicidal ideation, marked functional impairment or psychomotor retardation, or prolonged duration are not characteristic of **uncomplicated bereavement**).

Subgroups of Major Depressive Disorder
With Psychotic Features

Usually, there will be mood-congruent **hallucinations or delusions** (e.g., delusions of guilt, sin, poverty, or deserved punishment, somatic delusions of illness). These occur in approximately 15% of patients with major depressive disorder. Age of onset is usually in the fifth decade and there is a strong familial pattern. In these patients there is increased severity of illness, higher rates of relapse, chronicity, comorbidity, hospitalization, suicide attempts, and completed suicide. Combined antidepressant/antipsychotic pharmacotherapy is much more effective than either treatment alone. Electroconvulsive therapy (ECT) is probably the most effective and best tolerated treatment.

With Melancholic Features

These patients are characterized by loss of pleasure or interest in activities, as well as lack of reactivity to pleasurable activities or events. There is significant psychomotor retardation or agitation. A patient will awaken very early each day, and generally the depression will be worse during the morning hours (diurnal variation). There also may be signs of significant anorexia or weight loss, with excessive or inappropriate guilt. The presence of melancholic features increases the likelihood of response to somatic therapies (antidepressants and ECT).

With Atypical Features

These patients are typified by mood reactivity and "reverse" vegetative disturbances of hypersomnia, increased appetite, and weight gain. They experience a pattern of hypersensitivity to interpersonal rejection and severe fatigue with a heavy, "leaden" feeling in their arms and legs. Marked anxiety and phobic symptoms are often noted. Onset occurs at a younger age than in other depressive subtypes.

There is a better response to selective serotonin reuptake inhibitors (SSRIs), serotonin-norepinephrine reuptake inhibitors (SNRIs), and monoamine oxidase inhibitors (MAOIs) than to tricyclic antidepressants (TCAs).

With Seasonal Pattern

There is a regular temporal pattern between the onset and remission of a recurrent mood disorder and seasonal change, and it is more common in northern latitudes. The most common pattern involves the onset of depression (frequently with atypical features) beginning in the fall and remitting in the spring (occasionally with hypomanic symptoms). Artificial light therapy, using bright, full-spectrum light (2500–10,000 lux) for 30 minutes per day (usually in the morning), has been demonstrated to be a safe, effective treatment for mild to moderately severe seasonal depression. Phototherapy generally has few side effects but can cause headaches, eyestrain, insomnia, and irritability with some patients. Patients with more severe mood disorders benefit from other somatic therapies in conjunction with phototherapy.

With Postpartum Onset

Major depression with postpartum onset is different from the typical "**baby blues**" that normally occur in 50–80% of women; postpartum blues is characterized by tearfulness, irritability, and labile mood that generally resolves in 3–7 days postpartum with support and reassurance. The onset of postpartum depression is usually 2–4 weeks after delivery, but can occur up to 6 months. In addition to other symptoms of major depression, feelings of inadequacy as a mother are common. Thoughts of harming the infant, if present, are ego-dystonic and not usually acted upon. Major depression with postpartum onset is common in women with recurrent depression whose antidepressants were discontinued during pregnancy. In addition to a prior history of depression and anxiety disorders, other risk factors include negative life events, marital conflict, and poor social support.

Postpartum depressive or manic episodes may also include **psychotic symptoms** (1–2 per 1000 deliveries), especially delusions regarding the child (e.g., the infant has special powers or is possessed by an evil force). Infanticide is most often associated with postpartum psychotic episodes but may occur in nonpsychotic postpartum mood disorders. Postpartum psychotic mood disorders are more common in women with previous postpartum mood disorders or bipolar I disorder; the risk of subsequent postpartum psychotic episodes is 30–50%. Frequent symptoms include crying spells and mood lability, severe anxiety including panic attacks, insomnia, and disinterest in the baby.

Bipolar Disorder

Epidemiology and Clinical Course

Every patient presenting with depression should be screened for symptoms and a family history of bipolar disorder. Misdiagnosis not only delays appropriate therapy, but antidepressants prescribed as a single agent can induce mania or rapid cycling in bipolar depressed patients. Bipolar I disorder affects men and women equally; bipolar II disorder is more common in women. There is a lifetime prevalence of approximately 1% for bipolar I and 2–3% for bipolar II. First-degree relatives of patients with bipolar disorder have a 12% chance of developing a bipolar disorder and another 25% will have major depression or other mood disorders. Mean age at onset is the early 20s. The first episode in men is more likely to be manic; the first episode in women is more likely to be depressive; 90% of patients with bipolar disorder have a recurrent course, and there is a 50% incidence of comorbid alcohol or substance abuse.

Diagnostic Criteria (DSM-IV-TR)

Bipolar disorders are characterized by episodes of major depressive disorder interspersed with episodes of mania (type I) or hypomania (type II). Criteria for a **manic episode** include the following:

1. A distinct period of abnormally and persistently elevated, expansive, or irritable mood, lasting at least 1 week (or any duration if hospitalization is required), and at least three of the following symptoms (four if the mood is only irritable).
2. Inflated self-esteem or grandiosity.
3. Decreased need for sleep.

4. More talkative than usual or pressured speech.
5. Flight of ideas or subjective racing thoughts.
6. Distractibility.
7. Increase in goal-directed activity (socially, at work or school, sexually) or psychomotor agitation.
8. Excessive involvement in pleasurable activities that have a high potential for painful consequences (e.g., spending sprees, promiscuity, foolish financial investments).

In **manic episodes**, the symptoms are severe enough to cause marked impairment in usual social or occupational functioning or relationships with others, or are associated with psychotic features, or require hospitalization to prevent harm to self or others. **Hypomanic episodes** are characterized by the same symptoms as a manic episode, but are less severe, generally of brief duration, and by definition do not cause severe functional disability and do not have psychotic features.

Subgroups of Bipolar Disorder

In a **mixed episode**, the criteria are met for both a manic episode and major depression (except for duration) nearly every day for at least a week. **Rapid cycling** bipolar disorder refers to the occurrence of at least four episodes of major depression, hypomania, or mania within a 12-month period. An episode **with psychotic features** is characterized by hallucinations or delusions consistent with the manic themes of inflated worth, power, knowledge, identity, or special relationship to a deity or famous person. Bipolar disorders may also demonstrate seasonal patterns, postpartum onset, and catatonic features (e.g., mutism, posturing, motor immobility or purposeless motor activity, stupor).

Other Mood Disorders

Dysthymic disorder is a chronic (2 years in adults, 1 year in children and adolescents), low-grade, nonpsychotic depressive disorder. It usually begins in childhood; if it begins after an episode of major depression, it may represent partial remission of a depressive episode.

Dysthymic patients frequently go on to develop major depressive disorder (referred to as "double depression"). In addition to increased risk for depression and other psychiatric illnesses, patients with dysthymic disorder demonstrate significant impairments in occupational and social functioning, poorer general health, and increased health care expenditures. Antidepressants are effective in a significant number of dysthymic patients.

Cyclothymic disorder is the subsyndromal, chronic form of bipolar disorder, characterized by numerous episodes of hypomania and depressive symptoms that do not meet the full criteria for major depression.

Mood disorder due to a general medical condition is diagnosed when the mood disorder (depressed, manic, or mixed) is judged to be due to the direct physiologic effects of a medical illness (Table 8.1)

Table 8.1. Medical conditions frequently associated with mood disturbance.

	Depression	Mania
Infectious	Acquired immune deficiency disease (AIDS)	AIDS
	Mononucleosis	Viral encephalitis
	Viral hepatitis	Tertiary syphilis
	Tertiary syphilis	
Endocrinologic	Hyper-/hypothyroidism	
	Hyperthyroidism	
	Diabetes mellitus	
	Hyper-/hypoparathyroidism	
	Cushing's disease	
	Addison's disease	
Rheumatologic	Systemic lupus erythematosis (SLE)	Rheumatic chorea
	Rheumatoid arthritis	
	Fibromyalgia	
	Chronic fatigue syndrome	
Neurologic	Multiple sclerosis	Multiple sclerosis
	Parkinson's disease	Huntington's chorea
	Complex partial seizures	Complex partial seizures
	Post-head trauma	Post-head trauma
	Cerebrovascular disease/ Wilson's disease stroke	
	Tumors	Tumors
	Sleep apnea	Migraine
	Early dementias	Chronic pain syndromes
	Deficiencies of vitamin B_{12}, folate, niacin, thiamine, vitamin C	Deficiencies of vitamin B_{12}, folate, niacin, thiamine
Neoplastic	Pancreatic cancer	
	Disseminated carcinomatosis	
Cardiac	Coronary artery disease	
	Postcardiac transplantation	
	Postmyocardial infarction	

1. Medical disorder may cause psychiatric symptoms; treatment is directed toward the medical illness.
2. Depression and medical illness may be comorbid conditions; independent recognition and treatment of both disorders are indicated.

Substance-induced mood disorders are due to the direct physiologic effects of a substance, including drugs of abuse, prescription medications, or toxic exposure. They may produce either depressive or manic symptoms and may occur during intoxication or withdrawal from the substance (Table 8.2).

Premenstrual dysphoric disorder (PMDD) is characterized by symptoms that occur during most menstrual cycles within the past year, were present most of the time during the last week of the luteal phase, began to remit within a few days after the onset of the follicular phase, and were absent in the week postmenses. At least five of the following symptoms are present:

1. Depressed mood, hopelessness, or self-deprecating thoughts.
2. Marked anxiety, tension, or feeling "keyed up," or "on edge."
3. Marked mood swings or affective lability.
4. Anger, irritability, or increased interpersonal conflicts.

Table 8.2. Substances commonly associated with mood disturbances.

Depression	Mania
Corticosteroids	Corticosteroids
Anabolic steroids	Levodopa
Oral contraceptives	Bromocriptine
Levonorgestrel (Norplant)	Cocaine
Reserpine	Amphetamines
Alcohol	Methylphenidate
Sedative-hypnotics/benzodiazepines	Antidepressants
Neuroleptics	
α-Methyldopa	
Amphetamine/cocaine withdrawal	
Cimetidine	
Metoclopramide	
Nonsteroidal antiinflammatory drugs	
Insecticides, thallium, mercury	
Cycloserine, vincristine, vinblastine	

5. Decreased interest in the usual activities.
6. Subjective difficulty with concentration.
7. Lethargy, fatigue, significant lack of energy.
8. Change in appetite, overeating, or specific food cravings.
9. Hypersomnia or insomnia.
10. Subjective sense of being overwhelmed or out of control.
11. Other physical symptoms, such as breast tenderness or swelling, head-aches, joint or muscle pain, bloating, and weight gain.

Only 4–7% of women meet the criteria for PMDD, while 65–75% have some symptoms of **premenstrual syndrome (PMS)**. Of women with PMDD, 30% have a previous history of major depression, and women with PMDD are at higher risk for a future episode of major depression. Other psychiatric disorders are to be considered (e.g., mood and anxiety disorders, psychosis, bulimia, substance use disorders, personality disorders), and general medical conditions (e.g., seizures) may be exacerbated in the pre-menstrual period. The etiologies of PMDD and PMS are unknown. Despite the obvious relationship between the symptoms of PMDD and the phase of the menstrual cycle, the relationship between female sex hormones and PMDD is not linear. No consistent abnormalities in hormonal patterns or levels of estrogens, progesterone, or androgens have been established. However, a number of research investigations have demonstrated the role of serotonin in the pathophysiology of PMDD. Other studies have found high heritability of PMS/PMDD, the role of stressful life events, cultural differ-ences ("menstrual socialization"), and a high frequency of past sexual abuse in women with severe symptoms.

Treatment of PMS/PMDD includes the following:

1. Education and life-style modification: decrease salt, refined sugar, caffeine (especially coffee), red meat, and alcohol; increase aerobic exercise and stress reduction techniques including relaxation training, yoga, or meditation.

2. Vitamin and mineral supplements: large studies have shown benefits from vitamins B_6 (100 mg) and calcium (1200 mg); there is also good support for the efficacy of supplementation with vitamins C and E, and magnesium.

3. For women who do not respond to conservative treatments, SSRIs are the treatment of choice. Currently fluoxetine, sertraline, and par-oxetine are Food and Drug Administration (FDA) approved for PMDD. Most studies have found that intermittent dosing (i.e., taking the medication only during the 2-week luteal phase) is as effective as continuous dosing.

4. Diuretics and prostaglandin synthesis inhibitors [e.g., nonsteroi-dal antiinflammatory drugs (NSAIDs)] may provide symptomatic relief of bloating and dysmenorrhea; evening primrose oil (Efamol), a prostaglandin synthesis precursor containing γ-linoleic acid and vitamin E, has been shown to decrease premenstrual depressive symptoms.

5. Oral contraceptives, progesterone supplementation (oral or vaginal), gonadotropin-releasing hormone (GnRH), danazol, and bromocriptine have been shown to be effective for some patients with severe PMS, but some patients experience a worsening of symptoms and severe side effects of the drugs.

Treatment of Depression

General Principles of Management

Management of the depressed patient includes a thorough assessment of the patient's symptoms, significant medical and psychosocial history (stressors and supports), and treatment preference. Treatment consists of **acute phase** (initial remission of symptoms), a **continuation phase** (continued remission), and a **maintenance phase** (relapse prevention). Psychotherapeutic and somatic interventions need to be tailored to the individual patient.

Psychopharmacology: General Considerations and Gender Differences

Several studies suggest that gender is a significant factor in response to antidepressant treatment. Although psychosocial factors such as social roles, social status, and stressful life events (e.g., trauma or abuse) may contribute to the 2 : 1 differential rate of depression in women compared to men, the difference in prevalence is most likely related to neurobiological factors. As mentioned before, the difference in prevalence of mood disorders between women and men is noted only during child-bearing years, suggesting an important role for reproductive hormones in mood regulation. The most clinically significant research to date has focused on estrogen–serotonin interactions. Specifically, decreases in estrogen levels are associated with decreases of brain serotonin activity. This is consistent with the clinical observation of increased risk for mood disturbance during times of lower estrogen such as the premenstrual period, puerperium, and perimenopausal. The estrogen–serotonin interaction probably also accounts for some of the gender differences in symptoms and comorbidity between women and men. Women more often present with the so-called "atypical" pattern of hypersomnia, hyperphagia, carbohydrate craving, weight gain, extreme fatigue, anxiety, and somatic complaints such as muscle pain, migraine headaches, irritable bowel syndrome, interstitial cystitis, and pelvic pain. Likewise, women more often have comorbid "serotonin" disorders such as anxiety (especially panic attacks and phobias), eating disorders, seasonal affective disorder (SAD), and of course, PMDD. In contrast, men have a higher incidence of alcoholism, substance abuse, and attention-deficit hyperactivity disorder (ADHD), disorders more often associated with the norepinephrine/dopamine/opiate systems of the brain.

Not surprisingly, evidence has begun to emerge to suggest a differential gender response to classes of medications. Most of the evidence to date suggests that women have a better antidepressant response with the SSRIs and SNRIs than with the TCAs, which are predominantly norepinephrine reuptake inhibitors. Similarly, women may have a better response with MAOIs than TCAs. These studies also suggest that gender differences in response to antidepressants are less significant in older women; in particular, antidepressants that have noradrenergic effects might convey added benefit for older (i.e., lower estrogen) women.

Pharmacotherapy is the treatment of choice for depressions that are severe (e.g., associated with suicidal thinking), chronic, recurrent, or associated with psychotic or melancholic features. Medication choice is based on side effect profile, history of prior response, family history of response to a particular medication, type of depression, and the potential for adverse interactions with other prescribed medications or concurrent medical illnesses. Noncompliance can be a major factor in poor clinical outcomes; factors influencing noncompliance include acute and long-term side effects of medication, negative attitudes about medication, complexity of dosage regimen, and cost.

Severely depressed patients need to be seen frequently (e.g., at least weekly) to provide support and education, monitor adherence, and assess treatment progress, side effects, as well as the emergence of symptoms indicating a need for more intensive treatment.

Antidepressants are the most common drugs used in attempted and completed suicide overdoses; however, successful antidepressant treatment decreases suicidal thinking in addition to other depressive symptoms. Antidepressant response is typically observed after 10–14 days on a therapeutic dose, but the full effect may not occur for 6 weeks. Patients with major depression should continue antidepressants 6–12 months after remission of the first episode; maintenance pharmacotherapy is indicated for patients with recurrent depression (see below).

Heterocyclic Antidepressants

Indications include acute treatment and long-term prophylaxis for major depression. These antidepressants are also used in treatment of panic or phobic disorders, dysthymia, attention deficit disorder, narcolepsy, chronic pain, migraine, and eating disorders (Table 8.3).

Anticholinergic effects are the primary limiting side effect of heterocyclic antidepressants; most commonly, these effects are relatively minor and easily managed, such as dry mouth, constipation, blurred vision, and tachycardia. Urinary retention or hesitancy responds to bethanechol. The most serious anticholinergic side effect is delirium (altered sensorium, hot, dry skin, dilated pupils, and decreased or absent bowel sounds), most common in the elderly, in intentional or accidental overdose, or in patients taking other drugs with anticholinergic effects.

Antihistamine effects include daytime sedation, weight gain, and potentiation of the effects of alcohol and other sedatives. α-Adrenergic blocking effects account for postural hypotension, dizziness, and tachycardia. In patients without preexisting cardiac dysfunction, serious cardiovascular prob-

Table 8.3. Heterocyclic antidepressants.

Drug	Dose (mg/day)	Cardiac effects	Sedative effects	Anticholinergic hypotension	Orthostatic conduction delays
Imipramine	75–300	++	++	++	++
Amitriptyline	75–300	+++	+++	+++	++
Desipramine	75–300	+	+	+	++
Doxepin	75–300	+++	++	+++	++
Nortriptyline	30–150	+	+	+	++
Maprotiline	75–200	++	+	+	++
Protriptyline	15–60	+	+++	+	++
Trimipramine	75–300	+++	++	+	++
Amoxapine	75–300	++	++	+	++
Clomipramine	125–300	+++	+++	++	++
Trazodone	150–500	+++	0	+	+

lems are uncommon (except in overdose). Bundle branch block, the post-myocardial infarction period, and patients on quinidine are relative contraindications. Heterocyclic antidepressants have a quinidine-like effect, and patients with ventricular conduction delays need to be closely monitored. They generally are started at a low dose (e.g., 25–50 mg, usually in a single evening dose) and gradually titrated to therapeutic levels as tolerated.

Other side effects of heterocyclic antidepressants include lowered seizure threshold and sexual dysfunctions including delayed or inhibited orgasm and retrograde ejaculation. Measurements of plasma concentrations may be useful when patients fail to respond, suffer toxic side effects, or have a suspected abnormality in absorption or metabolism.

Heterocyclic overdose, potentially life-threatening, is characterized by cardiac arrhythmias, hypotension, seizures, and coma. Ingestion of a 10-day supply of medication may be fatal. Withdrawal symptoms, including nausea, dizziness, headache, malaise, increased perspiration, and sweating, have been reported with abrupt discontinuation of heterocyclics; gradual reduction of dosage is recommended to avoid this anticholinergic rebound.

Clomipramine has potent serotonin reuptake activity and is indicated for obsessive–compulsive disorders. Amoxapine has dopamine receptor blocking effects, and is useful for psychotic depression. Side effects may include dystonia, pseudoparkinsonism (tremor, bradykinesia, cogwheel rigidity, shuffling gait, masked facial expression), akathisia (subjective restlessness or need to be in motion), tardive dyskinesia, gynecomastia or galactorrhea, and neuroleptic malignant syndrome. Trazodone is safer in overdose than are the other heterocyclics; 1 in 800 men experience priapism.

Monoamine Oxidase Inhibitors

MAOIs are not first-line drugs for treating depressive illness but offer an important therapeutic alternative for some patients who fail to respond to other classes of antidepressants. They are particularly effective for depression with atypical features, as well as panic and phobic disorders (Table 8.4). Patients on MAOIs should be advised that a hypertensive crisis and possible death can occur if they are taken concurrently with certain drugs (e.g., stimulants) or foods high in tyramine content (e.g., aged cheeses or smoked meat).

More common side effects include symptoms of orthostatic hypotension (including lightheadedness, headache, and syncope), sleep disturbances (both insomnia and hypersomnia), fatigue, weakness, paresthesias, weight gain, pedal edema, and sexual dysfunctions (anorgasmia and ejaculatory disturbances). MAOIs are contraindicated for patients who are unable to comply with the dietary restrictions, consume excessive amounts of alcohol, have severe cardiovascular, hepatic, or renal disease, or have a pheochromocytoma.

A 2-week "washout" interval should generally be allowed when switching from an MAOI to another antidepressant. In rare cases of treatment for refractory depression, combined MAOI/heterocyclic treatment may be effective, but in combination with selective serotonin inhibitors may be fatal.

Selective Serotonin Reuptake Inhibitors

SSRIs are the most commonly prescribed antidepressants due to efficacy, safety, ease of dosing, and favorable side effect profile; compliance is greater with SSRIs than heterocyclics (Table 8.5). SSRIs are accepted first-line treatments in major depression, panic disorder, obsessive-compulsive disorder (OCD), social anxiety disorder, posttraumatic stress disorder (PTSD), bulimia, generalized anxiety disorder (GAD), and PMDD. Side effects are generally mild and transient; the most common include gastrointestinal (GI) disturbance (nausea, diarrhea, heartburn), sexual dysfunction (decreased libido, delayed or absent ejaculation or orgasm), insomnia or sedation, and headache. Anticholinergic,

Table 8.4.   Monoamine oxidase inhibitors.

Drug	Dose (mg/day)	Cardiac effects	Sedative effects	Anticholinergic hypotension	Orthostatic conduction delays
Phenylzine	30–90	+	+	+++	0
Tranylcypromine	10–60	0	+	+++	0

antihistaminic, and cardiac effects are almost absent. In addition, SSRIs are safer in cases of overdose than heterocyclics or MAOIs. Pending further studies, the FDA has recently recommended close monitoring for the emergence of suicidal thoughts or behaviors in patients (especially children and adolescents) who have recently been started on SSRIs (and other antidepressants) or have had the dose increased.

Serotonin augmenting agents (SSRIs and SNRIs) with shorter half-lives (e.g., paroxetine, fluvoxamine) may be associated with a **withdrawal syndrome** upon abrupt discontinuation. Symptoms include agitation, insomnia, anxiety, rebound depression, malaise, nausea, dizziness, and "electrical" paresthesias. These symptoms typically begin 1–5 days after discontinuation and may persist up to 2 weeks. This problem can be avoided by a gradual tapering of the dose or a switch to fluoxetine. **Serotonin syndrome** is marked by agitation, tachycardia, myoclonus, and hyperthermia and can progress to delirium, seizures, coma, and death. It is a rare complication of SSRI overdose, but is most commonly observed as the result of the interaction with MAOIs and other serotonin-enhancing agents.

Newer Atypical Antidepressants

There are several new drugs that offer first- or second-line antidepressant alternatives for patients who cannot tolerate the side effects of or do not respond to SSRIs, and they generally have more favorable side effect profiles than heterocyclics (Table 8.6).

Venlafaxine is an **SNRI** that has been increasing in popularity since the introduction of a once-a-day XR (extended release) form. There is growing evidence that dual-action antidepressants (i.e., affect both serotonergic and noradrenergic systems) are more effective in achieving **complete remission** of depressive symptoms, as opposed to antidepressant response (defined as a 50% reduction in symptoms). Potential consequences of failing to achieve complete remission of depression include increased risk of relapse and treatment resistance, continued functional psychosocial limitations, and sustained morbidity and mortality of other conditions. Dual-action antidepressants such as venlafaxine (and the soon-to-be-released duloxetine) appear to be more effective than SSRIs in alleviating the physical symptoms (e.g., headache, back pain, diffuse musculoskeletal pain, stomach problems) that are present in approximately 70% of depressed patients. Venlafaxine was the first antidepressant to be FDA approved for generalized anxiety disorder, and other studies have demonstrated its effectiveness in ADHD and hot flashes associated with menopause or tamoxifen therapy.

Bupropion has a unique mechanism of action compared to other currently available antidepressants. It inhibits the neuronal reuptake of norepinephrine and dopamine, and has no clinically significant effect on serotonin. Enhancement of dopamine appears related to improved attention (and benefit with attention deficit disorders), interest, and pleasure, and probably accounts for the benefit with smoking cessation. Noradrenergic effects increase

Table 8.5. Selective serotonin reuptake inhibitors.[a]

	Fluoxetine (Prozac, Prozac Weekly, Serafem, Symbyax[b])	Sertraline (Zoloft)	Paroxetine (Paxil, Paxil CR)	Escitalopram (Lexapro)
Side effects	Anxiety, insomnia, nausea, agitation, akathisia, anorexia, weight loss, dizziness, drowsiness, mania, rash, sweating, tremor, sexual dysfunction	Somnolence, fatigue, nausea, dry mouth, diarrhea, dyspepsia, insomnia, sweating, tremor, agitation, decreased libido, ejaculatory/orgasm delay	Nausea, headache, somnolence, dry mouth, diarrhea, constipation, blurred vision, sweating, asthenia, decreased libido, ejaculatory/orgasm delay	Nausea, insomnia, ejaculation disorder, somnolence, sweating, fatigue, decreased libido, anorgasmia
Dosage	10–80 mg/day (single AM dose)	50–200 mg/day (single AM or PM dose)	CR: 12.5–75 mg/day (single hs dose)	10–20 mg/day (single AM or PM dose)
Drug interaction	Increases levels of heterocyclics, antipsychotics, phenytoin, diazepam, carbamazepine, type IC antiarrhythmics, closely monitor	Increases levels of heterocyclics, antipsychotics, diazepam, carbamazepine, type IC antiarrhythmics, closely monitor	Contraindicated with thioridazine. Increases levels of heterocyclics, antipsychotics, type IC antiarrhythmics,	Fewer clinically significant interactions than other SSRIs. Caution with heterocyclics and

Other	PT/PTT in patients on NSAIDs, ASA, heparin, warfarin	PT/PTT in patients on NSAIDs, ASA, heparin, warfarin	closely monitor for PT/PTT in patients on NSAIDs, ASA, heparin, warfarin	anticoagulants
	FDA approved for depression in adults and adolescents, OCD, bulimia, PMDD	FDA approved for depression, PMDD, panic disorder, OCD in adult and pediatric, social anxiety disorder	FDA approved for depression, panic disorder, social anxiety disorder, PMDD	FDA approved for depression and generalized anxiety disorder
	5-week washout for MAOI	14-day washout for MAOI	14-day washout for MAOI	14-day washout for MAOI
	No withdrawal syndrome due to long half-life	Minimal anorectic effect	Most sedative SSRI	Low drop-out rates due to adverse side effects
			Highest incidence of withdrawal syndrome	

[a] PT/PTT, prothrombin time/partial thromboplastin time; NSAIDs, nonsteroidal antiinflammatory drugs; ASA, aminosalicylic acid; OCD, obsessive-compulsive disorder; PMDD, premenstrual dysphoric disorder; MAOI, monoamine oxidase inhibitors; SSRI, selective serotonin reuptake inhibitors.

[b] Symbyax is fluoxetine and olanzapine combined, for psychotic depression.

Table 8.6. Newer atypical antidepressants.

	Venlafaxine (Effexor, Effexor XR)	Bupropion (Wellbutrin, Wellbutrin SR, Wellbutrin XL, Zyban)	Mirtazipine (Remeron)	Nefazodone (Serzone)
Side effects	Nausea, dizziness, sedation, abnormal ejaculation, sweating, dry mouth, gas, blurred vision, nervousness, insomnia, anorexia, constipation, agitation, tremor, yawning, palpitations	Headache, dry mouth, nausea, constipation, insomnia, dizziness, pharyngitis, anorexia, weight loss (lowest drop-out rate due to side effects of all antidepressants)	Dry mouth, sedation, somnolence, weight gain, increased cholesterol and triglycerides, orthostatic blood pressure changes, dizziness	Dizziness, asthenia, dry mouth, nausea, constipation, somnolence, postural hypotension, weakness, blurred vision, confusion, hepatotoxicity and rare liver failure
Dosage	XR: 75–375 mg/day (single AM or PM dose)	XL: 300–450 mg/day (single AM dose)	30–45 mg/day (single hs dose)	300–600 mg/day (bid)

Drug interaction	Few clinically significant drug interactions	Few clinically significant drug interactions / Contraindicated with history of seizure disorder, bulimia or anorexia nervosa, or undergoing abrupt discontinuation of alcohol or sedatives	Few clinically significant drug interactions / Added sedative effects with other central nervous system depressants	Few clinically significant drug interactions / Increases levels of alprazolam, estazolam, carbamazepine, calcium channel blockers / Contraindicated with terfenidine, astemizole, cisapride
Other	FDA approved for depression, generalized anxiety disorder, social anxiety disorder / 7-day washout for monoamine oxidase inhibitor (MAOI) / Increased risk of hypertension with doses >225 mg/day / Taper off to avoid withdrawal syndrome	FDA approved for depression, smoking cessation (Zyban) / 14-day washout for MAOI / Seizure risk dose related (0.4% at 450 mg/day) / Minimal sedation, weight gain, or sexual side effects	FDA approved for depression / 14-day washout for MAOI / Minimal nausea and other gastrointestinal side effects / Minimal sexual side effects / Less sedation and weight gain with higher doses	FDA approved for depression / 7-day washout for MAOI / Does not suppress REM sleep / Minimal sexual side effects

energy and alertness, and decrease appetite. Bupropion has fewer sedation, weight gain, and sexual side effects than other antidepressants, side effects that not uncommonly lead to noncompliance (and relapse) with long-term antidepressant therapy. It is commonly added to SSRIs to augment the antidepressant response (creating a "dual-action" effect) and to treat sexual side effects of SSRIs (see below). Bupropion has a low incidence of mania induction and is an effective alternative to stimulants in the treatment of ADHD. The risk of seizures is dose related and appears to be less with the once-a-day XL form that avoids spikes of serum bupropion levels.

Mirtazipine enhances both serotonin and norepinephrine release via α_2-adrenergic antagonism and α_1-adrenergic receptor stimulation on 5-hydroxytryptamine (5-HT) cell bodies; there is no specific neurotransmitter reuptake inhibition. Sedation and weight gain are the primary side effects, both of which are less with higher doses. Advantages include anxiolytic effects, minimal GI and sexual side effects, minimal rapid eye movement (REM) suppression, and few clinically significant drug–drug interactions. Its unique pharmacology makes mirtazipine a useful agent in combination with other antidepressants in the treatment refractory depression.

Nefazodone is chemically related to trazodone; its primary mechanism of antidepressant effect appears to be antagonism of the postsynaptic $5\text{-}HT_2$ receptor, although reuptake inhibition of serotonin and norepinephrine may be involved. Nefazodone is helpful with anxious patients, promotes good sleep without REM suppression like many of the other antidepressants, has fewer GI side effects and weight gain than the SSRIs, and is unlikely to cause sexual side effects. Unfortunately, the sedation requires a gradual dosage titration and a twice-a-day dosage schedule, and monitoring of hepatic function is necessary given the black box warning about rare (1/300,000 patient years) liver failure and death.

Indications for Maintenance Pharmacotherapy

1. Three or more episodes of depression.
2. Patients older than 50 years at first depression.
3. Patients with a second episode of depression and
   - a first-degree relative with recurrent depression or bipolar disorder
   - relapse of depression within 1 year of stopping medication
   - first episode of depression before age 20 years
   - episodes of depression are severe, sudden, or life-threatening.

Prophylactic antidepressant therapy is most effective if dosage is maintained at the level that produced an initial treatment response.

Electroconvulsive Therapy

ECT is the most effective treatment modality for moderate to severe depression, and has the most rapid onset of therapeutic effect, often after the first or second treatment. Indications include psychotic depression, catatonia, severe suicidality, a previous preferential response to ECT, a failure of response to other treatments, and an acute manic episode.

The usual course of ECT involves 6–12 treatments; unilateral treatments are associated with less postictal confusion and anterograde/retrograde memory interference, but may be less effective than bilateral ECT. ECT has an excellent safety record, although there is some risk associated with the brief general anesthesia. Cognitive impairment generally resolves within a few weeks; rarely, patients may report a more persistent and pervasive memory disturbance.

Psychotherapy

Supportive therapy is a critical component of the treatment of all depressed patients, and includes maintaining a therapeutic relationship that provides support, accurate empathy, education regarding the illness and treatment, and an increased sense of hope for recovery. It may involve interaction with significant others or aspects of the patient's environment (e.g., providing a leave of absence from work or enlisting the assistance of others).

Certain specific forms of psychotherapy [cognitive-behavioral therapy (CBT) and interpersonal therapy (IPT)] are as effective as pharmacotherapy in the acute treatment of depression. CBT and IPT may be considered first-line treatments for mild to moderate depression. Psychotherapy alone may be a treatment option for more severely depressed outpatients who wish to pursue it and who are able to work productively in therapy.

Group, family, and marital therapies have been shown to be effective interventions with depressed patients, particularly if interpersonal problems are a major factor. Treatment of concurrent substance abuse disorders is essential (e.g., Alcoholics Anonymous meetings).

Combined pharmacotherapy and psychotherapy work at least as well, and in some cases better, than either modality alone. In combined treatment, each treatment offers distinct advantages; pharmacotherapy tends to produce a more rapid response, particularly with somatic symptoms; psychotherapy affects cognitive, social, and interpersonal functioning, and improves long-term remission rates. Combined treatment has a lower dropout rate than single modality approaches. However, there is no evidence that long-term psychoanalytic therapy is effective for the treatment of major depressive disorder.

Cognitive-Behavioral Therapy

This therapy is based on the finding that depressed patients have a persistent negative bias in thinking and distortions in appraisal of self (worthlessness), world (helplessness), and future (hopelessness): the negative cognitive triad. CBT is an active, highly structured, short-term treatment approach in which the therapist engages the patient in identification, revision, and modification of dysfunctional cognitions and depressive behaviors.

Behavioral techniques include scheduling activities that provide the patient with enjoyment or a sense of accomplishment; graded task assignments to assist patients in overcoming anxiety, avoidance tendencies, and behavioral inertia; and homework assignments to continue self-help work outside of therapy sessions.

Cognitive strategies are designed to help the patient identify and test the validity of depressive automatic thoughts, cognitive distortions and errors (e.g., all or nothing thinking, overpersonalization, overgeneralization), and underlying depressogenic schemas (e.g., "I must be loved by this person for my life to have meaning"). Therapy is focused primarily on "here and now" issues and symptom reduction.

Interpersonal Therapy

Interpersonal therapy is based on the observation that depressive episodes are often precipitated by disturbances of interpersonal relationships, including loss and grief (e.g., death of a family member), disputes with significant others (e.g., marital problems), role transitions (e.g., loss of a job), and interpersonal deficits (e.g., social isolation); it is also a structured, short-term, active, "here and now" form of therapy.

The therapist guides the patient to complete an interpersonal inventory, an assessment of significant relationships, expectations of each party, satisfactory/unsatisfactory aspects of the relationship, and development of goals for change. Therapeutic techniques include ventilation and mourning, analysis of communication styles and repetitive patterns in relationships (and in the therapeutic relationship), and the development of conflict resolution skills; the therapist encourages the formation of new relationships and social support systems.

Treatment of Bipolar Disorders
General Principles and Goals of Management

General principles and goals of management from the Revised APA Practice Guidelines of 2002 include the establishment and maintenance of a supportive therapeutic alliance with the following:

1. Monitor changes in patient's psychiatric status.
2. Provide education regarding bipolar illness (patient and family).
3. Enhance compliance with treatment.
4. Promote regular patterns of activity and wakefulness.
5. Assist understanding of and adaptation to the psychosocial effects of illness.
6. Help the patient and family to identify new episodes early.
7. Reduce morbidity and sequelae of bipolar disorder.

Psychopharmacology: General Considerations

Mood stabilizers are a critical component in the treatment of patients with bipolar disorder. Lithium carbonate, divalproex, carbamazepine, lamotrigine, and the second-generation (atypical) antipsychotics are effective in the acute episode, as well as in the prevention of future episodes of depression and mania. Only 50–60% of patients have an adequate response to one of the mood stabilizers alone; the use of multiple medications is often necessary.

Antidepressants may be indicated (in combination with mood stabilizers) in bipolar depression; however, antidepressants have been associated with an increased incidence of manic activation and mixed affective states, especially in bipolar type I patients. Recent research suggests that the risk of antidepressant-induced rapid cycling is less significant than previously thought. Benzodiazepines (e.g., clonazepam and lorazepam) are effective adjunctive agents for acute agitation, anxiety, and insomnia, but their use involves the risk of dysphoria, disinhibition, and dependency.

Lithium

Lithium is generally very well tolerated if plasma concentrations are monitored and maintained (0.75–1.5 mEq/liter for acute manic episode, 0.4–1.0 mEq/liter during the maintenance phase of therapy); the usual maintenance dose is 900–1200 mg/day (bid or tid dose).

Common side effects include nausea, diarrhea, fatigue, fine tremor (responsive to β-blockers), polydipsia, polyuria, edema, weight gain, and occasionally cognitive slowing.

Lithium toxicity (levels >2.0 mEq/liter) is characterized by severe nausea and vomiting, ataxia, dysarthria, coarse tremor, choreoathetoid movements, confusion, seizures, and cardiac arrhythmias; levels >4.0 mEq/liter can cause coma, renal failure, and death; impaired renal function, and extracellular volume depletion. Most diuretics and NSAIDs can result in higher serum levels and toxicity; caution is advised for patients with cardiac, neurologic, or renal disease, decreased sodium intake, and the elderly.

Other infrequent side effects include goiter, hypothyroidism, nephrogenic diabetes insipidus, benign leukocytosis, acne, and other dermatologic effects such as induction or exacerbation of psoriasis. Lithium use is associated with cardiac and other birth defects; contraceptive counseling for females of childbearing age is essential (see below).

Divalproex

Divalproex is effective with all subtypes of mania, including classic, mixed, and rapid-cycling. It is often effective with lithium-unresponsive bipolar patients. The FDA has approved its use for seizures and migraine in addition to treatment of bipolar disorder. Cimetidine, erythromycin, phenothiazines, fluvoxamine, fluoxetine, aspirin, ibuprofen, and topirimate may increase levels of valproate. Rifampin, carbamazepine, phenobarbital, oxcarbazepine, and lamotrigine can reduce serum levels. Divalproex is metabolized by hepatic oxidation and conjugation, is highly protein bound, takes 1–3 days to steady state, and has a therapeutic range of 50–125 μg/ml; the usual therapeutic dose is 750–2000 mg/day (bid or tid dose; an extended release form is available for once a day dosing).

Common side effects include mild abdominal cramps and diarrhea, menstrual disturbances, bruising, temporary alopecia (benefit from selenium and zinc supplements), nausea and vomiting, tremor, and weight gain. Hepatotoxicity, the most serious side effect, usually occurs in the first few months of treatment and is characterized by fever, anorexia, vomiting, lethargy, and elevated liver enzymes; fatal hepatotoxicity has occurred in 1 in 40,000 cases, almost exclusively in children aged 2 years and under with seizures and other metabolic disorders. Pancreatitis is also a rare but serious side effect. Baseline liver functions and periodic (e.g., twice a year) monitoring is recommended. Since divalproex is teratogenic, carrying a 1–2% risk of neural tube defects, contraceptive counseling is essential. It should be discontinued and folate prescribed if pregnancy occurs (see below).

Carbamazepine

FDA-approved as an anticonvulsant, carbamazepine is also used for other neurologic syndromes, such as chronic neurogenic pain (e.g., trigeminal neuralgia), and impulsive behavior disorders. Numerous drug interactions include the following:

1. Serum levels of antidepressants, benzodiazepines, antipsychotics, oral contraceptives, and anticoagulants are decreased.
2. Carbamazepine levels are increased by fluvoxamine, fluoxetine, divalproex, erythromycin, isoniazid, cimetidine, diltiazem, doxycycline, fluconazole, prednisolone, propoxyphene, and grapefruit juice.
3. Carbamazepine levels are decreased by phenytoin and phenobarbital.

Most common side effects include dizziness, sedation, ataxia, and nausea. Leukopenia, thrombocytopenia (approximately 2%), or aplastic anemia (approximately 0.002%) can occur, and baseline and periodic monitoring of complete blood count (CBC) are indicated, particularly with unexplained fever or rash. It is teratogenic (see below).

Lamotrigine (Lamictal)

Lamotrigine is indicated for the maintenance treatment of bipolar disorders. It is effective in decreasing manic, hypomanic, and mixed episodes, but is a particularly effective first-line treatment for the bipolar depressed phase; it is sometimes referred to as a "bottom-up" mood stabilizer. It has a more limited role in acute treatment of mood episodes because a slow titration of dosage is required to reduce the risk of serious rashes including Stevens–Johnson syndrome (0.08% monotherapy, 0.13% adjunctive therapy). The incidence of these serious rashes is higher in adult epileptics (0.3%), with coadministration of divalproex (requiring even slower titration), and in pediatric patients.

Second-Generation Antipsychotics

The second-generation antipsychotics (SGAs), sometimes referred to as "atypical" antipsychotics, have largely replaced the "typical" neuroleptics such as chlorpromazine and haloperidol in clinical practice. The SGAs (risperidone, olazapine, quetiapine, ziprasidone, aripiprazole, clozapine) have a substantially lower risk of extrapyramidal symptoms (dystonia, pseudoparkinsonism, akathisia, tardive dyskinesia) than traditional agents. In addition to antipsychotic actions (that appear to be mediated by antagonism/modulation of dopamine receptors), the SGAs have other pharmacologic actions that account for their antimanic, antidepressant, and mood-stabilizing properties, alone or in combination with other drugs. The SGAs (especially olanzapine and clozapine) are associated with an increased risk of weight gain, glucose dysregulation including diabetes, and increases of cholesterol and triglycerides.

Psychotherapy

Social skill-based family therapy, IPT, and CBT are effective adjuncts to pharmocologic treatments. Goals of therapy include modifying social risk factors, enhancing compliance with medications, and increasing the patient's and family's acceptance of the illness. Comorbid conditions, particularly substance abuse, need to be addressed for treatment of the mood disorder to be successful.

Special Clinical Situations
Evaluation of Suicidal Risk

Most suicides are depression-related: 15% of patients with affective disorders commit suicide, accounting for 16,000 suicide deaths annually, with the highest rate among the elderly.

- Suicide attempts: 3:1 female:male.
- Completed suicide: 3:1 male:female.

Risk Factors

Risk factors include hopelessness, general medical illness, family history of suicide, substance abuse, prior suicide attempts, living alone, bipolar disorder and psychotic symptoms, organic brain syndromes, availability of weapon or other means of suicide, and specific plan or intent.

Not every patient with suicidal ideation needs to be hospitalized; however, all patients with mood disorders need to be evaluated regularly for the emergence of suicidal thoughts and changes in the intensity of ideation. If a patient is unable to participate in outpatient treatment or to agree to contact the physician if suicidal thoughts increase, has active substance abuse or psychotic symptoms, or reports strong impulses to act on the self-destructive thoughts or profound sense of hopelessness, then hospitalization needs to be seriously considered.

Psychopharmacology, Pregnancy, and Breastfeeding

Contrary to previous beliefs that pregnancy offered a protective effect against depression, recent studies indicate that approximately 10% of pregnant women suffer from clinically significant depression. The risk of obsessive-compulsive disorder may increase, and mania and psychosis may occur or worsen during pregnancy. Psychotropic medications are indicated during pregnancy when the potential risk to the fetus from exposure to the drugs is outweighed by the risk of untreated maternal psychiatric illness. Complications of untreated maternal mood disorders include observed negative behavioral effects on the neonate, impairment of maternal–infant bonding, and the risks associated with poor maternal nutritional intake and self-care.

If nonpharmacologic treatments (e.g., CBT or light therapy) are not effective or if depression is severe (e.g., the patient is suicidal, psychotic, or not eating), medication is indicated. There is no strong evidence that heterocyclics (nortriptyline, desipramine), SSRIs (fluoxetine, sertraline, citalopram, escitalopram), SNRIs (venlafaxine), or bupropion (Pregnancy Category B) are associated with teratogenic effects. Most studies of women taking fluoxetine through pregnancy have found no risk of obstetric complications, though there have been a few reports of lower birth weight, preterm birth, and altered neurobehavioral adaptation in newborns exposed *in utero*. This risk is difficult to interpret as untreated depression has been found to triple the risk of preterm delivery and small-for-gestational age and low-birthweight infants. There have also been reports of a transient withdrawal or discontinuation syndrome (irritability, tachypnea, temperature instability, poor feeding) in newborn infants following third trimester exposure to SSRIs including fluoxetine, sertraline, and paroxetine. Women with a history of severe recurrent depression or prior postpartum depression may benefit from reintroduction of antidepressants in the third trimester or during the early puerperium. ECT has an excellent record of safety during pregnancy, and it has proved effective for both depressive and manic episodes.

The management of women with bipolar disorder is complicated by the teratogenic effects of the mood stabilizers:

1.   Lithium (Pregnancy Category D) exposure during the first trimester is associated with a 4–12% risk of congenital abnormalities, particularly cardiac abnormalities (0.1% risk of Ebstein's anomaly). Neonatal toxicity and a "floppy baby" syndrome (hypotonicity and cyanosis) have been described. Women on lithium are more prone to hypothyroidism, and neonatal hypothyroidism and diabetes insipidus have been reported.

2.   Neural tube defects have been reported with both valproate (2–5%) and carbamazepine (1–3%); craniofacial defects, fingernail hypoplasia, microcephaly, cardiac defects, and developmental delays have also been described with first-trimester exposure. Both valproate and carbamazepine are Category D.

3.   First-trimester exposure to benzodiazepines has been implicated in an increased incidence of cleft palate (<0.1%); *in utero* exposure during the last trimester or during labor can lead to hypotonicity, failure to feed, low

Apgar scores, and withdrawal symptoms (clonazepam may be the safest benzodiazepine in pregnancy).

   4.   First-generation neuroleptic exposure (e.g., chlorpromazine, haloperidol) may be associated with a slight increase in congenital abnormalities and transient extrapyramidal side effects in newborns. All second-generation atypical antipsychotics are Category C except clozapine (Category B). The potential risks of weight gain and glucose dysregulation with these drugs are of particular concern during pregnancy.

General Guidelines for Bipolar Women

   1.   Discuss pregnancy and medication risks with all bipolar women as early as possible.

   2.   If possible, gradually taper and discontinue mood stabilizers prior to pregnancy (rapid discontinuation is associated with an increased risk of relapse).

   3.   In women with a history of severe bipolar episodes, attempt to discontinue medication for a period coinciding with embryogenesis or switch to a lower-risk drug during pregnancy; consider reintroduction of mood stabilizers or neuroleptics if clinical deterioration occurs.

   4.   If medications are necessary, close monitoring of serum levels is necessary throughout pregnancy; risk counseling and monitoring of fetal development (e.g., fetal echocardiogram and high-resolution ultrasound, α-fetoprotein levels) are indicated. High-dose folate supplementation (3–4 mg/day) may reduce the risk for neural tube defects in women who continue valproate or carbamazepine.

   Most psychotropic agents used in the treatment of mood disorders are excreted in breast milk and often can be detected in the breast-fed infant; however, psychotropic medication is not an absolute contraindication for breastfeeding. Antidepressants (heterocyclics, SSRIs, SNRIs, and the other new generation antidepressants) have not been associated with any serious ill effects in infants studied, but MAOIs are contraindicated. Nevertheless, the American Academy of Pediatrics has classified antidepressants as "drugs for which the effect on nursing infants is unknown but may be of concern." Many experts recommend sertraline as first-line antidepressant treatment for breast-feeding women because of its relatively low risk.

   Anticonvulsants may lead to vitamin K deficiency, produce drowsiness, and result in feeding problems or inadequate weight gain. Some experts consider lithium to be a contraindication for breastfeeding (e.g., American Academy of Pediatrics); others believe that breastfeeding may be attempted if the infant is closely monitored for restlessness or other signs of toxic effects. Benzodiazepines may accumulate in the infant and lead to lethargy. Neuroleptics are generally not associated with observable ill effects, although a few reports of lethargy have been reported; phenothiazines may increase jaundice.

Management of Antidepressant-Induced Sexual Dysfunction

Although physicians often do not specifically inquire about sexual side effects, recent studies have established that 30–40% of patients on antidepressants (including heterocyclics, MAOIs, SSRIs, and SNRIs) have sexual dysfunction, most commonly decreased libido and impaired ejaculation and orgasm. The differential diagnosis of sexual dysfunction includes symptoms of depressive disorder, complications of concomitant medical disorders (e.g., diabetes), or primary sexual dysfunction. Treatment alternatives include the following:

1.   Wait for the development of tolerance; this may take several months and probably occurs only in a small percentage of cases.

2.   Prescribe a lower dosage of antidepressant or periodic drug holidays; although this approach is occasionally effective, there is a risk of subtherapeutic antidepressant levels and relapse of depressive disorder.

3.   Switch to a different antidepressant; bupropion, nefazodone, and mirtazipine appear to be associated with significantly less sexual dysfunction than other antidepressants.

4.   Continue antidepressants and treat sexual dysfunction with another pharmacologic agent (often contraindicated with MAOIs), e.g., bupropion (75–150 mg/day), sildenafil (50–200 mg), yohimbine (5.4 mg tid or prn 2 hours prior to coitus), or cyproheptadine (4–12 mg/day or 1 hour prior to coitus); other agents that have been reported to be effective include buspirone, bromocriptine, methylphenidate, amantidine, ginkgo biloba, and panax ginseng.

Antidepressants do not invariably have adverse effects on sexual functioning. Trazodone (sometimes in combination with yohimbine) is a safe and often effective treatment for psychogenic impotence, and SSRIs have been successfully used in some cases of premature ejaculation. A small percentage of men and women report increased libido and enhanced arousal and orgasm; a few cases of spontaneous orgasm associated with yawning have been reported with clomipramine and fluoxetine.

Indications for Psychiatric Consultation and Referral

Indications include the following:

1.   Diagnostic confusion or comorbidity (e.g., another psychiatric disorder requiring special treatment, such as substance abuse or a complex medical condition that may complicate treatment with antidepressants).
2.   Failure or partial response to two acute phase trials of antidepressants. Severe, recurrent, or psychotic depression.
3.   Presence of suicidal ideation.
4.   Need for hospitalization or ECT.
5.   Need for psychotherapy (may be effectively provided by nonmedical mental health professionals in many cases).
6.   Request by patient or family.

Suggested Reading

Altshuler LL, Cohen L, Szuba MP, et al. Pharmacologic management of psychiatric illness during pregnancy: dilemmas and guidelines. *Am J Psychiatry* 1996;153:592–606.

Altshuler LL, Cohen LS, Mount ML, et al. The Expert Consensus Guideline Series: Treatment of Depression in Women 2001. *Postgrad Med* Special Report, March 2001.

American Psychiatric Association. Practice guideline for the treatment of patients with major depressive disorder (Revision). *Am J Psychiatry* 2000; 157(suppl 4):1–45.

American Psychiatric Association. Practice guideline for the treatment of patients with bipolar disorder (Revision). *Am J Psychiatry* 2002;159(suppl 4):1–50.

American Psychiatric Association. *Diagnostic and Statistical Manual of Mental Disorders, Fourth Edition, Text Revision.* Washington, DC: American Psychiatric Press; 2000.

American Psychiatric Association Task Force on Electroconvulsive Therapy. *The Practice of Electroconvulsive Therapy.* Washington, DC: American Psychiatric Press; 1990.

Balon R. The effects of antidepressants on human sexuality: diagnosis and management. *Primary Psychiatry* 1995;2(8):2–10.

Beck AT, Rush AJ, Shaw BF, Emery G. *Cognitive Therapy of Depression.* New York: Guilford Press; 1979.

Chaudron LH, Pies RW. The relationship between postpartum psychosis and bipolar disorder: a review. *J Clin Psychiatry* 2003;64:1284–92.

Cohen LS, Friedman JM, Jefferson JW, et al. A reevaluation of risk of in utero exposure to lithium. *JAMA* 1994;271:146–50.

Gitlin MJ, Pasnau RO. Psychiatric syndromes linked to reproductive function in women: a review of current knowledge. *Am J Psychiatry* 1989;146: 1413–22.

Klerman GL, Weissman MM, Rounsaville BJ, Chervon ES. *Interpersonal Psychotherapy of Depression.* New York: Basic Books; 1984.

Miller LJ. Postpartum depression. *JAMA* 2002;287(6):762–64.

Persons JB, Thase ME, Crits-Cristoph P. The role of psychotherapy in the treatment of depression. *Arch Gen Psychiatry* 1996;53:283–90.

Ross LE, Steiner M. A biopsychosocial approach to premenstrual dysphoric disorder. *Psychiatr Clin N Am* 2003;26(3):529–46.

Schatzberg AF, Cole JO, DeBattista C. *Manual of Clinical Psychopharmacology*, 4th ed. Washington DC: American Psychiatric Publishing; 2003.

Sloan DME, Kornstein SG. Gender differences in depression and response to antidepressant treatment. *Psychiatr Clin N Am* 2003;26(3):581–94.

Wright JH, Schrodt GR Jr. Combined cognitive therapy and pharmacotherapy. In *Handbook of Cognitive Therapy*. Freeman A, Simon MK, Arkowitz H, et al. (eds). New York: Plenum Press; 1989.

Yonkers KA, Wisner KL, Stowe Z, et al. Management of bipolar disorder during pregnancy and the postpartum period. *Am J Psychiatry* 2004; 161:608–20.

9

Breast Disease

William H. Hindle

Background Information

Evaluation of breast symptoms and complaints may be appropriately managed by obstetrician-gynecologists in the ambulatory setting. Furthermore, surveillance for signs of breast cancer by mammography and physical examination is the responsibility of the primary health care physician for women, usually the ob/gyn. Diagnosed breast cancer and other breast problems beyond the expertise of the primary care physician should be suitably referred but must be continuously followed to be certain proper treatment is given and the clinical problem is resolved satisfactorily. In most cases, the patient will return to her primary care physician on whom she may rely for lifelong follow-up after her treatment is completed.

Knowledge of the natural history of breast lesions, technology for evaluation of the breast, and therapy of breast lesions have been dramatically transformed in the past 30 years, resulting in diverse improved diagnostic and treatment options for physicians and their patients. With the availability of local breast-oriented physician consultants in cytology, mammography, surgical oncology, and plastic surgery, the office settings of primary care physicians can function as breast diagnostic centers, supplying medical information about breast health and care and coordinating therapy for women with breast problems that require specialized medical attention.

Establishing a Diagnosis
Breast Evaluation Techniques

The basic techniques of breast evaluation consist of (1) a breast-oriented medical history, (2) clinical breast examination (CBE), (3) mammography, and (4) fine-needle aspiration (FNA) of a persistent palpable breast mass (the latter three being known as the "Diagnostic Triad"). After receiving supervised training in these techniques, obstetrician-gynecologists can readily perform breast evaluations in their offices. Otherwise, women with breast problems should be referred to a physician trained and experienced in breast-evaluation techniques.

Breast-Oriented Medical History

The essentials of a breast-oriented medical history are listed in Table 9.1. This information should be given to the mammographer when a mammogram is ordered and to the cytopathologist when FNA slides are submitted. A new patient's complete medical history should be obtained and the pertinent facts recorded. At this time, a patient may ask about risk factors for breast cancer, a relative's breast problems, the effects of hormone therapy on the breast and on breast cancer risk, and screening mammography. In response, current evidence-based medical data should be objectively given in understandable lay terms.

Clinical Breast Examination

A thorough, bilateral breast examination should be performed when a woman presents with a breast problem and annually for asymptomatic women. Medico-legal issues make it mandatory that a clear notation of the breast examination be

Table 9.1.   The patient's medical history and basic clinical information.[a]

Patient's breast-oriented history
Presenting complaint
  Mass
  Pain
  Nipple discharge
Age
Last menstrual period
Family history of breast cancer—particularly first-degree relatives
Personal history of breast cancer
Breast surgeries
Last mammogram—date performed and results
Hormone therapy—current or past

---

[a]This should be recorded and given to the mammographer or other consultants.

noted in the patient's medical record. Any breast abnormality should be explicitly described and the absence of a palpable mass noted as well. Drawings are useful for the depiction of a palpable mass, an area of patient concern, or the exact site of a procedure, e.g., FNA. The steps of a CBE are illustrated in Fig. 9.1.

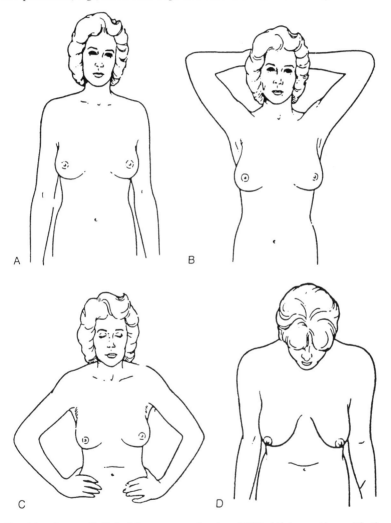

Fig. 9.1. Steps of clinical breast examination (CBE): (A) inspection with the patient erect; (B) inspection with the patient's arms raised over her head; (C) inspection with the patient pressing her hands on her hips; (D) inspection with the patient leaning forward.

Continued.

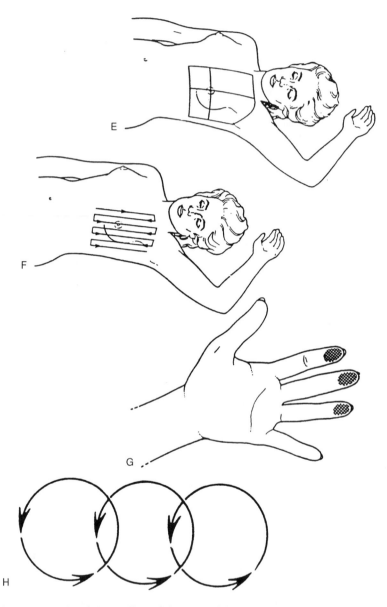

Fig. 9.1. *Continued.* (E) outline of the area of the entire anterior chest wall to be palpated; (F) diagram of the vertical strip method of systematically palpating the anterior chest wall; (G) pads of the middle three fingers used for palpation; (H) rotary, dime-sized motions used for palpation with the finger pads.

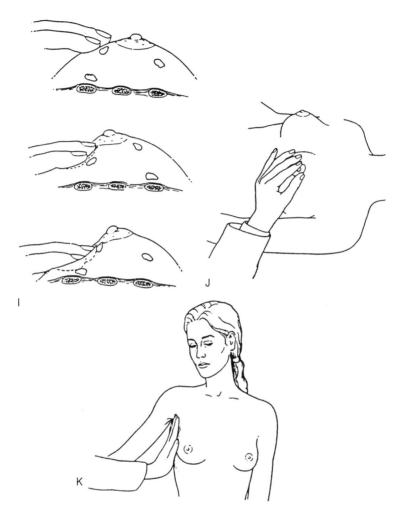

Fig. 9.1. *Continued.* (I) light, medium, and firm pressure used to palpate masses at variable depths within the breast; (J) gentle compression of the nipple after palpation of the subareolar area; and (K) palpation of the axillary area. (From Hindle W. The diagnostic evaluation. Obstet Gynecol Clin N Am 1994; 21(3): 504–11. W.B. Saunders, Philadelphia, September 1994. By permission.)

Fine-Needle Aspiration

The equipment required for FNA is listed in Table 9.2. Various techniques of FNA are illustrated in Figs. 9.2, 9.3, and 9.4. Normally, cytology slides are prepared in the same manner as hematology slides and then fixed in the same

Table 9.2.   Fine-needle aspiration.

Stabilization of a breast mass prior to fine-needle aspiration: locating the mass with the index and middle finger of the nondominant hand and stabilization of the mass over a rib with the taut skin tented over the mass

Fine-needle aspiration equipment
Alcohol (or equivalent antiseptic) skin wipe
22-gauge 1-in. needle with transparent hub
10-ml syringe
Sterile 4 × 4-in. gauze pad
Band-Aid optional

way as Pap smears. However, as the methodology of slide preparation, fixation, and staining may vary with the training and experience of the cytopathologist, the clinician just beginning FNAs should personally contact the consultant cytopathologist and learn his or her preferences. The goal is to obtain an abundant well-preserved cell sample for cytologic interpretation. An alternative collection method is the utilization of liquid-based media and mechanical slide preparation such as ThinPrep (CYTYC Corp., Boxborough, MA).

FNA is no more painful and takes no longer to perform than a venipuncture. When it is explained that the FNA cell sample has the same potential clinical value as a Pap smear, patients readily consent to the procedure.

The indication for FNA is a persistent, palpable, dominant breast mass; there are no contraindications. Complications (when FNA is performed with the mass fixed over a rib) are ecchymoses and, rarely, hematoma forma-

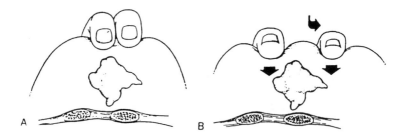

Fig. 9.2.   Stabilization of a breast mass prior to fine-needle aspiration: (A) locating the mass with the index and middle finger of the nondominant hand; (B) stabilization of the mass over a rib with the taut skin tented over the mass. (From Hindle W. The diagnostic evaluation. *Obstet Gynecol Clin N Am* 1994;21(3):504–11. WB Saunders, Philadelphia, September 1994. By permission.)

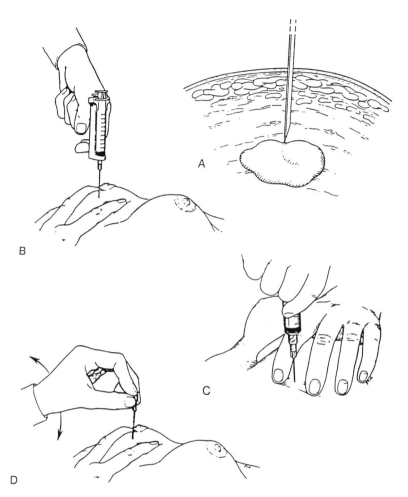

Fig. 9.3. Illustrations of the steps in breast fine-needle aspiration and various techniques: (A) initial exploration with attention to tissue resistance and texture; (B) use of a pistol-type syringe holder, which maintains negative pressure; (C) use of a syringe alone to maintain negative pressure; and (D) use of a needle alone without negative pressure. (From Hindle W. The diagnostic evaluation. Obstet Gynecol Clin N Am 1994; 21(3): 504–11. W.B. Saunders, Philadelphia, September 1994. By permission.)

tion. Because of the latter possibility, mammography is optimally performed prior to FNA or at least 2 weeks after the FNA since a hematoma within the breast tissue can simulate a mammographically "suspicious" lesion. More vigorous FNA techniques, e.g., radial aspirations within the breast tissue and

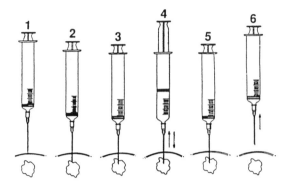

Fig. 9.4. Sequential steps when using a syringe for aspiration cytology of a solid mass. Negative pressure within the syringe is applied *only* during step 4. (From Hindle W. The diagositc evaluation. Obstet Gynecol Clin N Am 1994; 21(3): 504–11. W.B. Saunders, Philadelphia, September 1994. By permission.)

multiple aspirations at the same site, increase the potential for ecchymosis and hematoma formation. Pressure for at least 2 minutes over the aspiration site, using a 4 × 4-in. sterile gauze pad folded in quarters, usually provides hemostasis and avoids ecchymoses. Figure 9.5 is an algorithm for the evaluation of a persistent, palpable, dominant, solid breast mass.

Percutaneous tissue core-needle biopsy, with or without ultrasound guidance, is becoming popular for the histologic diagnosis of a palpable breast mass and is replacing stereotactic needle localization open surgical biopsy for nonpalpable (usually mammographically detected) breast lesions.

FNA Cytology

As many as 90% of breast neoplasms can be specifically diagnosed by FNA cytology. Cancers are usually readily diagnosed by FNA because of the abundance of cellular material and the characteristic malignant cellular pattern. The cytologic "sine qua non" of breast adenocarcinoma are well-preserved single cells with reversal of the nuclear cytoplasmic ratio and malignant (e.g., pleomorphic) nuclei. The malignant cells have a "discohesive" pattern, and there is a "dirty" background. However, as the cancers are often vascular, blood in the aspirate is common and it interferes with the cytologic interpretation. Bloody smears should not be discarded as all the smears from a carcinoma may be grossly bloody. FNA cytology cannot definitely diagnose carcinoma as *in situ* but can give an impression of "consistent with invasive carcinoma." Some surgical oncologists will perform definitive surgical therapy on the basis of an FNA cytologic diagnosis of "adenocarcinoma"; others will perform a frozen section for confirmation immediately prior to definitive surgical therapy. When the cytopathologist is uncertain of the diagnosis or there is a question of cellular atypia or malignancy, a surgical biopsy is indicated.

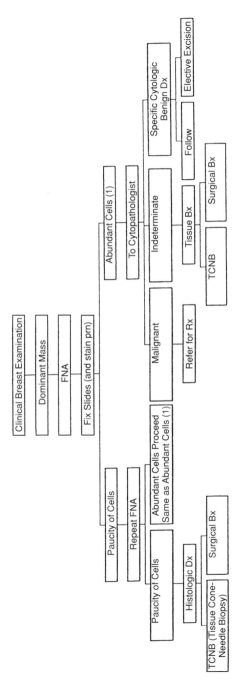

Fig. 9.5. A clinical algorithm for the evaluation of a persistent, dominant, solid breast mass. Bx, biopsy; CBE, clinical breast examination; Dx, diagnosis; FNA, fine-needle aspiration; Rx, treatment; TCNB, tissue core-needle biopsy. (From Hindle W. The diagnostic evaluation. *Obstet Gynecol Clin N Am* 1994;21(3):504–11. WB Saunders, Philadelphia, September 1994. By permission.)

Fibroadenoma Cytology

Because of their highly cellular composition, fibroadenomas are readily diagnosed by FNA cytology. There are established, definite cytologic diagnostic criteria for the diagnosis of breast fibroadenoma. Cohesive sheets of benign ductal cells, so-called naked bipolar nuclei, and benign stroma are cytologically characteristic of a fibroadenoma. The "naked" nuclei are thought to be from the benign myoepithelial (contractile) cells around the single cell layered ducts.

Nonneoplastic Cytology

FNA of normal breast tissue usually yields a paucity of cells with some stroma and adipose tissue. Benign ductal cells are uniform and appear as cohesive segments of ducts or terminal duct lobular units. When fibrocystic changes are present, FNA reveals foamy histiocytes and apocrine change in the appearance of some benign ductal cells.

When the FNA cytologic diagnosis is in doubt (either by the cytopathologist, clinician, or patient) or if atypical cells are noted, an open surgical biopsy (or tissue core needle biopsy) should be done to obtain a specific histologic diagnosis.

FNA of Cysts

Cysts are readily diagnosed by FNA when gross fluid (not blood) is obtained. Figure 9.6 is a clinical algorithm for the evaluation of a palpable cyst. All the cyst fluid should be aspirated with a syringe, and then the fluid can be discarded because cyst fluid cytology is not cost effective. However, grossly bloody (nontraumatic) cyst fluid can be a sign of the rare intracystic carcinoma. After aspiration of a cyst, the patient can be managed by the ob-gyn if (1) palpation of the area shows no residual or underlying mass, (2) the fluid is not grossly bloody, and (3) reexamination within 3 months determines that the cyst has not refilled. The patient should be referred to a breast specialist if there is a residual mass, the fluid is grossly bloody, or the cyst refills after a second aspiration.

Diagnostic Mammography

Diagnostic mammography is the third component of the diagnostic triad for breast lesions. When a nonpalpable abnormality is perceived on a mammogram (whether diagnostic or screening), the mammographer should make a mammographic evaluation and give a specific recommendation such as (1) annual repeat mammogram, (2) interval (6 months) repeat mammogram, (3) stereotactic or ultrasound guided tissue core needle biopsy, or (4) mammographically guided needle localization and open surgical excision biopsy. For women with mammographically dense breasts, particularly young women, ultrasound as a focused examination of the area in question may be a useful adjunct to mammography. Ultrasound is as accurate in differentiating a cyst from a solid mass

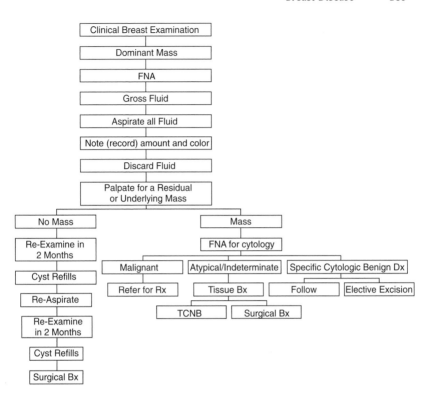

Fig. 9.6. A clinical algorithm for the evaluation of a palpable breast cyst. For abbreviations see legend of Fig. 9.5. *Grossly bloody (atraumatic) aspirated fluid should be smeared, fixed, and sent for cytologic evaluation as a malignancy can yield grossly bloody fluid. (From Hindle W. The diagnostic evaluation. *Obstet Gynecol Clin N Am* 1994;21(3):504–11. WB Saunders, Philadelphia, September 1994. By permission.)

in the breast as it is in the ovary. Breast imaging reports are required to follow the American College of Radiology's Illustrated Breast Imaging Reporting and Data System (BI-RADS^t). This BI-RADS format provides an assessment of breast mammographic density, a succinct diagnosis, and a definite recommendation as well as a precise category "score," which is a reliable clinical guideline.

In spite of the substantial cost of the equipment and installation, many radiology centers are switching from film-screen mammography to digital mammography for both diagnostic and screening breast imaging. Digital mammography offers the advantages of (1) shorter procedure time, (2) computer-aided diagnosis, (3) computer manipulation of the images, (4) telecommunication of the images, and (5) elimination of the problems of film storage and retrieval.

Common Problems
Fear of Breast Cancer

Most women who see a doctor because of a lump, pain, or nipple discharge have a profound underlying fear of breast cancer. Primary care physicians should be sensitive to the emotional aspects associated with breast problems. The patient's family and near relatives are usually personally concerned and have their own related anxieties. It is useful to have the patient's partner be present during breast evaluations, and many physicians request that someone close to the patient be present when the diagnosis and management of a patient's breast cancer are being discussed.

Dominant Breast Mass

A persistent, dominant breast mass must be definitively diagnosed. Optimally, the diagnosis can be established quickly and options of treatment thoroughly discussed. If a menstruating woman is thought to have a "totally benign" or vague breast mass, it is acceptable to reexamine the patient over the course of one or two menstrual cycles. However, if the mass persists, even if it seems the same size or smaller, the diagnostic triad should be applied and a definitive diagnosis obtained.

Screening for Breast Cancer

Mammography is the only proven effective method of screening for nonpalpable breast cancer. CBE is required in addition to mammography for detecting palpable breast cancer. About 10% of palpable breast cancers are not perceived with mammography. Multiple studies have demonstrated reduced breast cancer mortality when population-based screening mammography is performed. Recent data verify a statistically significant reduction in breast cancer mortality for women aged 40–70 years who have routine screening mammography.

Multidisciplinary Treatment Planning Conference

Optimum treatment planning for a woman diagnosed with breast cancer is performed by a multispecialty conference team composed of a surgical oncologist, medical oncologist, radiation oncologist, plastic surgeon, pathologist, mammographers, and other therapeutic and support personnel. Primary care physicians should continue to follow their breast cancer patients, offer compassionate support to the patient and her family, and respond to their requests for information and medical advice.

The technique of axillary sentinel node mapping and biopsy is replacing the traditional axillary lymph node dissection in the treatment of invasive breast cancer. Lumpectomy following the NSABP (National Surgical Adjuvant Breast and Bowel Project) protocol has replaced simple surgical excision of undiagnosed and malignant breast masses. Adjuvant radiation therapy is known to decrease the incidence of local recurrence of breast cancer. Adjuvant polychemotherapy has been demonstrated in clinical trials to prolong the life of women with invasive breast cancer. The therapeutic plan for a woman with diagnosed invasive breast cancer should be individualized to that particular patient and the various therapeutic options explained to the patient by the members of the multidisciplinary treatment planning conference. Primary care providers for women, e.g., ob-gyns, can assist in giving current pertinent information and in responding appropriately to the patient's questions.

Ductal Carcinoma *in Situ*

Ductal carcinoma *in situ* (*DCIS*) is usually nonpalpable and not associated with any specific breast symptoms. Thus, DCIS is most commonly detected by the perception of irregular dense branching microcalcifications on screening mammograms. After a complete breast imaging evaluation, the diagnosis must be histologically confirmed, usually by needle/wire localization excision biopsy. Tissue diagnosis is essential to rule out invasive carcinoma. The traditional treatment of DCIS is mastectomy, which has a near 99% "cure rate." However, recent studies have indicated that breast conserving surgery (lumpectomy) can be effective treatment in selected cases. Adjuvant tamoxifen therapy and/or irradiation appear to significantly reduce recurrences when clear surgical margins are obtained with lumpectomy.

Clinical Intervention and Treatment

Treatment of Fibroadenoma

If the FNA cytology diagnosis is "fibroadenoma," the lesion can be followed or electively excised at a time convenient to the patient. Many women will decide to have the fibroadenoma surgically removed. However, since fibroadenomas are clinically related to estrogen levels, the lesions tend to shrink in the postmenopausal years and can become nonpalpable and/or calcify with a typical mammographic pattern.

Mastalgia

Pain of any etiology in the anterior chest is often thought by the patient to be "breast pain" and can be emotionally linked to the fear of breast cancer. A primary care physician, by careful history and examination, should ascertain that the breast pain is true mastalgia. The patient's description of the pattern (e.g., cyclic, intermittent, or constant) and the distribution (e.g., diffuse or localized) of the pain is particularly important. Cyclic mastalgia is pathophysiologic and not a sign of a clinically significant intrinsic breast lesion. Diffuse breast pain was once a symptom of cancer at a time when breast cancers were often at an advanced stage when first evaluated. Currently, mastalgia alone (i.e., without an associated palpable mass) is rarely a sign of breast cancer. Following a complete breast evaluation, most women with breast pain are satisfied when reassured that there is no evidence of a serious breast condition. While analgesia may be helpful in some cases, specific pharmacologic therapy is seldom necessary. Figure 9.7 is an algorithm for the evaluation of breast pain. Table 9.3 is the stepwise therapy for mastalgia. Multiple double-blind crossover studies have demonstrated that methylxanthines (e.g., caffeine) are not etiologic agents for mastalgia, and the treatment of mastalgia by the elimination of methylxanthines is not based on medical evidence.

Nipple Discharge

Most women can express discharge from the nipple on repeated squeezing. However, pathologic nipple discharge is spontaneous, usually unilateral, and

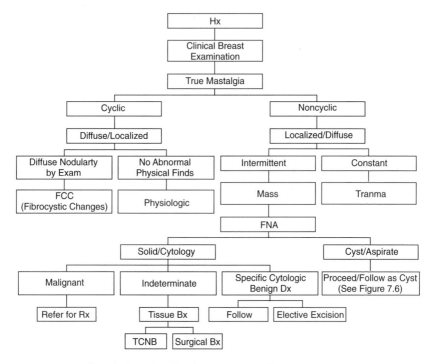

Fig. 9.7. A clinical algorithm for the evaluation of pain within the breast. CBE, clinical breast examination; FCC, fibrocystic changes; FNA, fine-needle aspiration; Hx, patient's medical history; TCNB, tissue core-needle biopsy. (From Hindle W. The diagnostic evaluation. *Obstet Gynecol Clin N Am* 1994;21(3):504–11. WB Saunders, Philadelphia, September 1994. By permission.)

Table 9.3.   Stepwise therapy for mastalgia.[a]

Reassurance that there is no evidence of any serious breast problem (after complete evaluation)

Mechanical measures (e.g., changing an underwire or ill-fitting bra)

Premenstrual salt restriction (avoiding diuretics)

Intermittent nonsteroidal analgesia

A trial of oral contraceptive therapy (low estrogen dose)

Danazol

---

[a] If the patient is not satisfied after the first step or if she requests further therapy, proceed to the next therapeutic step.

usually from a single duct opening on the nipple (except for galactorrhea and periductal mastitis).

Galactography (ductogram) is effective in identifying intraluminal lesions as the cause of pathologic spontaneous nipple discharge from a single duct opening. All intraluminal lesions should be surgically excised in order to diagnose histologically the rare intraductal papillary carcinoma. The most common etiology of pathologic nipple discharge is benign intraductal papilloma. Figure 9.8 is the algorithm for the evaluation of nipple discharge. Ductal lavage and ductoscopy are investigational techniques being evaluated for clinical assessment of nipple discharge.

Galactorrhea is not caused by intrinsic breast pathology. It is an endocrine disturbance that may be related to a pituitary prolactin-secreting adenoma, but more commonly it is related to psychotropic medications or is idiopathic. Periductal mastitis (mammary duct ectasia) occurs in perimenopausal women who typically have dark, greenish discharge from multiple duct openings on the nipple. A Hemostix or similar test tape can differentiate the dark discharge from old blood. Antibiotics are not effective for the treatment of periductal mastitis. When the diagnosis is confirmed, and if the patient insists on eradication of the discharge, the therapy is surgical.

Mastitis

Breast infections should be treated as soon as suspected and then reevaluated every 3 days (see Table 9.4). Those antibiotics that are effective against *Staphylococcus aureus* (e.g., dicloxicillin) are indicated as initial therapy and are usually effective. If the infection does not respond, the antibiotic should be changed. Dermal biopsy (e.g., skin punch biopsy) should be considered if the lack of clinical response persists. The rare inflammatory carcinoma, with extensive invasion of the dermal lymphatics, can mimic diffuse mastitis but does not respond to antibiotic therapy (see Fig. 9.9).

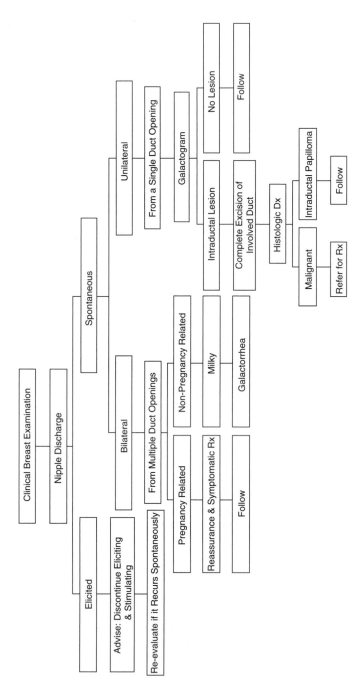

Fig. 9.8. A clinical algorithm for the evaluation of nipple discharge. CBE, clinical breast examination; Dx, diagnosis; Rx, treatment. (From Hindle W. The diagnostic evaluation. *Obstet Gynecol Clin N Am* 1994;21(3):504–11. WB Saunders, Philadelphia, September 1994. By permission.)

Table 9.4. **Appropriate initial antibiotic therapy for mastitis.**

Puerperal mastitis
   Dicloxacillin 500 mg po four times a day for 7 days
   (for patients sensitive to penicillin: vancomycin 125 mg po four times a
      day for 7 days)
Nonpuerperal mastitis
   Acute: amoxicillin/clavulanate 400 mg po four times a day for 7 days
   Chronic: dicloxacillin 500 mg and metronidazole 500 mg both po four
      times a day for 10 days

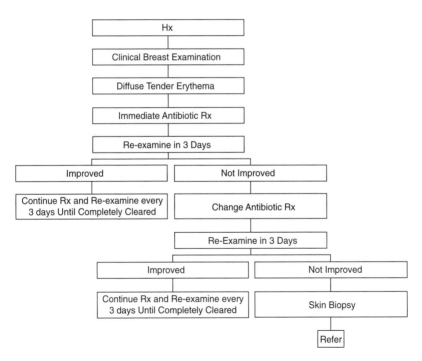

Fig. 9.9. A clinical algorithm for the evaluation of breast infections. Bx, biopsy; Hx, patient's medical history; CBE, clinical breast examination. If there is suspicion of abscess formation, aspiration of the center of the involved area, looking for pus, or focused ultrasound should be performed. (From Hindle W. The diagnostic evaluation. *Obstet Gynecol Clin N Am* 1994;21(3):504–11. WB Saunders, Philadelphia, September 1994. By permission.)

Breast Abscess

If there is clinical evidence or suspicion of abscess formation, needle aspiration (under local anesthesia using an #18-gauge needle) should be performed and all the purulent material aspirated. The patient should be reevaluated every 3 days and the aspiration may have to be repeated several times until all clinical evidence of infection subsides.

Hormone Therapy and Breast Cancer Risk

There are no consistent clinically meaningful data linking oral contraceptive therapy with increased relative risk of breast cancer. Although some epidemiologic studies have shown a "weak association" between estrogen therapy (ET) and hormone therapy (HT) and increased relative risk of breast cancer, clinically meaningful data are lacking. Furthermore, there are no published, prospective, randomized clinical trials proving the relationship of ET, HT and breast cancer. However, some recent studies, e.g., The Women's Health Initiative, have shown a statistical increased relative risk of breast cancer with long-term HT and have questioned the "benefit" of HT. In overview perspective, the published relative risk of breast cancer data should not alter the medical indications for ET. However, a profound fear of breast cancer may inhibit an individual patient's compliance, even after full explanation of ET.

Each estrogen-deficient woman should make her own informed choice about ET.

Summary

All women presenting with a breast problem should undergo a complete breast evaluation, be given appropriate therapy and advice, and be followed until the problem is resolved. Even after apparent clinical resolution, the patient should be instructed to perform monthly breast self-examination (BSE), to continue annual CBE and screening mammography according to current ACOG guidelines (Table 9.5), and to return immediately if symptoms or signs recur. The frequency

Table 9.5.   ACOG guidelines for screening mammography for women with no known increased relative risk factors for breast cancer.

Asymptomatic women aged 40 through 49 years
    Every 1 or 2 years at the physician's discretion
Asymptomatic women aged 50 years and older
    Annually

The following recommendations are based on limited and inconsistent scientific evidence.
Source: Breast cancer screening. ACOG Practice Bulletin No. 42. American College of Obstetricians and Gynecologists. Obstet Gynecol 2003; 101: 821–32.

and the usually indolent progress of breast cancer make it possible for the patient and/or her physician to mistake a malignancy for a benign or even physiologic process. Whenever doubt on the part of the patient or her physician persists, the patient should be referred immediately to a breast specialist for consultation. The primary care physician should confirm that the patient is seen by the breast specialist and that appropriate evaluation and/or therapy is carried out. In all cases, the primary care physician should continue to follow up on the case.

Suggested Reading

ACOG Committee Opinion, Committee on Gynecologic Practice, No. 186, September 1997. *Role of the Obstetrician-Gynecologist in the Diagnosis and Treatment of Breast Disease*. Washington DC: American College of Obstetricians and Gynecologists; 1997.

ACOG Committee Opinion, Committee on Gynecologic Practice, No. 224, October 1999. *Tamoxifen and the Prevention of Breast Cancer in High-Risk Women*. Washington DC: American College of Obstetricians and Gynecologists; 1999.

ACOG Practice Bulletin, No. 42, April 2003. *Breast Cancer Screening*. Washington DC: American College of Obstetricians and Gynecologists; 2003.

American College of Radiology (ACR). *Illustrated Breast Imaging Reporting and Data System (BI-RADS^{TM})*, 3rd ed. Reston, VA: American College of Radiology; 1998.

Bush TL, Whiteman M, Flaws JA. Hormone replacement therapy and breast cancer: a qualitative review. *Obstet Gynecol* 2001;98:498–508.

Fisher B, Jeong J-H, Anderson S, et al. Twenty-five-year follow-up of a randomized trial comparing radical mastectomy, total mastectomy, and total mastectomy followed by irradiation. [NSABP B-04] *N Engl J Med* 2002;347:567–75.

Fisher B, Dignam J, Bryant J, et al. Five versus more than five years of tamoxifen for lymph node-negative breast cancer: updated findings from the National Surgical Adjuvant Breast and Bowel project B-14 randomized trial. *J Natl Cancer Inst* 2001;93:684–90.

Fisher B, Land S, Mamounas E, et al. Prevention of invasive breast cancer in women with ductal carcinoma in situ: an update of the national surgical adjuvant breast and bowel project experience. *Semin Oncol* 2001;28:400–18.

Fisher B, Costantino JP, Wickerham DL, et al. Tamoxifen for prevention of breast cancer: report of the National Surgical Adjuvant Breast and Bowel Project P-1 study. *J Natl Cancer Inst* 1998;90:1371–88.

Giuliano AE, Jones RC, Brennan M, et al. Sentinel lymphadenectomy in breast cancer. *J Clin Oncol* 1997;15:2345–50.

Grimes DA, Lobo RA. Perspectives on the Women's Health Initiative trial of hormone replacement therapy. *Obstet Gynecol* 2002;100:1344–53.

Hindle WH, ed. *Breast Disease for Gynecologists*. Norwalk, CT: Appleton & Lange; 1990.

Hindle WH, ed. *Breast Care*. New York: Springer-Verlag; 1999.

Hindle WH. Breast cancer: introduction. *Clin Obstet Gynecol* 2002;45(3): 738–45.

Hindle WH. Breast cancer: prevention and surveillance. *Clin Obstet Gynecol* 2002;45(3):778–83.

Hindle WH. Breast in situ carcinoma—diagnosis and treatment. *Clin Obstet Gynecol* 2002;45(3):774–77.

Hindle WH. Breast mass evaluation. *Clin Obstet Gynecol* 2002;45(3): 750–57.

Hindle WH. Mammography—screening and diagnosis. *Clin Obstet Gynecol* 2002;45(3):746–49.

Hindle WH. Treatment of invasive carcinoma. *Clin Obstet Gynecol* 2002; 45(3):767–69.

Hindle WH, Arias RD, Florentine B, Whang J. Lack of utility in clinical practice of cytologic examination of nonbloody cyst fluid from palpable breast cysts. *Am J Obstet Gynecol* 2000;182:1300–05.

Hindle WH, Arias RD, Felix J, Sueda A. Adaptation of FNA to office practice. *Clin Obstet Gynecol* 2002;45(3):761–66.

Margolese R, Poisson R, Shibata H, et al. The technique of segmental mastectomy (lumpectomy) and axillary dissection: a syllabus from the National Surgical Adjuvant Breast Project workshops. *Surgery* 1987;102:828–34.

Morrow M, Strom EA, Bassett LW, et al. Standard for the management of ductal carcinoma in situ of the breast (DCIS). *CA Cancer J Clin* 2002;52:256–76.

Morrow M, Strom EA, Bassett LW, et al. Standard for breast conserving therapy in the management of invasive breast carcinoma. *CA Cancer J Clin* 2002;52:277–300.

Nanda K, Bastian LA, Schulz K. Hormone replacement therapy and the risk of death from breast cancer: a systematic review. *Am J Obstet Gynecol* 2002;186:325–34.

Tabar L, Vitak B, Chen HH, et al. The Swedish Two-County Trial twenty years later. Updated mortality results and new insights from long-term follow-up. *Radiol Clin N Am* 2000;38:625–51.

Weiss LK, Burkman RT, Cushing KL, et al. Hormone replacement therapy regimens and breast cancer risk. *Obstet Gynecol* 2002;100:1148–58.

10

Cardiovascular Hypertension

Dayton W. Daberkow II and Thomas E. Nolan

Background Information

The primary role of the obstetrician/gynecologist in the management of hypertension in the past was obstetrical-related hypertension. The role of the gynecologist in overall health care maintenance and disease prevention is expanding and the recognition and treatment of hypertension should be considered in this role. Hypertension is a primary cause of cardiovascular disease, which remains a significant cause of morbidity and mortality in women. More than 60 million persons in the United States have some degree of hypertension, with an incidence of 65% between the ages of 65 and 74 years. The contribution of hypertension to overall cardiovascular morbidity and mortality in women has been considered less important than in men, but this absence of data may be the result of gender bias. Cardiovascular disease is in many cases the manifestation of multiple risk factors including obesity, hyperlipidemia, hypertriglyceridemia, type 2 diabetes, and hyperinsulinemia. Hypertension continues as the most prevalent associated factor in cardiovascular disease and in many cases coexists with other risk factors. Hypertension awareness has resulted in the lowering of average blood pressure in the United States over the past several decades.

    The approach to disease states is changing from primarily recognition and treatment to a focus on wellness and risk assessment. For many years, hypertension was considered a diagnosis alone in treatment paradigms. Current recommendations, workup, and therapy consider other disease variables in the aggressiveness used to lower blood pressure. Hypertension significantly contributes to other causes of morbidity in women, primarily cerebrovascular and renal. Women have a higher incidence of hypertension than men after age 50 years. This interesting statistic is thought to reflect the impact of earlier cardiovascular disease in men that results in premature death. Gender and race are important variables in the effect of hypertension on longevity. Male sex and black race are poor prognosticators for many of the common complications of hypertension (e.g., congestive heart failure, coronary artery disease, and renal failure) in the United States.

The impact of culture on the incidence of hypertension is interesting. There is a relative lack of hypertensive diseases found among native Africans, which is in direct contradistinction to African-Americans. Operative factors may be multifactorial. In rural native African populations, physical labor (hence, "exercise") is important in daily existence. The diet is high in complex carbohydrates, vegetable protein, and potassium. In Western populations, however, caloric intake is high with increased simple carbohydrates, animal protein, fats (both saturated and unsaturated), sodium, phosphorus, dairy, and processed food.

Treatment of hypertension should be evaluated in an overall management scheme of wellness, which includes modification of diet, aerobic exercise, identification and control of hyperlipidemias, and elimination of cigarette smoking.

Epidemiology

The incidence of hypertension increases with age. More than 95% of cases of hypertension have an unknown etiology and are classified as "essential." Certain factors are important in the overall incidence and long-term sequelae. African-American patients, regardless of sex, have approximately twice the incidence of hypertension as whites. Genetic factors are described in the animal model, but data are lacking in human beings. Family history has been found in many studies as a risk factor. In addition, the role of body mass index and obesity in families may contribute to the finding of hypertension, as it does in type 2 diabetes. Most evidence suggests that hypertension is a polygenic disease, but no specific gene(s) has been localized.

The Joint National Committee on prevention, detection, evaluation and treatment of high blood pressure (JNC 7) released their seventh report in 2003. The purpose was to provide an evidence-based approach to the prevention and management of hypertension. The key points of this report are:

- Systolic blood pressure (BP) in those older than 50 years of age is a more important cardiovascular risk factor than diastolic BP.
- Beginning at 115/75 mm Hg, CVD risk doubles for each increment of 20/10 mm Hg.
- Those who are normotensive at 55 years of age will have a 90% lifetime risk of developing hypertension.

- Patients with prehypertension (systolic blood pressure 120–139 mm Hg or diastolic blood pressures 80–89 mm Hg) require health-promoting lifestyle modifications to prevent the progressive rise in blood pressure and CVD.
- For uncomplicated hypertension, a thiazide diuretic should be used in drug treatment for most, either alone or combined with drugs from other classes for hypertensive patients unresponsive to lifestyle changes as shown in Figure 10.1.
- This report delineates specific high-risk conditions that are compelling indications for the use of other antihypertensive drug classes (angiotensin-converting enzyme inhibitors, angiotensin-receptor blockers, beta-blockers, calcium channel blockers). These conditions are heart failure, post-myocardial infarction, high coronary disease risk, diabetes, chronic kidney disease, or stroke.
- Two or more antihypertensive medications will be required to achieve goal BP (<140/90 mm Hg, or <130/80 mm Hg) for patients with diabetes or chronic kidney disease.
- For patients whose BP is more than 20 mm Hg above systolic BP goal or more than 10 mm Hg above the diastolic BP goal, initiation of therapy using two agents, one of which will be a thiazide diuretic, should be considered.
- Regardless of therapy or care, hypertension will be controlled only if patients are motivated to stay on their treatment plan.

Pathogenesis of Hypertension

Several important theories on pathophysiology have been proposed for the etiology of hypertension and a basic understanding of these proposed mechanisms will help determine which therapies may have the greatest benefits in certain individuals. Sodium in the diet is thought to have an effect on pressure volume receptors involved in renal sympathetic nerve activity and has been suggested as a possible mechanism for hypertension, especially in immigrants. The effect of sodium on hypertension in many studies is directly related to the individual response. Factors that may influence sodium response are genetic background, age, gender, race, weight, the renin–angiotensin–aldosterone system, baroreflex sensitivity, and other electrolyte concentrations, specifically related to dietary intake of calcium, potassium, chloride, and magnesium. This partial list of variables emphasizes the difficulty in establishing the effect of a single agent as the etiology of essential hypertension. Studies on the role of minerals are limited and at times conflicting. Interestingly, levels of potassium in the diet may have an effect on hypertension. Individuals who consume high-potassium diets were noted to have a decrease in blood pressure, while individuals who consume low potassium diets had a slow but progressive increase in blood pressure.

Other dietary issues have been evaluated and the most extensively studied is alcohol use. Most studies have found that heavy use of alcohol

Measure Blood Pressure

Patient should:

- Rest for 5 minutes prior to performing
- No smoking or caffeine for 30 minutes prior to measurement
- Sitting in chair, feet flat on floor, back and arm supported, arm at level of heart

Clinician should:

- Make sure cuff size appropriate for patient's arm size
- Periodically assure that office cuffs are calibrated
- Average 2 or more readings with at least 2 minutes between measurements

Primary Prevention (Healthy Lifestyle Choices)

- Quit Smoking
- Lose weight if appropriate
- Restrict sodium to 2 grams per day
- Limit alcohol to 1-2 drinks per day
- 30-45 minutes of aerobic activity on most days
- Maintain adequate potassium, calcium and magnesium intake

Set Patient Goal (Remember to look at risk factors, TOD/CCD)

- Blood pressure decrease to 140/90 mm Hg if uncomplicated hypertension
- With Diabetes, set goal of < 130/85 mm Hg
- With renal insufficiency and proteinuria > 1 gram per 24 hours, set goal of 125/75 mm Hg

Treatment

- Begin with lifestyle modifications (should be implemented regardless of final therapy!)
- Start with diuretic or beta-blocker unless compelling reason to use other agent. Start low and titrate upward.
- If no response, try different class or add second agent (usually a diuretic)
- If still no response, refer to an internist

Adherence

- Continue lifestyle modifications
- Involve patient and family in therapy, continue communications
- Integrate lifestyle with daily activities
- Use once a day formulations, combinations if necessary
- Use generics and scored formulations to decrease expense
- Modify as needed and use nurse case management if possible

Fig. 10.1. Algorithm for the Drug Choices for Hypertensive Patients Unresponsive to Lifestyle Changes. Goal BP is <140/90 mm Hg, or <130/80 mm Hg for those with diabetes or chronic kidney disease. (Modified from *The Seventh Report of the Joint National Committee on Prevention, Detection, Evaluation, and Treatment of High Blood Pressure (JNC VII)*. JAMA. 2003;289:2560–2572.)

◄───────────────────────────────────────

(defined as more than five drinks daily) is associated with elevated blood pressure in most patients. One large prospective study showed a "U"-shaped distribution of hemorrhagic stroke in women. That is, women who were moderate drinkers (5–14 g daily) had fewer strokes than women in the other extremes, that is, nondrinkers and heavy drinkers. Obesity and increased body weight remain the most important predictors of hypertension. Currently, weight reduction (via exercise) and alcohol reduction to two drinks daily are mainstays in the initial treatment of hypertension. Despite the widespread perception of the role of fats and fish oil in the diet, they have not been associated with any beneficial or harmful changes in blood pressure.

Establishing the Diagnosis of Hypertension

Obstetricians and gynecologists should not interpret blood pressure with the same criteria they have learned for preeclampsia and eclampsia. Blood pressure levels of less than 220/120 mm Hg *are not* a medical emergency that requires hospitalization and immediate therapy! Essential facts and documentation that should be determined in the history and physical examinations are found in Table 10.2. Patient age is important in the initial evaluation: the young patient who has a diastolic blood pressure of greater than 105 mm Hg should be closely

Table 10.1. Blood Pressure Classification. (Adults 18 years and older)

Category	Systolic BP (mm Hg)		Diastolic BP (mm Hg)
Normal	<120	and	<80
Prehypertension	120–139	or	80–89
Stage 1 Hypertension	140–159	or	90–99
Stage 2 Hypertension	≥160	or	≥100

Modified from the *The Seventh Report of the Joint National Committee on Prevention, Detection, Evaluation, and Treatment of High Blood Pressure (JNC VII)*. JAMA. 2003;289:2560–2572.

Table 10.2. Important historical points in the evaluation of hypertension.

History of prior elevated blood pressure readings, evaluation, and treatment (lifestyle changes, medication, doses, and side effects)
- Other medical conditions or evidence of end organ damage, including visual changes, chest pain syndromes, myocardial infarction, prior stroke, and renal disease
- Assessment of other known cardiovascular risk factors, including smoking history in pack-years (packs per day multiplied by number of years), cholesterol measurements, obesity, and diabetes mellitus
- Family history of cardiovascular disease (primarily myocardial infarction or coronary ischemia) before age 55 years in parents or siblings; if first degree relative died, age and cause of death
- Dietary history to evaluate fad diets or excessive use of sodium
- The four Ps of pheochromocytoma (Pain, Palpitations, Pallor, and Perspiration)
- Analgesic abuse, including nonsteroidal antiinflammatory drugs
- Alcohol use, specifically more than two drinks daily
- Medication use (and primarily overuse) of adrenocorticosteroids and sympatho-mimetic amines found in "cold preparations" and nasal decongestants

Source: Adapted from The Seventh Report of the Joint National Committee on Prevention, Detection, Evaluation, and Treatment of High Blood Pressure (JNC VII). JAMA. 2003; 289: 2560–2572.

evaluated for secondary (correctable) causes of hypertension. Blood pressure readings determine the frequency of follow-up and whether dietary or medical interventions are necessary. For instance, a single elevated diastolic blood pressure reading of less than 90 mm Hg does not require therapy and should be rechecked within 2 months. When the diastolic pressure is greater than 110 mm Hg, consider follow-up in 2–4 weeks or consult with an internist. Other reasons for early referral include the following:

- Poor control of hypertension with two drugs; an initial diastolic pressure of greater than 100 mm Hg.
- A diastolic blood pressure greater than 140 mm Hg with papilledema (malignant hypertension). This is a medical emergency that requires hospital admission.
- Evidence of end organ damage (renal insufficiency or congestive heart failure).

Among women who initially have elevated blood pressure, 20–33% will have a reduction into the normal range during an observation period after examination. A gynecologic office visit, especially with the expectation of a pelvic examination, is one of the most stressful encounters in medicine. The elevation induced by the stress of seeing a health care provider is labeled "white coat" hypertension, which is a well-characterized clinical syndrome. The issue of treating systolic hypertension was controversial for years. Recent evidence and guidelines recommend that patients with systolic hypertension be treated. Patients treated for systolic hypertension experience significantly fewer cerebral vascular accidents, including stroke.

Baseline laboratory evaluations are recommended in the initial evaluation of patients who have hypertension to rule out secondary or reversible causes. The initial battery of tests is presented in Table 10.3. Abnormal results require additional workup or possible referral to an internist. Urinalysis findings of red cell casts or albuminuria may indicate an underlying renal disease, such as nephrotic syndrome or collagen vascular disease manifesting as a hypertension disorder. Patients with elevated blood urea nitrogen or creatinine may have long-standing renal disease with some degree of renal insufficiency. Anemia may be a clue to an underlying chronic disease, such as a carcinoma or connective tissue disease. Hypokalemia may be indicative of congenital adrenal syndromes or altered aldosterone states from tumors or renal vascular hypertension. Another important cause of hypokalemia is secondary to hypomagnesium from alcohol abuse.

Overall assessment of patients who have hypertension and the approach to therapy require the role of covariables that contribute to significant morbidity and mortality. Measurement of lipids and cholesterol is important in assessing additional risks for cardiovascular disease. Important variables in the overall risk assessment for cardiovascular morbidity include the cofactors of tobacco abuse, lipid disorders, and glucose intolerance. When all three are present, morbidity is especially high. Hypercholesterolemia with a strong family history of cardiovascular events at an early age requires at a minimum dietary intervention and usually medical therapy. Because diuretics and

Table 10.3.   Minimal laboratory workup for hypertension.

Dipstick urinalysis for protein and glucose (microscopic is indicated if any abnormalities)

- Hemoglobin or hematocrit
- Levels of creatinine or blood urea nitrogen, potassium, and fasting glucose
- Levels of total cholesterol, high-density lipoprotein cholesterol, and fasting triglycerides
- Electrocardiogram to evaluate hypertensive changes, such as left ventricular hypertrophy or previous evidence of myocardial infarction
- Chest radiographs (optional)

Source: Adapted from The Seventh Report of the Joint National Committee on Prevention Detection, Evaluation, and Treatment of High Blood Pressure (JNC VII). JAMA. 2003; 289: 2560–2572.

β-blockers have a negative impact on serum cholesterol level, many experts have recommended other agents for blood pressure control.

A low level of high-density lipoprotein (HDL) cholesterol is *associated* with atherosclerotic disease but by itself is not indicative of atherosclerosis. Many patients and physicians assume that a low level of HDL cholesterol is causative for myocardial or cardiovascular disease. A low HDL cholesterol in isolation is not causative of atherosclerotic cardiovascular disease (ASCVD). However, if other risk factors are present, the overall likelihood of atherosclerosis is increased. The electrocardiogram (ECG) is probably the least sensitive test in the initial evaluation but when suggestive of left ventricular hypertrophy, prior silent infarctions or conduction disturbances may change the approach to therapy.

The major causes of secondary hypertension are listed in Table 10.4. Patients who have secondary hypertension are usually younger than 35 or older than 55 years of age. In younger patients, consideration should be given

Table 10.4.   Secondary causes of hypertension.

Renal
  Renal vascular disease (including fibromuscular dysplasia in the young woman),
    congenital vascular abnormalities, atherosclerotic disease
  Polycystic kidney disease (family history important)
  Collagen vascular disease
  Renin secreting tumors
Endocrine
  Adrenal (primary aldosteronism, congenital adrenal hyperplasia, Cushing's
    syndrome, pheochromocytoma)
  Hyperparathyroidism
  Acromegaly
Cardiac
  Coarctation of the aorta (found in association with aortic stenosis, primarily a
    disease of men)
Medications
  Glucocorticoids and mineralocorticoids
  Sympathomimetics, such as phenylpropanolamine commonly found in over-the-
    counter preparations such as nasal sprays, combination "cold" remedies; other
    common preparations include phenylephrine, pseudoephedrin, and ephedrine
Caffeine
Nicotine

Source: Adapted from the Seventh Report of the Joint National Committee on Prevention, Detection, Evaluation, and Treatment of High Blood Pressure (JNC VII). JAMA. 2003; 289: 2560–2572.

to metabolic etiologies and congenital anomalies, whereas atherosclerosis or carcinoma is more common in elderly patients. If the initial blood pressure measurements are (>180 systolic and >110 diastolic), then secondary causes should be aggressively sought.

Measurement of Blood Pressure

The most important variable in the evaluation and management of hypertension is the performance of blood pressure measurement. Unfortunately, most health care providers are unaware of the variables involved or perform with a lack of precision. Multiple studies have reinforced the need to standardize measurements. There are two major ways to measure blood pressure: the traditional sphygmomanometer with stethoscope and, recently, ambulatory blood pressure devices. Regardless of the method used, office measurements of blood pressure should be standardized. With the advent of ambulatory monitoring techniques, home monitoring by the patient may be worthwhile in many cases. Problems of reliability with commercial devices and patient interpretation skills remain variables to be considered with home measurements.

Blood pressure measurements in the office should be standardized and all personnel taking measurements need to be educated and periodically reevaluated. Several important variables must be considered: the woman should be relaxed; the cuff should be applied properly, deflated slowly, and placed at the level of the heart; and an adequate time interval should be allowed between measurements.

For reproducible measurements, the following guidelines should be instituted in the office. The patient should be allowed to rest for 5 minutes in a seated position, and, if possible, the right arm should be used. The right arm, for unknown reasons, has higher readings than the left arm and therefore is preferred for determinations. Cuff placement on the arm and the cuff size are important variables, and lack of attention to detail may result in false readings, both high and low. Most commercially available cuffs are marked with "normal limits" for the size arm they can accurately accommodate. The most common clinical problem is to use too small a cuff on an obese patient, which results in "cuff hypertension." The cuff should be applied 20 mm above the bend of the elbow, with the arm parallel to the floor. The cuff should then be inflated to 30 mm Hg above the disappearance of the brachial pulse, or to 220 mm Hg. The cuff should be deflated slowly at a rate of no more than 2 mm Hg/second. The following common problems affect blood pressure measurement:

- Falsely high readings: the cuff is too narrow or short, wrapped too loosely, deflated too slowly, or the arm is too high in relationship to the heart
- Falsely low readings: the cuff is too wide or long, or the arm is too low in relationship to the heart
- Korotkoff's sounds are difficult to hear: falsely high diastolic or a falsely low systolic reading

- Cuff is released too rapidly: falsely high diastolic or a falsely low systolic reading

The most accurate, device for measurement is the stethoscope with a mercury sphygmomanometer. Mercury devices are bulky and relatively immobile and environmental concerns of spills from these devices have limited their popularity. Other commonly used devices are aneroid manometers (bellows and lever systems) and automated devices. All have problems with long-term accuracy and should be calibrated every 6 months. The automated devices are currently becoming more popular and may prove to be the most accurate. Cost is a major concern in implementing these devices.

At the turn of the twentieth century, Korotkoff characterized sphygmomanometer sounds by using a stethoscope and occluding cuff and hence these sounds were named after him. Most problems with reporting of measurements are in the interpretation of phase IV (muffled sounds) and V sounds (all sounds disappear). Most experts in the study of hypertensive diseases advocate the use of phase V Korotkoff sounds.

Blood pressure is dynamic and responds to exercise, sleep, and diurnal and daily activity. In the 1960s, devices that allowed for ambulatory blood pressure measurement over 24 hours were invented. During the past 3 decades, these machines have become lighter, more compact, and more accurate. They are beginning to move from the research to the clinical environment. The accuracy of these devices depends on the range of blood pressure measured, with discrepancies at the higher and lower ranges. Finally, the end points of target organ damage, strokes, and myocardial infarctions have not been assessed with these devices. The use of automated devices eliminates human discrepancies in measurements. At least two observations should be obtained with less than a 10 mm Hg disparity to be regarded as adequate measures. Repeated assessments should be performed with at least 2 minutes of rest between measurements. Because blood pressure has a diurnal pattern (highest at midday and lowest between 12 and 4 AM), determinations should be performed at the same time of day. If the patient is receiving medication, then the time of the last dose should also be recorded.

Automated sphygmomanometers are readily available. Unfortunately, there are no national standards that control the manufacture or standards of these devices. Physicians may consider recommending one particular model in their practices in an attempt to standardize. Patients who use these devices should be required to demonstrate their use in the office to a health care provider. Office readings should be correlated with the home device to assess the accuracy of the devices. Once the bias of the machine is known, its use may facilitate trends in the patient's blood pressure and allow for more accurate interventions, if necessary. Anxious and less sophisticated patients may be poorly suited for home monitoring because of device misuse or their own anxiety.

Therapy

Nonpharmacologic Interventions

A trend in the treatment of hypertension that evolved over the past decade assesses overall risk factors (such as diet, weight, and alcohol use) and then attempts to modify lifestyle rather than initiate early pharmacologic therapy. These broad lifestyle changes have effects not only on hypertension, but other disease entities, including diabetes and obesity. Much of the morbidity from side effects of antihypertension therapy may be avoided. In evaluating the patient, multiple aspects of lifestyle should be assessed to better approach changes. Nonpharmacologic interventions should be used for initial therapy, unless diastolic blood pressure is persistently greater than 100 mm Hg.

Cigarette smoking, unfortunately, has increased in women and is probably the single most important variable for an increase in prevalence of cardiac disease. Paradoxically, cigarette smokers have less hypertension because they tend to weigh less. An isolated report using ambulatory monitoring showed that blood pressure levels may be normal in the office environment but elevate when the patient was smoking. The effect of caffeine with smoking may be additive in blood pressure elevation. When counseling patients in cigarette cessation, implementation of exercise is important to mediate weight gain.

Obesity is an epidemic in the United States and is the most common independent variable in the prevalence of hypertension. Blood pressure elevations are not just limited to the morbidly obese but are quantitatively increased in direct relationship to body fat. When evaluating data on obesity, cofactors of left ventricular hypertrophy, dyslipidemia, and glucose with insulin intolerance are important in assessing overall cardiovascular risk. The role of moderate exercise in overall well-being (preventive in cardiovascular disease and diabetes) is currently receiving attention and has an important effect on obese patients. Studies in men have shown that by limiting caloric intake and beginning an exercise program, hypertension can be controlled without medication. The effect of weight reduction in obese patients with reduction of salt intake may be synergistic in reducing blood pressure. Alcohol use has a paradoxical effect, especially in women. At low usage, there is evidence it is protective against coronary artery disease and stroke. At lower (less than two drinks per day) or higher usage (greater than five drinks per day), these effects are ameliorated (the so-called U effect). In addition, alcohol use may increase weight, thereby leading to obesity. The role of sodium with heavy alcohol use (defined as more than six drinks daily) is controversial. Current recommendations are to limit alcohol intake to moderate levels (approximately two drinks daily) and to encourage heavier users to decrease consumption.

The role of dietary salt as an independent variable in the control of hypertension is extremely controversial, with multiple contradictory studies. The largest available study reveals a weak association between hypertension and salt intake; however, this association is eliminated when such variables as basal metabolic index, alcohol intake, and potassium excretion are considered. In general, in populations that culturally have heavy use of salt, such as users of soy sauce, a trial of decreased intake of salt may be useful.

After 3–6 months of nonpharmacologic intervention, medical therapy should be initiated if repeat blood pressure levels remain above 140 mm Hg systolic and 90 mm Hg diastolic. Therapeutic schemes that relied on two or three medications have changed during the past 20 years because of the explosion of new medications. The so-called step therapies (start with diuretics; if they didn't work, add second-step drugs and then third-step drugs) are no longer recommended. The therapeutic goal is to lower blood pressure into the "normal range" or a systolic pressure of less than 140 mm Hg and a diastolic pressure of less than 85 mm Hg.

Pharmacologic Interventions

Diuretics

Diuretics have been commonly used for years to control essential hypertension. The scope of this review is limited to thiazide diuretics; loop diuretics are reserved for complicated cases with advanced disease, such as individuals with renal insufficiency. Thiazide-like drugs are mostly sulfonamide derivatives that are transported to the proximal tubule. Primarily these drugs interfere with sodium chloride reabsorption in the distal tubule, which results in the excretion of potassium and water. A cascade of physiologic changes takes place, including decreased plasma volume, which in turn causes decreased venous return, cardiac output, blood pressure, and, finally, peripheral resistance. The loss of extracellular fluid, magnesium, and potassium results in a "contraction" alkalosis and electrolyte imbalance, primarily hypokalemia. The addition of potassium-sparing agents, such as amiloride, triamterene, and spirolactone, reverses the loss of potassium. These drugs may also contribute to glucose intolerance and hyperlipidemias. Because of the metabolic side effects, the popularity of these drugs has decreased. The initial dose of thiazides should be 12.5 mg and should rarely exceed 50 mg. The greatest response to diuretics has been observed in elderly patients and in combination with angiotensin-converting enzyme inhibitors, β-blockers, and calcium channel blockers. In addition, women tolerate these drugs better than men.

Angiotensin-Converting Enzyme Inhibitors (ACE Inhibitors)

ACE inhibitors have rapidly become the first-line class of drugs for hypertensive therapy. The mechanism of action is complex and not fully understood, but several theories have been offered. These agents interfere with sympathetic transmission of ACE at the presynaptic level, which has an effect on sodium transport at the vascular wall level, resulting in a direct effect on various tissues with cardiovascular regulation. A unique characteristic of this class of medications is their ability to affect peripheral vasodilatation without reflex sympathetic activation. These drugs are classified by the zinc ligand associated with the parent compound. There is an association between the specific ligand and the relative strength and half-life of these drugs. Metabolism differs between compounds and is primarily hepatic or renal, which may influence medication choice in certain patients.

ACE inhibitors are relatively safe and have few side effects such as occasional hypotension with the first dose (especially if the patient has relative hypovolemia), blood dyscrasias, and a chronic cough. An important attribute of these medications is that they rarely interfere with a patient's quality of life. Other relatively rare side effects include rashes, loss of taste, fatigue, and headaches. With the newer formulations, the incidence of cough is decreased. ACE inhibitors should not be considered for younger patients who could become pregnant because they are contraindicated in pregnancy. An additional benefit of this class of medications is that they can be used with other antihypertensive agents, such as diuretics, β-blockers, and calcium channel antagonists. Unlike β-blockers, ACE inhibitors are not contraindicated with common medical conditions, including asthma, chronic obstructive airway disease, and depression, They are less effective in African-Americans unless a diuretic is added.

Calcium Channel Blockers

Calcium channel blockers or calcium antagonist drugs were initially used in the treatment of angina in coronary artery disease. The mechanism of action is to block calcium uptake in calcium-sensitive tissues, which results in dilation. This effect is important in peripheral vascular disease and coronary vessels. The original formulations required multiple dosing, which limited compliance. Short-acting preparations in high dosage have been implicated in inducing myocardial ischemia. Longer-acting formulations have helped overcome compliance problems and have decreased some troublesome side effects such as myocardial ischemia and constipation associated with verapamil. These drugs are especially effective in elderly and African-American patients. Patients who suffer with migraines may have a relative amelioration of symptoms with this class of drugs.

β-Blockers

β-Blockers have been extensively used and proven effective for more than 40 years in the treatment of hypertension and coronary artery disease. The mechanism of action is a competitive inhibition of endogenous or exogenous catecholamines at the α-adrenergic site. α-Adrenergic responses are divided into two major types: β_1-receptors, which control heart rate (by blocking these receptors, the heart rate slows down), and β_2-receptors, which primarily work at peripheral sites and the vessel wall. It has recently been shown that tissues have a varying number of both receptors and do not consist purely of one type, but a combination of the two. Early drugs in this class were not β-receptor specific, which resulted in certain disturbing side effects that ultimately affect compliance. For instance, the first popular formulation propranolol is highly lipid soluble, which caused fatigue, cold extremities, and, in some patients, depression, sleep disturbances (nightmares in elderly patients), and constipation.

Angiotensin-Receptor Blockers

The angiotensin-receptor blockers (ARBs) like losartan and valsartan are drugs that interfere with the binding of angiotensin 2 to AT 1 receptors. They are effective like the ACE inhibitors in lowering blood pressure without causing the side effect of coughing. ARBs like ACE inhibitors have demonstrated favorable effects on the progression of kidney disease in diabetics and non-diabetics as well as heart failure.

Newer formulations (e.g., atenolol) were developed that are water soluble and β_1 selective (i.e., the effect of lower heart rate is less pronounced) and hence have fewer side effects. The water-soluble formulations are poorly transported across the brain–blood barrier. Water-soluble drugs have longer half-lives and most only require a single daily dose, an important consideration in compliance. Multiple metabolic changes have been associated with use of β-blockers and include a mild increase in serum levels of potassium, a mild increase in levels of blood sugar, an increase in lipid levels of triglycerides, very low-density lipoprotein (VLDL) cholesterol, neutral effect on levels of total cholesterol and LDL cholesterol, and a decrease in levels of HDL cholesterol. The lipid changes have raised concerns regarding the use of these medications, especially if preexisting coronary artery disease is present.

Contraindications to the use of β-blockers include asthma, chronic obstructive pulmonary diseases, and conduction abnormalities of the heart, such as sick sinus syndrome. Patients who have angina may have a rebound phenomenon of ischemia, which could lead to myocardial infarction if discontinued acutely. Despite these limitations, β-blockers continue to be useful because of their reasonable cost and long history of effectiveness.

Vasodilators

Vasodilators are rarely used with the advent of newer medications; however, two major vasodilators, hydralazine and minoxidil, are occasionally used in specific clinical situations. The mechanism of action is the direct relaxation of arterial wall smooth muscle. The major side effects are related to their sympathetic actions, causing headaches, tachycardia, and fluid retention. Vasodilators are commonly used in combination with β-blockers to minimize the tachycardia and headaches without compromising the blood pressure lowering effects. Hydralazine has been implicated in drug-induced lupus, but this complication is rare when normal therapeutic doses (25–50 mg three times/day) are used. Minoxidil, because of its potency, is rarely used except in specific individuals (renal failure, difficult to control hypertension) and is further limited in women because of beard growth and hypertrichosis. Other drugs in this class are used only in IV formulations and include nitroprusside and diazoxide. These drugs are not used in the ambulatory environment.

α_1-Adrenergic Blockers

α_1-Adrenergic drugs are effective peripheral dilators that have a beneficial effect on serum lipids and insulin sensitivity. When used as a single agent, they decrease levels of total cholesterol and LDL cholesterol, while increasing levels of HDL cholesterol. The mechanism of action for these medications is to decrease peripheral vascular resistance by blocking postganglionic norepinephrine vasoconstriction in vascular smooth muscle beds. Prazosin, terosin, and doxazosin are the most popular preparations available in this group; labetalol has both adrenergic blocker and nonselect β-blocker effects. These formulations may have limited usefulness in women because they alter urethral tone and may induce stress urinary incontinence. Another unique side effect is the "first-dose effect," which may occur in up to 40% of patients. The first dose effect is most commonly seen in elderly patients and consists of severe orthostasis after receiving the initial dose. This effect is more evident in the shorter-acting preparation (prazosin) than the longer-acting formulation (doxazosin). Patients should be started on the lowest possible initial doses, which should be given in bed at bedtime for several days before increasing the dose. Side effects that may limit usage include tachycardia, weakness, dizziness, and mild fluid retention.

Central-Acting Agents

Central acting α_2-agonist medications (methyldopa and clonidine) are well known for their use in obstetrics. The mechanism of action of these medications is thought to be mediated through catecholamine metabolism centrally in the brain. The advantages of this class of medication are primarily cost and their neutral effects on glucose and lipid metabolism, and cardiorespiratory physiology (they have been rarely implemented in coronary ischemia and hypotension). The side effects profile, which includes taste disorders, nasal stuffiness, dry mouth, and frequent dosing (except for the transdermal form of clonidine), limits the popularity of these drugs. Clonidine also causes drowsiness when suddenly withdrawn and may cause severe rebound hypertension. It should therefore be reserved for patients who are reliable and compliant. The introduction of new classes of drugs with better side effect profiles has resulted in less usage of these drugs, however, clonidine still is widely used in difficult to control hypertension.

Combination Therapy

Certain patients will not respond to a single agent and will require combination therapy. Referral to an internist should be considered for patients in whom monotherapy or simple combination therapy (adding a diuretic to an ACE inhibitor) is ineffective. Causes of refractory therapy, such as other underlying diseases (renal insufficiency, systemic lupus erythematosis) or

Table 10.5. Combinations for control of essential hypertension.

Angiotensin-converting enzyme (ACE) inhibitor
    Consider adding a diuretic
Calcium channel blockers
    Consider adding a diuretic or β-blocker
α-Blockers
    Consider adding a diuretic or β-blocker
Diuretic
    Consider adding either a calcium channel blocker or ACE inhibitor

Source: Adapted from The Seventh Report of the Joint National Committee on Prevention, Detection, Evaluation, and Treatment of High Blood Pressure (JNC VII). JAMA. 2003; 289: 2560–2572.

secondary hypertension, should be considered. Common combinations are listed in Table 10.5. Concurrent medical conditions should be considered in the evaluation for therapy because certain medications may be useful in combination with an underlying disorder. For example, patients who have migraine syndromes may do best with either a β-blocker (first choice) or a calcium channel blocker.

Monitoring Therapy

Once the decision is made that antihypertensive therapy is indicated, monitoring should be initiated. Patients who have nonpharmacologically controlled hypertension or mild hypertension should have measurements performed at least monthly until blood pressure either normalizes or therapy is begun. Many companies have an industrial nurse who can perform this task, or it can be performed in the physician's office. Individuals capable of home monitoring should perform their measurements at least twice a week and at the same time of day. Regardless of where the readings are done, results should be charted for review when evaluating therapy.

If pharmacologic therapy is necessary, a return appointment should be scheduled in 2–4 weeks. Before initiating therapy, common side effects of the chosen medication should be discussed so that the patient is alerted and does not discontinue without calling the practitioner. At return visits, blood pressure response and side effects should be noted. Table 10.6 summarizes follow-up intervals during the initial assessment. Once the woman reaches a steady state, then office visits for review of blood pressures may be performed at 3 month intervals. At the annual examination, blood chemistries should be considered to monitor renal function and hyperlipidemias, if present. If side effects are intolerable for the woman, then a different class of medications should be initiated.

Table 10.6.   Recommended follow-up in monitoring of hypertension.

Initial screening blood pressure (mm Hg)		
Systolic	Diastolic	Follow-up recommended
<130	<85	Recheck in 2 years
130–139	85–89	Recheck in 1 year, diet, etc.
140–159	90–99	Confirm in 2 months
160–179	100–109	Evaluate or refer in 1 month
180–209	110–119	Evaluate or refer in 1 week
≥210	≥120	Refer immediately

Source: Adapted from the Joint National Committee: The detection, evaluation, and treatment of high blood pressure. *Arch Intern Med* 1993;153: 154–83.

Case Study

A 41-year-old obese patient (5 feet 4 inches, 290 pounds) presents with blood pressures of 140/100 mm Hg and 146/98 mm Hg in the past 3 months. Her physical examination is unremarkable and she does not smoke or have a family history of coronary artery disease. She also complains of migraine headaches and nasal stuffiness. She periodically takes over-the-counter medications for her sinuses and nonsteroidal antiinflammatory drugs (NSAIDs) for migraines. You order various tests and suggest the following:

- She should lose weight and begin an American Diabetes Diet. Make sure that the laboratory work ordered is done in a fasting state so that (1) you do not have to reorder blood work if her glucose is high and (2) you get an accurate understanding of her lipid status. Even though lipids may not be that important with a normal family history, it may affect the choice of medications.
- Take a further history on her headaches to make sure she has migraines. If she does and fails nonpharmacologic interventions, a good first choice would be β-blockers as long as she does not have asthma and her blood sugar is normal
- Spend time to try and get the patient to start an exercise program and stress the many benefits including cardiovascular, prevention of diabetes, and general wellness.

- This is a good patient for a nurse educator if your office has one. A plan for all hypertensive patients could be started and the nurse would be the individual that is getting the readings and following weight, etc.
- Finally, if the patient is amenable, she should buy a blood pressure (BP) cuff and monitor her own pressure. Nothing helps compliance like patient participation!

The textbook answer to management of this patient would be as follows: The diagnosis and management of hypertension are based on the classification of blood pressure readings and the risk group stratification. Laboratory tests and procedures that are recommended in the initial evaluation of uncomplicated hypertension are found in Table 10.3. For patients with stage 1 hypertension and no compelling indications like heart failure, post-myocardial infarction, high coronary disease risk, diabetes, chronic kidney disease, or stroke a thiazide diuretic should be started in most patients

Summary

The gynecologist is competent to perform an initial evaluation workup and, in many women, institute therapy. The concept of wellness in the primary care model is important in designing therapy, and risk factors should be weighed. For uncomplicated hypertension, a thiazide diuretic should be used in drug treatment for most, either alone or combined with drugs from other classes.

Referral should be considered if concerns of secondary hypertension exist or abnormal laboratory values or other systemic diseases are present. In addition, if the woman does not respond to monotherapy, or a simple combination, then referral to an internist should be considered. Patients who have markedly elevated systolic (e.g., greater than 160 mm Hg) or diastolic (e.g., greater than 110 mm Hg) pressure should be referred early in the evaluation. A summary of these findings is found in the algorithm in Figure 10.1.

Suggested Reading

Anastos K, Charney P, Charon RA, et al. Hypertension in women: what is really known. *Ann Intern Med* 1991;115:287–93.

Cappuccio FP, Siani A, Strazzullo P. Oral calcium supplementation and blood pressure: an overview of randomized controlled trials. *J Hypertens* 1989; 7:941–46.

Cubeddu LX, Aranda I, Singh B, et al. A comparison of verapamil and propranolol for the initial treatment of hypertension: racial differences in response. *JAMA* 1986;256:2214–21.

Dwyer PL, Teele IS. Prazosin: a neglected cause of genuine stress incontinence. *Obstet Gynecol* 1992;79:117–21.

Folsom AR, Luepker RV, Gillum RF, et al. Improvement in hypertension detection and control from 1973–74 to 1980–81: the Minnesota Heart Survey experience. *JAMA* 1983;250:916–21.

Frishman WH. Beta-adrenergic blocker withdrawal. *Am J Cardiol* 1987;59: 26F–32F.

Frost CD, Law MR, Wald NI. By how much does dietary salt reduction lower blood pressure? II. Analysis of observational data within populations. *BMJ* 1991;302:815–18.

Gillum RF, Prineas RI, Ieffery RW, et al. Nonpharmacological therapy of hypertension: the independent effect of weight reduction and sodium restriction in overweight borderline hypertensive patients. *Am Heart J* 1983;105:128–33.

Havlik RI, Hubert HB, Fabsitz RR, et al. Weight and hypertension. *Ann Intern Med* 1983;98:855–59.

Karvonen M, Ormo E, Keys A, et al. Cigarette smoking, serum cholesterol, blood pressure and body fitness: observations in Finland. *Lancet* 1959; i:492–94.

Krishna GC, Miller E, Kapoor S. Increased blood pressure during potassium depletion in normotensive men. *N Engl J Med* 1989;320:1177–82.

Lesniak KT, Dubbert PM. Exercise and hypertension. *Curr Opinion Cardiol* 2001;16:356–9.

Liu K, Ruth K, Flack I, et al. Ethnic difference in 5-year blood pressure change in young adults: the CARDIA study. *Circulation* 1992;85:6A.

Mancia G, Bertinieri G, Grassi G, et al. Effects of blood pressure measurement by the doctor on patient's blood pressure and heart rate. *Lancet* 1983; ii:695–98.

Marmot M, Brunner E. Alcohol and cardiovascular disease: the status of the U shaped curve. *BMJ* 1991;303:565–68.

Marmot MG, Rose G, Shipley MI, et al. Alcohol and mortality: a U-shaped curve. *Lancet* 1981;i:580–83.

McAlister FA, Campbell NRC, Zarnke K, Levine M, Graham ID. The management of hypertension in Canada; a review of current guidelines, their shortcomings and implications for the future. *CMAJ* 2001;164(4): 517–22.

McAlister FA, Straus SE. Evidence based treatment of hypertension. Measurement of blood pressure: an evidence based review. *BMJ* 2001;322:908–11.

McCarron DA, Henry HI, Morris CD. Human nutrition and blood pressure regulation: an integrated approach. *Hypertension* 1992;4:2S–13S.

Medical Research Council Working Party on Mild to Moderate Hypertension. Adverse reactions to bendrofluazide and propranolol in the treatment of mild hypertension. *Lancet* 1981;ii:539–43.

Morris MC, Sacks FM. Dietary fats and blood pressure. In *Textbook of Hypertension*. JD Swales (ed). Oxford, England: Blackwell Scientific; 1994, pp 605–18.

O'Brien E, Atkins N, Mee F, et al. Comparative accuracy of six ambulatory devices according to blood pressure levels. *J Hypertens* 1993;11:673–75.

Pan WH, Nanas S, Dyer A, et al. The role of weight in the positive association between age and blood pressure. *Am J Epidemiol* 1986;124:612–23.

Pool JL, Lenz ML, Taylor AA. Alpha:1-adrenoceptor blockade and the molecular basis of lipid metabolism alterations. *J Hum Hypertens* 1990;4:23–33.

Psaty BM, Heckbert SR, Koepsell TD, et al. The risk of myocardial infarction associated with antihypertensive drug therapies. *JAMA* 1995;274:620–25.

Roberts I, Maurer K. Blood pressure levels of persons 6–74 years, United States, 1971–74. Vital and Health Statistics, Series 11, 203. National Center for Health Statistics. Washington, DC: US Government Printing Office, 1977, DHEW Publication No. (HRA) 78-1648.

Selby IV, Friedman GD, Quesenberry CP Jr. Precursors of essential hypertension: the role of body fat distribution pattern. *Am J Epidemiol* 1989; 129:43–53.

Seventh Report of the Joint National Committee on Prevention, Detection, Evaluation, and Treatment of High Blood Pressure (JNC VII). *JAMA* 2003;289:2560–72.

Sever PS, Poulter NR. A hypothesis for the pathogenesis of essential hypertension: the initiating factors. *J Hypertens* 1989;7:9S–12S.

SHEP Cooperative Research Group. Prevention of stroke by antihypertensive drug treatment in older persons with isolated systolic hypertension. *JAMA* 1991;265:3255–64.

Siani A, Strazullo P, Giogione N, et al. Increasing dietary potassium intake reduces the need for antihypertensive medication. *Am J Hypertens* 1990; 3:110A.

The sixth report of the Joint National Committee on prevention, detection, evaluation, and treatment of high blood pressure. *Ach Intern Med* 1997; 157:2413–46. NIH publication No. 98-4080.

Stampfer MI, Colditz GA, Willard WO, et al. A prospective study of moderate alcohol consumption and the risk of coronary disease and stroke in women. *N Engl J Med* 1988;319:267–73.

Swales JD. Angiotensin-converting enzyme inhibitors. In *Textbook of Hypertension*. JD Swales (ed). Oxford, England: Blackwell Scientific; 1994, pp 1115–27.

Truswell AS, Kennelly BM, Hansen IDL, et al. Blood pressure of Kung bushmen in northern Botswana. *Am Heart J* 1972;84:5–12.

11

Chronic Pelvic Pain

Arnold P. Advincula and Arleen Song

Introduction

The practicing gynecologist sees many patients in the office with complaints of chronic pelvic pain. The evaluation and treatment of these patients can often be daunting and evoke a visceral response of angst in the practicing physician. This can be avoided by approaching patients in a structured framework that addresses issues in a multifactorial fashion. The purpose of this chapter is to present some of the more common causes of chronic pelvic pain. This will begin with a brief overview followed by a discussion of an approach to history and physical examination, laboratory and diagnostic studies, differential diagnosis, and finally treatment options.

Overview

Chronic pelvic pain is a significant problem facing primary care providers. Approximately 14–16% of patients presenting to primary care practices report experiencing significant pelvic pain during the past 6 months. Pelvic pain is the major indication for approximately 12% of the nearly 600,000 hysterectomies performed annually in the United States as well as 15–40% of laparoscopies. Laparoscopy is commonly performed to both diagnose and treat pelvic pain. The majority of these cases occur during the reproductive years.

Despite knowledge that certain disease entities such as endometriosis, uterine fibroids, and adhesions are common causes of pelvic pain, such pathology does not cause pain in all women. Variations in the stimulus provided by the pathology itself as well as the individual woman's response to the painful stimulus require an integrated approach. Use of a biopsychosocial model yields a more effective treatment plan than the classic mind–body split. Psychosocial history with particular attention to past history of sexual and/or physical abuse should be included. Many studies suggest that histories of abuse are more common in women referred to specialty clinics for pelvic pain. Abuse prevalence rates can range from 48% to 56%. Care must be taken to place a history of abuse in the proper context to avoid overemphasizing the relationship between the patient's pain and her past abuse. Working within a biopsychosocial model can help avoid this problem and thereby prevent the possibility that overemphasis of the psychological will postpone timely medical or surgical attention.

History

Chronic pelvic pain is generally defined as pain present in the pelvis for 6 months or longer. Many women who have had pain for this long may begin to experience emotional and behavioral changes consistent with a chronic pain syndrome. The clinical hallmarks listed in Table 11.1 are useful for detecting the development of a chronic pain syndrome. The causes of chronic

Table 11.1. Chronic pain syndrome characteristics.

Duration of 6 months or more
Incomplete relief by previous treatments
Pain out of proportion to tissue damage
Vegetative signs of depression
Loss of physical function
Altered family dynamics

pelvic pain can often be diagnosed on the basis of a careful, detailed clinical history and physical examination with very little need for additional studies. A good rule of thumb is that if substantial uncertainty exists regarding the differential diagnosis after the initial encounter, more historical questions need to be asked.

The history of the present illness should include questions regarding the character, intensity, location, radiation, and duration of the pain. In particular, it is useful to pay attention to the precise chronology of the addition of each component of the pain. Understanding the timing of the onset of each component may help the clinician distinguish between primary causes and superimposed aggravating factors.

Unique to the pelvic pain history is the inclusion of detailed sexual and menstrual histories. The presence or absence of menstrual pain and dyspareunia as well as the method of contraception should be addressed in this history. When dyspareunia is present, distinction should be made between the superficial and deep varieties. Superficial dyspareunia tends to indicate a vulvar inflammatory process or a problem with introital muscle control, whereas deep dyspareunia can suggest endometriosis or pelvic adhesive disease. Previous surgeries, pelvic infections, cervical dysplasia, infertility, and past obstetric experiences may be significant clues to discerning the cause of chronic pelvic pain. Whenever possible old operative reports from previous abdominal and pelvic surgeries should be reviewed.

Also of importance is the effect the pain has had on the patient as an individual, on her relationships, and on her ability to function in day to day activities. This type of information enables the clinician to determine the extent of impact the pain has had on the patient. Such a detailed history, in some instances, will require more than one visit. Psychometric instruments and/or psychological or psychiatric consultation can serve as an aid.

Physical Examination

The differential diagnoses that emerge from history taking will help guide the physical examination. For example, posture, stance, gait, and sitting behavior can all provide clues toward a possible musculoskeletal explanation for chronic abdominal pain. Abdominal examination should begin by first asking the patient to point to the area of pain. Use of a single finger tends to indicate more of a discrete source than a sweeping motion of the whole hand. Simple drawings may be used to aid with site identification.

The actual physical examination of the abdomen should begin with inspection particularly for the presence of any deformities, scars, hernias, or masses. After auscultation, the abdominal wall should be systematically palpated by the examiner's index finger in an effort to identify focal spots of tenderness, or myofascial trigger points. Evaluation of the abdominal wall with the patient's head raised off the table, and the rectus muscles tensed can help distinguish between abdominal and intraabdominal pathology. Pain of visceral origin usually diminishes with this maneuver, while myofascial pain or trigger points will increase.

Similarly, the pelvic examination should be carried out in a systematic fashion. This should begin with inspection and sensory examination of the vulva using a light touch with a cotton swab. The presence of an anal wink and bulbocavernosus reflex documents an intact pudendal nerve. Focal tenderness of the posterior vestibule may indicate the presence of vestibulodynia. The use of vulvoscopy or colposcopy may aide in the diagnosis of vulvar lesions.

A unimanual (single-digit) technique is employed to palpate the introitus and then the pelvic floor, particularly the levator and piriformis muscles. The unimanual technique is used to maximize the clinician's ability to determine the source of discomfort. The single-digit technique will decrease the potential for examination discomfort to be confused with true tenderness. The anterior vaginal wall, urethra, and bladder are examinationined next. Focused digital examination may elicit clues leading toward a presumptive diagnosis of urethral diverticulum, chronic urethritis/trigonitis, or interstitial cystitis. Cystoscopy may aide in confirming the diagnosis.

The unimanual examination is then carried more cephalad to the paravaginal tissues, cervix, uterus, and adnexa. If the uterus and cervix are surgically absent, a detailed examination of the vaginal apex for intrinsic tenderness must be performed. Once systematic palpation of the pelvis with the single-digit technique is complete, the abdominal hand is added to the examination. Within the limitations imposed by the patient's body habitus, this will allow the examiner to pick up pelvic masses and clearly define the uterus and adnexal structures if present.

Rather than following a rigid sequence, speculum examination should be done at a time when it makes the most sense. This will depend on the type of pain under consideration. Lastly, a rectovaginal examination is performed. This allows the posterior cul-de-sac, uterosacral ligaments, and rectum as well as pelvic floor to be evaluated. Abnormalities detected by this examination include endometriosis, rectocele, enterocele, and adnexal abnormalities. Table 11.2 summarizes some of the typical history and physical examination findings for various disease states.

Laboratory and Diagnostic Studies

Following the history and physical examination, the clinician will usually be able to narrow down the list of possible diagnoses. The need for laboratory studies, if any, should be tailored to the individual patient's symptomatology. Pregnancy as a cause for abdominal pain in a reproductive aged woman must always be ruled out with either a urine or serum pregnancy test. If the test is positive, ectopic pregnancy must be definitively ruled out with ultrasound.

Table 11.2. Typical history and physical findings for various disease states.

History	Examination Findings	Disease state
Progressively worsening dysmenorrhea • Deep dyspareunia	• Tenderness in implant areas • Uterosacral ligament nodularity	Endometriosis
• Symptom onset 3–6 months after surgery • Tugging and pulling sensation in abdomen or pelvis	• Diminished mobility of the pelvic viscera	Pelvic adhesive disease
• Abnormal uterine bleeding • Dysmenorrhea	• Enlarged, firm, irregular uterus	Leiomyoma
• Pain on arising, climbing stairs, driving car	• Pain on external rotation of thigh, which is palpated transvaginally or externally	Piriformis muscle spasm
• Frequency and urgency • Urethral or bladder pain	• Bladder tender to palpation	Interstitial cystitis

Additional laboratory studies may include a urinalysis and/or cultures if a pelvic or bladder infection is suspected.

The need for imaging studies should also be determined by the data obtained on history and physical examination. A common reflex response by many practitioners is to order an ultrasound. This imaging study is often useful in evaluating acute pain but it rarely sheds any light on the etiology of chronic pain. It is most useful for confirming anatomy in the setting of an inadequate or inconclusive pelvic examination. X-ray studies such as intravenous pyelograms and barium enemas, although useful when specific signs relating to an organ system are present, serve no purpose in the general evaluation of chronic pelvic pain. Specialized imaging studies such as computed tomography or magnetic resonance imaging may be considered only after a careful review of the individual patient's symptomatology and physical examination. Utilization of these specialized imaging studies in the absence of a clear question is inappropriate.

Another modality available in the clinician's diagnostic armamentarium is the use of trigger-point injections. Trigger-point injections have been well established as a diagnostic and therapeutic technique. Various types of local anesthetics are employed to inject abdominal wall and pelvic trigger points. These injections are especially helpful in distinguishing visceral from musculoskeletal pain. As noted previously, psychometric instruments are often helpful. Questionnaires such as the Symptom Checklist-90-R and the Beck Depression Inventory can provide a baseline evaluation of the patient's functional and emotional status. Psychological evaluation may be useful in determining an appropriate care plan and in establishing a baseline to measure response to treatment.

Endoscopic studies, in selected cases, may be helpful in the evaluation of causes of chronic pelvic pain. Cystoscopy and hydrodistention can aid in making the diagnosis of interstitial cystitis in suspected cases. Similarly, colonoscopy should be reserved for those patients with specific indications warranting evaluation of the gastrointestinal tract.

Although hysteroscopy is of little value in the evaluation of chronic pelvic pain, laparoscopy may be helpful. This is particularly true in the setting of abnormal pelvic findings or failure of initial therapy. Laparoscopy potentially affords the clinician the ability to make a diagnosis and effect therapy at the same time. Recent technological advances characterized by the development of small-caliber fiberoptic endoscopic equipment have spawned the age of microlaparoscopic pelvic pain mapping. Use of conscious sedation with these procedures allows patient and physician to communicate regarding potential cause and effect relationships thereby enhancing the evaluation of chronic pelvic pain.

Gynecologic Causes of Chronic Pelvic Pain
Dysmenorrhea

Dysmenorrhea is defined as painful cramping in the lower abdomen that occurs just prior to or during menses. Cramping may also occur in the lower back and upper thighs. Prevalence has been cited as anywhere from 3% to 90% with the best estimate being 75%. Dysmenorrhea has significant personal and public health implications, and accounts for approximately 600 million work hours of absenteeism per year in the United States.

Dysmenorrhea is classified as primary when there is no pelvic pathology evident as the cause of pain. This is a diagnosis of exclusion that is generally made in women under 20 years of age. Primary dysmenorrhea is thought to be due to the release of the prostaglandins $F_{2\alpha}$ and E_2 from the endometrium during menses. This abnormal increase in prostaglandin levels leads to excessive uterine contractions that contribute to pain. Other factors that are associated with dysmenorrhea are family history, early menarche, increased duration of menses, and smoking.

Primary dysmenorrhea usually begins 6–12 months after menarche at the initiation of ovulatory cycles. Pain symptoms range from cramping to a dull throb that is usually located in the lower abdomen and can radiate to the back and thighs. Patients may also experience nausea, headache, vomiting, diarrhea, and fatigue. These symptoms last from 48 to 72 hours and can start 1–2 days prior to the onset of menses.

Secondary dysmenorrhea presents similarly to primary dysmenorrhea, but tends to start at a later age. Obtaining a history of prior cervical surgery, menorrhagia, or excessive vaginal discharge can help determine secondary causes of dysmenorrhea. Timing of the onset of pain can also help determine the cause of dysmenorrhea. Secondary dysmenorrhea is diagnosed when there is pelvic pathology that is believed to be the etiology of pain with menstruation and is more common in women over 20 years old. Common causes of secondary dysmenorrhea are endometriosis, cervical stenosis, adenomyosis, leiomyomas, congenital malformations (e.g., imperforate hymen), pelvic infections, or intrauterine device (IUD) use.

Physical examination should assess uterine size, presence of masses, and tenderness. Rectovaginal examination is essential to determine if there is nodularity of the uterosacral ligaments or cul-de-sac. Any abnormal findings on examination are more consistent with secondary dysmenorrhea. There are no laboratory tests that are useful for diagnosing either primary or secondary dysmenorrhea with the exception of cervical cultures to rule out cervical infection. Ultrasonography can be used to evaluate the pelvis for leiomyomata or adnexal masses. Laparoscopy is the most useful diagnostic tool to assess pelvic pathology such as endometriosis.

Oral contraceptive pills (OCPs) are first line medical management of primary dysmenorrhea. OCPs suppress ovulation, which decreases prostaglandin release as well as uterine activity. This treatment is ideal, especially in women desiring contraception. Nonsteroidal antiinflammatory drugs (NSAIDs) that inhibit prostaglandin synthetase have also played a significant role in the treatment of dysmenorrhea. In a review of 51 trials it was found that 72% of patients had relief with NSAIDs as compared to 15% of patients using placebo. NSAIDs are started at the onset of pain and continued on a regular schedule until the pain ends. Initially NSAIDs should be taken on an as needed basis, however, in those cases in which pain is inadequately controlled, it may be more useful to proceed with a trial of scheduled dosing. There are several different NSAIDs that have been found to be effective, and if a patient is not responding to one brand, it is worthwhile to consider changing to another (Table 11.3). A trial of 3–6 months is usually necessary to assess for relief of symptoms. Side effects include heartburn, gastrointestinal irritation, nausea, vomiting, headache, and allergic reactions.

The cyclooxygenase (COX) pathway is one of the major routes of conversion of arachidonic acid to prostaglandins. This is mediated by COX-1

Table 11.3. Antiinflammatories: dosing for primary dysmenorrhea.

Nonsteroidal antiinflammatory drugs (NSAIDs)	Cyclooxygenase-2 inhibitors (COX-2 inhibitors)
Ibuprofen 400–800 mg po q 6–8 hours	Celecoxib 400 mg po loading dose first day followed by 200 mg po bid maintenance dose
Naproxen sodium 275–500 mg po q 6–8 hours	Rofecoxib 25–50 mg po q day
Mefenamic acid 250–500 mg po q 6–8 hours	Valdecoxib 20 mg po q day

and COX-2 enzymes. They are similar in structure, but COX-1 is involved in hemostasis while COX-2 is involved in pain pathways and inflammation. Prostaglandins produced by COX-1 play a role in maintaining normal platelet and kidney function, in addition to maintaining the integrity of the gastrointestinal mucosa. NSAIDs inhibit both enzymes, and can have adverse effects on the gastrointestinal (GI) tract. The development of COX-2 specific inhibitors has allowed for effective analgesia with fewer GI side effects (Table 11.3).

There are other nonpharmacologic methods that have been found to be useful in managing primary dysmenorrhea. Transcutaneous electrical nerve stimulation (TENS) relieves pain by blocking pain impulses through the dorsal nerve horns. Acupuncture is another nonpharmacologic method that has been used to treat primary dysmenorrhea, likely through similar methods.

Endometriosis

Endometriosis is one of the most enigmatic gynecologic diagnoses. Prevalence rates in the general population have been estimated to be 7–15% in studies of asymptomatic multiparous women who undergo laparoscopic sterilization. Studies have shown that these prevalence rates increase to 30–40% in women undergoing laparoscopy for pain and infertility. Although extensive research has been done in the area of endometriosis, this disorder continues to present difficulties with diagnosis and management.

Several theories have been proposed in an attempt to explain the pathogenesis of endometriosis. One theory involves coelomic metaplasia in which mesothelial cells undergo metaplastic transformation into endometrial cells as a result of some unspecified stimulus. Another theory relates to lymphatic or vascular transport of endometrial fragments. A third hypothesis suggests that embryonic rests of Müllerian tissue respond to estrogenic stimulation and differentiate into functional glands and stroma.

The most popular and widely accepted theory is that of Sampson, who proposed that during menstruation, viable endometrial cells reflux through the fallopian tubes and implant on the surrounding pelvic viscera. Most normally menstruating women, however, experience some retrograde menstruation with each cycle so the theory requires modification to explain why some women are predisposed and others protected. Some experts have proposed a genetic predisposition to implantation and others a dysfunction of the immune system.

Although it occurs most frequently in the pelvis, endometriosis and its painful sequelae have been found in most areas of the body. These include the GI, urinary, and pulmonary systems as well as deep within the posterior cul-de-sac. Interestingly, a poor correlation exists between extent of disease and pain symptoms. The symptoms of endometriosis may vary with location, stage of disease, and type of lesion.

Patients will typically give a history of progressively worsening dysmenorrhea. Premenstrual pain manifesting in the abdomen and/or pelvis may then appear, ultimately followed by pain present for all of the menstrual month but with continuing premenstrual and menstrual exacerbations. Severe dysmenorrhea during adolescence with worsening in early adult life should also suggest endometriosis. Deep dyspareunia may join the picture at any time along with dysuria or dyschezia.

Physical examination may not detect any abnormalities early in the disease process. As endometriosis gradually progresses to a point where severe dysmenorrhea and deep dyspareunia are present, the pelvic examination may reveal focal tenderness in the posterior cul-de-sac and nodularity of the uterosacral ligaments. Other physical findings may include a fixed retroverted uterus, palpable adnexal mass suggesting an endometrioma, or generalized pelvic tenderness.

Although clinical history and physical examination may lead an individual to the presumptive diagnosis of endometriosis, a definitive diagnosis can be made only by direct visualization of the pelvis. Laparoscopy is therefore the procedure of choice. This modality establishes a diagnosis and permits concurrent surgical treatment in the form of electrocoagulation, laser ablation, or excision of endometriotic implants.

Many clinicians will often initiate medical management for a presumptive diagnosis of endometriosis without performing laparoscopy. See Table 11.4 for a list of various medical treatment options. A reasonable start to medical management is with active OCPs taken continuously to avoid dysmenorrhea. NSAIDs or COX-2 inhibitors are often also used in conjunction with OCPs. Additional medical therapies include danazol, continuous high-dose progestins, and gonadotropin-releasing hormone (GnRH) agonists though these agents incur significantly greater costs, side effects, and disruption of the normal endocrinologic milieu. For these reasons, many clinicians advocate laparoscopic confirmation of the diagnosis before embarking on medical therapies with the potential for adverse effects.

Table 11.4. Hormonal treatments for endometriosis.

Drug	Dose	Side effects
Combination oral contraceptive pill	Taken continuously	• Breakthrough bleeding • Nausea
Danazol	200–800 mg daily for 6 months	• Masculinizing (androgenic effects)
High-dose oral progestins *Medroxyprogesterone acetate*	20–100 mg daily for 3–6 months	• Irregular vaginal bleeding • Nausea • Fluid retention
Gonadotropin-releasing hormone (GnRH) agonists *Luprolide*	3.75 mg IM monthly for 3–6 months	• Menopausal symptoms • Loss of bone density if >6 months use

Adenomyosis

Adenomyosis is a benign condition in which endometrial glands and stroma grow within the myometrium, usually without direct connection to the endometrium. The reported incidence of adenomyosis has ranged over the years from 6% to 70%. It is more common in parous women but does not appear to correlate with increasing parity. Most of the variation is likely due to the degree to which pathologists pursue the diagnosis. The pathogenesis of adenomyosis remains unknown but the current theory is that it develops as a result of the invagination of the basalis endometrium into the myometrium.

Approximately 35% of adenomyotic cases are asymptomatic. Symptomatic patients may present with menorrhagia and abdominal/pelvic pain that occurs before, during, and after menses. On physical examination, the uterus is enlarged in a globular configuration. Marked tenderness can often be elicited on bimanual palpation of the uterine contour. Cyclic changes in the size, consistency, and tenderness of the uterus can be demonstrated if a substantial amount of adenomyosis is present. These changes are most pronounced premenstrually. During this time the uterus can be enlarged as much as 1.5 times its baseline; examination shows the uterus to be extremely tender and much softer in consistency than normal.

In the past, the diagnosis was made only at hysterectomy. Advances in magnetic resonance imaging have increased the sensitivity enough to distinguish adenomyosis without requiring hysterectomy or myometrial biopsy.

Although hysterectomy remains the only definitive treatment for adenomyosis, medical management can be attempted with ovarian suppression. This can be accomplished with the use of continuous oral contraceptives, progestins, danazol, or GnRH agonists. Failure of medical management should prompt a search for other diagnoses (e.g., endometrial biopsy to exclude malignancy) before proceeding with surgery.

Leiomyomas

Leiomyomas ("fibroids") are the most common tumors found in the female genital tract. They are discovered in 25% of white women and 50% of black women. These tumors are benign and are made up predominantly of smooth muscle fibers as well as some fibrous connective tissue. Leiomyomas grow under the influence of cyclic estrogen and progesterone. They can vary in size from microscopic to large, multinodular uterine tumors that literally fill the patient's abdomen.

The majority of women with fibroids are asymptomatic. When present, the most common symptoms are pressure from an enlarging pelvic mass, abdominal/pelvic pain including dysmenorrhea, and abnormal uterine bleeding. Pain can occur secondary to degeneration of a fibroid, which results from alteration in the blood supply to the tumor. This may occur with rapid growth, torsion, or atrophy due to menopause or the use of GnRH agonists. Abnormal uterine bleeding is experienced by 30% of women with leiomyomas. These tumors may also produce urinary frequency and urgency by pressing on the bladder.

The diagnosis of leiomyomas is usually confirmed by palpating an enlarged, firm, irregular uterus during pelvic examination. Although laparoscopy may offer little additional diagnostic information, submucous myomas may be detected by ultrasound, particularly when combined with saline infusion sonography (SIS). This technique involves the instillation of several milliliters of normal saline into the uterus during pelvic ultrasound to better delineate the endometrial cavity.

Expectant management in the asymptomatic patient is recommended because the majority of women will not need any therapy. Symptomatic women on the other hand may be medically managed by suppressing ovarian function. GnRH agonists, sometimes with add-back hormonal therapy, have been used to shrink fibroids and induce amenorrhea. This treatment is short-lived; after cessation of therapy, myomas gradually resume their pretreatment size. Cost and hypoestrogenic side effects become significant factors if administration of GnRH agonists is continued.

Surgical management involves either myomectomy or hysterectomy. The choice between the two is usually determined by the patient's age and future reproductive plans. Advances in laparoscopy and hysteroscopy have allowed clinicians to resect some myomas in a minimally invasive fashion. Interventional radiologists have introduced uterine artery embolization for the treatment of fibroids. Long-term follow-up of this technique is awaited. The technique may not represent cost savings in view of high rates of recurrence. In addition, several deaths have been reported following the technique. Magnetic resonance imaging (MRI) cryoablation is a newer technique currently being evaluated.

Pelvic Adhesive Disease

The role of adhesions in chronic pelvic pain is controversial. Pelvic adhesive disease is commonly detected at the time of surgical exploration of patients with chronic pelvic or abdominal pain. The prevalence rate of adhesions in asymptomatic women undergoing laparoscopic tubal sterilization is approximately 12%. This figure is estimated to be between 6% and 51% in women undergoing laparoscopy for chronic pelvic pain.

Though adhesions may play an etiologic role in chronic pelvic and/or abdominal pain, they do not always produce pain. Adhesions may be more likely to play an etiologic role when they limit the mobility of intraperitoneal organs or when their location correlates with the location of the pain.

Unfortunately, the clinical diagnosis of adhesions is quite difficult. Nonsurgical methods of diagnosing adhesions have been largely unsuccessful. Although physical examination may suggest the presence of adhesions based on diminished mobility of the pelvic viscera, studies have found it to be a poor predictor of the presence and location of adhesions visualized during subsequent laparoscopy. Imaging studies have also proven unreliable. Diagnostic laparoscopy remains the gold standard for diagnosing pelvic adhesive disease. Laparoscopy also allows for initiation of surgical treatment of any adhesions that are believed to be clinically significant. The advent of microlaparoscopy under conscious sedation (pain mapping) has enhanced this diagnostic modality.

Studies to date of the effect of adhesiolysis on chronic pelvic pain leave many questions unanswered. Although studies have clearly demonstrated in an animal model that laparoscopy is more successful than laparotomy in treating postoperative adhesions, nevertheless, *de novo* adhesions can form to some degree after laparoscopy. Although laparoscopic adhesiolysis may not be an entirely innocuous procedure, it appears to result in improvement more often than does laparotomy. The prevention of *de novo* adhesions and adhesion reformation has been and continues to be the subject of much research.

Treatment of adhesions in some cases may play an important role in the management of chronic abdominal and pelvic pain. This must, however, be evaluated in the context of the placebo effect of surgery, the severity of adhesions, clinical history and physical examination, and psychological profile. Clinicians must remain aware that when adhesions are present, their role in producing a patient's pain must be constantly reevaluated.

Miscellaneous Gynecologic Causes of Chronic Pelvic Pain

Miscellaneous gynecologic causes of chronic pelvic pain are listed in Table 11.5.

Table 11.5.   Causes of chronic pelvic pain.

Pelvic congestion syndrome
Residual ovary syndrome
Ovarian remnant syndrome
Vaginal apex pain
Recurrent ovarian cysts
Vulvodynia

Pelvic Congestion Syndrome

This is a condition of chronic pelvic pain that occurs in the setting of pelvic varicosities, usually in the absence of other obvious pathologic causes. Historically this syndrome, and its many different names, has been discussed at length in the literature. Pelvic congestion has been controversial since it was first described by Taylor in 1949. Taylor found pelvic congestion to be, with few exceptions, a psychogenic complaint. Others were skeptical of his formulation because they noted dilated pelvic vessels at the time of surgery or during pregnancy in asymptomatic women. For pelvic congestion syndrome, like many of the diseases already discussed, the presence of the pathology does not necessarily mean that pain is present. Current technology provides ways to objectively diagnose and treat pelvic congestion.

Patients with pelvic congestion typically complain of steady dull pain and pressure low in the pelvis that becomes progressively worse throughout the day, but can have acute exacerbations. Deep dyspareunia and postcoital ache are common findings in women with pelvic congestion. Menstrual cycle abnormalities are common such as menorrhagia. Although these women commonly have a number of other complaints such as backache, headache, and urinary symptoms, bowel symptoms are uncommon. Interestingly, 60% have evidence of significant emotional disturbance.

Although physical examination lacks concrete findings, "ovarian point" tenderness is often found. This site is located at the junction of the upper and middle thirds of a line drawn from the anterior superior iliac spine to the umbilicus. Although "pathognomonic" for pelvic congestion when dilated vessels are present, tenderness in this area may be present in women without other evidence of this disorder. The pelvic examination may reveal a "doughy" consistency to the parametrial tissues on bimanual examination with the patient reporting these areas as the most sensitive in the pelvis.

Diagnostic laparoscopy, venography, and ultrasonography have all been employed to help make the diagnosis. Although helpful in excluding other abdominal and pelvic pathology such as endometriosis and pelvic adhesive disease, laparoscopy may miss the diagnosis of pelvic congestion. This may be due to emptying of the veins secondary to Trendelenburg positioning and increased intraabdominal pressure with pneumoperitoneum.

Various venographic techniques for imaging the dilated venous plexus have been described, including selective transfemoral ovarian venography and transcervical venography. The latter technique was first described by Heinen and Seigel in 1925 and has since been adopted by many researchers today. This approach involves injection of a water-soluble contrast directly into the muscle of the uterus followed by observation on a fluoroscopic screen. In a normal woman, all of the contrast disappears by 20 seconds after the injection, and the diameter of the ovarian vein is less than 4 mm. Women with pelvic pain from variceal congestion have evidence of dilated veins (>5 mm) as well as delayed disappearance and pooling of the contrast. Finally, ultrasonography has been used to document pelvic venous congestion. Vascular structures lateral to the uterus with a diameter of greater than 5 mm are typically indicative of pelvic varices.

Although few effective treatments have been developed, conservative medical management with medroxyprogesterone acetate at a dose of 30 mg per day has been efficacious. In fact, when combined with therapy aimed at stress management and education, one study showed ≥50% improvement in 75% of the women. Other hormonal therapies such as GnRH agonists and oral contraceptive pills have shown less promise. Surgical therapies have ranged from ovarian vein ligation to hysterectomy with bilateral salpingo-oophorectomy. Interventional radiologic embolization, which has previously been used successfully to treat testicular varicoceles in men, is now being used in women with some early reports of success.

Residual Ovary Syndrome

This syndrome was originally described by Grogan in 1958 and refers to the development of pain in one or both ovaries conserved at the time of hysterectomy. Grogan postulated that perioophoritis with a thickened ovarian capsule developed and led to pain from cyclical expansion of the ovary encased in adhesions.

This syndrome is thought to occur in approximately 3% of women who have undergone hysterectomy with ovarian conservation. The most common complaints are chronic lower abdominal pain, dyspareunia, and radiation of pain to the back and anterior thigh. During pelvic examination, a tender mass may be palpated. Although suppression of ovarian function may reduce the discomfort, treatment has typically been oophorectomy.

Ovarian Remnant Syndrome

Although this syndrome is uncommon, it is not as rare as previously thought. This syndrome may result from incomplete removal of ovarian tissue at the time of bilateral salpingoophorectomy and is associated with chronic abdominal and pelvic pain in premenopausal women. Incomplete removal of ovarian tissue may occur in the setting of extensive endometriosis or pelvic inflammatory disease. The presence of functioning ovarian tissue is suspected when serum levels of follicle-stimulating hormone (FSH) are within the premenopausal range (<30 m^{IU}/ml). In addition to serum levels of FSH, ultrasonography can help make the diagnosis.

The degree to which an ovarian remnant contributes to a patient's pain may be determined by suppression of ovarian function with GnRH agonists. This provocative test may also be therapeutic, particularly if the patient is nearing menopause. If the patient is far from menopause then surgery should be contemplated. Clomiphene citrate, an ovarian stimulant, can assist in both making an ultrasonographic diagnosis of ovarian remnant syndrome and in removing it surgically. Despite the best surgical techniques, there is a 10–15% chance of recurrence of the ovarian remnant after careful excision.

Vaginal Apex Pain

Occasionally, the vaginal apex may become intrinsically sensitive after hysterectomy. Granulation tissue is often the cause of this problem in the immediate postoperative period. Localized sensitivity, however, sometimes remains for years thereafter, even after all postoperative inflammation has disappeared. Patients will often complain of deep dyspareunia. This condition is detected during speculum examination by gently "walking" a cotton-tipped applicator over the vaginal apex. Typically one part of the vaginal apex will be sensitive, whereas other parts will be comfortable to palpation. Treatment with local anesthetic blocks or an intravaginal anesthetic jelly may provide relief. If this conservative approach fails, then surgical revision of the vaginal apex may be helpful in a procedure known as a vaginal cuff revision. This can often be performed laparoscopically.

Recurrent Ovarian Cysts

Adnexal masses are rarely a cause for pain. During each menstrual cycle the ovary normally produces a functional cyst. Frequently, however, patients with chronic abdominal or pelvic pain are led to believe that their normal ovarian cysts are causing pain. In the absence of torsion, enlargement with mass effect, or rupture with significant peritoneal irritation, functional ovarian cysts do not cause pain. In the case of cysts that do have characteristics that cause pain, they may be monitored for one or two menstrual cycles as tolerated by the patient. If the ovarian cyst is persistent, it may be approached laparoscopically. Barring the true symptomatic pelvic mass, clinicians must resist the temptation of treating normal functional ovarian cysts while still considering the risk of malignancy.

Vulvodynia

Vulvodynia is defined by the International Society for the Study of Vulvar Disease (ISSVD) as "chronic vulvar discomfort, especially that characterized by the patient's complaint of burning, stinging, irritation, or rawness." The prevalence of vulvodynia is difficult to assess, although it has been estimated that over 200,000 women in the United States have significant vulvar pain.

Patients with vulvodynia can present with varying symptoms that help classify them into different diagnostic categories. Vulvar vestibulitis or vestibulodynia is diagnosed when there is severe pain on palpation of the vestibule and a physical finding that is limited to vestibular erythema. Patients with vulvar vestibulitis typically present with complaints of dyspareunia on entry, persistent yeast infection, soreness, burning, or rawness. Tight clothing, prolonged sitting, or exercise may exacerbate these symptoms. Itching is rarely a symptom. On examination, palpation of the vestibule with a Q-tip in a clockwise fashion will cause reproduction of the pain. Patients with vulvar vestibulitis should discontinue the use of all soaps, douches, creams, or other potential irritants such as synthetic underwear. Topical agents such as vegetable oil or zinc oxide have been found to be useful. In addition, use of a local anesthetic can provide temporary relief. For patients with moderate to severe vestibulitis medical management with low-dose tricyclic antidepressants and gaba-pentin has had some success. Biofeedback, physical therapy, and relaxation training have also been found to improve symptomatology. Surgical treatment through vestibulectomy is a last resort. Although success rates for vestibulectomy have been reported as high as 95%, actual long-term success is much lower.

Dysesthetic vulvodynia, pudendal neuralgia, and essential vulvodynia are components of vestibulitis that are characterized by chronic continuous burning or pain. Dypareunia is not usually the primary complaint. Patients with these conditions develop hyperthesia that is likely due to the development of a sympathetically maintained pain-loop. Pain may be localized to branches of the iliohypogastric, ilioinguinal, genitofemoral, or pudendal nerves. The standard treatment is amitriptyline titrated up to 75–100 mg a day. Selective serotonin inhibitors have not been thoroughly studied but anecdotally have been found to be helpful.

Vulvar dermatoses are also a cause of vulvodynia and include dermatitis (cyclic vulvovaginitis), lichen planus, and lichen sclerosis. These conditions present with vulvar pain, burning, or dyspareunia and have skin changes noted on physical examination. Cyclic vulvovaginitis is characterized by recurrent itching and burning. Labial erythema and edema may be noted. Wet preps and cultures usually confirm candidiasis. Treatment consists of long-term systemic suppression with oral fluconazole or ketoconazole.

Lichen sclerosis is characterized by superficial mucosal ulceration and frequent fissuring with eventual stenosis and atrophy of the vulva. Depigmentation of the vulva, friability, loss of the labia minora, and introital narrowing may be seen on physical examination. Biopsy should be performed especially on areas of acanthosis as these areas may have epithelial atypia or malignancy. Treatment is with high-dose topical corticosteroids followed by an eventual transition to maintenance therapy with a low-dose topical corticosteroid.

Lichen planus is a chronic, shallow mucositis that may be accompanied by oral lesions and polygonal violaceous papules on the extremities. Colposcopic examination may show white, "lace-like" changes on the labial surface. Therapy is typically with high-dose topical corticosteroids. Dapsone, griseofulvin, and cyclosporine have also been used with variable results.

Vulvodynia is a chronic problem that can be frustrating for both the patient and the physician. It is a symptom complex that involves both physiologic and psychological factors, and treatment should focus on both aspects. Although it does not typically come to mind as a classic cause for chronic pelvic pain, its presence as a significant cause for pain and discomfort with the region of the pelvis is worth mentioning in the context of this chapter.

Urologic Causes of Chronic Pelvic Pain

Interstitial Cystitis

Interstitial cystitis is one of the most common bladder problems associated with chronic pelvic pain. Estimates of the prevalence of interstitial cystitis have varied from 60 to 450 women per 100,000. This may be due to the fact that this disorder lacks a precise definition. The diagnosis of interstitial cystitis is based upon criteria established by the National Institute of Arthritis, Diabetes, Digestive, and Kidney Disease (NIDDK). The criteria used for entry into NIH-funded research studies on interstitial cystitis are extensive and may identify only the most severe and advanced cases of interstitial cystitis (Table 11.6).

Patients typically present with chronic debilitating symptoms characterized by frequency, nocturia, urgency, urethral or bladder pain, and often abdominal, genital, or pelvic pain. Pain may range from mild burning to excruciating and debilitating. These symptoms tend to be cyclic in women of reproductive age with symptom flares the week prior to menses. There is no single feature of interstitial cystitis, but instead a constellation of symptoms that persist and worsen over the years. A thorough history and physical examination are required for diagnosis along with a cystoscopy under anesthesia with hydrodistention and biopsy. Before considering interstitial cystitis, the clinician must first check for chronic recurrent urinary tract infections including urethritis. Symptoms are similar to that of interstitial cystitis but a urinalysis along with clean-catch urine culture will diagnose many bacterial infections of the urinary tract.

As the etiology of this disorder is unclear, therapies are aimed at symptom relief. See Table 11.7 for a list of various medical and surgical treatment options. Currently, there are two FDA approved medications for the treatment of interstitial cystitis. Oral pentosan polysulfate sodium (PPS, Elmiron) has been shown to be effective and well-tolerated in patients with interstitial cystitis. Full effect is usually achieved with at least 6 months of therapy. Intravesical dimethyl sulfoxide (DMSO) is an antiinflammatory agent that acts as a muscle relaxant.

Because PPS can take several weeks before reduction in pain is noted, utilizing other methods such as hydrodistention to provide short-term relief can help control symptoms. In addition, antihistamines, anticholinergics, and selective serotonin reuptake inhibitors may also provide short-term relief. Lifestyle modifications, biofeedback, and electrical stimulation have also been shown to help relieve symptoms of interstitial cystitis.

Table 11.6.   NIH-NIDDK diagnostic criteria for interstitial cystitis.

Category A: At least one of the following findings on cystoscopy:
- Diffuse glomerulations (at least 10 per quadrant) in at least three quadrants of the bladder
- A classic Hunner's ulcer

Category B: At least one of the following symptoms:
- Pain associated with the bladder
- Urinary urgency

Exclusion criteria:
- Age <18 years[a]
- Urinary frequency while awake <8 times per day
- Maximal bladder capacity >350 ml while patient is awake
- Absence of an intense urge to void with bladder filled to 150 ml of water with medium filling rate (30–100 ml/minute) during cystometry
- Involuntary bladder contractions on cystometry using medium filling rate
- Duration of symptoms <9 months[a]
- Symptoms relieved by antimicrobial agents (antibiotics, urinary antiseptics), anticholinergics, or antispasmodics[a]
- Urinary tract infection in the last 3 months[a]
- Active genital herpes
- Vaginitis[a]
- Uterine, cervical, vaginal, or urethral cancer within the past 5 years[a]
- Bladder or ureteral calculi[a]
- Urethral diverticulum[a]
- History of cyclophosphamide or chemical cystitis or tuberculous or radiation cystitis
- Benign or malignant bladder tumors

[a] Relative exclusion criteria.
Source: National Kidney and Urologic Diseases Information Clearinghouse (NKUDIC) NIH Publication No. 05-3220 June 2005.

Table 11.7.   Treatment modalities in interstitial cystitis.

Behavioral techniques	Intravesical agents	Oral agents	Surgery
Biofeedback • Bladder retraining exercises • Kegel exercises • Electrical stimulation	• Dimethyl sulfoxide (DMSO) • Heparin • Silver nitrate • Oxychlorosene sodium (Chlorpactin) • Corticosteroids • Bupivacaine	• Amitriptyline • Hydroxyzine • Sodium pentosan polysulfate (Elmiron)	• Hydrodistention • Transurethral resection and fulgaration • Bladder augmentation procedures • Urinary diversion

Gastroenterologic Causes of Chronic Pelvic Pain
Irritable Bowel Syndrome

Irritable bowel syndrome (IBS) is one of more than 20 functional GI tract disorders. It is defined as chronic abdominal pain (usually in the lower segment) and disturbed defecation in the absence of structural or biochemical abnormalities. Over the years, terms such as spastic colon and mucous colitis have been applied to what is now known as IBS. The pathophysiology of IBS remains unclear, however, several research-generated insights have allowed for an improved understanding of this complicated syndrome. The physiologic mechanisms underlying the abdominal pain and altered bowel habits of IBS patients are thought to be a result of the dysregulation of brain–gut interactions leading to altered perceptions of pain. Recent studies using positron emission tomography scans have shown that patients with IBS have a different cerebral response to pain compared to controls. This suggests that selective activation of one area of the brain over another may represent a form of brain–gut dysfunction that leads to a centrally mediated hyperalgesic state. In addition, biochemical factors such as 5-hydroxytryptamine (5-HT), cholecystokinin (CCK), substance P, neurotensin, and cytokines are also potential participants in transmission of painful and nonpainful sensations and in the regulation of mood and behavior.

Psychosocial factors such as early life experiences, conditioning factors, physical stress, personal and social coping systems, and psychological stress influence the expression of symptoms and illness behavior. Numerous studies indicated that psychosocial disturbances affect illness experience and

Table 11.8.   Rome II diagnostic criteria for irritable bowel syndrome (IBS).

At least 12 weeks, which need not be consecutive, in the preceding 12 months, of abdominal discomfort or pain that has two of three features
- Relieved with defecation
- Onset associated with a change in frequency of stool
- Onset associated with a change in form (appearance) of stool

The following symptoms are not essential for the diagnosis, but their presence increases confidence in the diagnosis and may be used to identify subgroups of IBS
- Abnormal stool frequency (>3/day or <3/week)
- Abnormal stool form (lumpy/hard or loose/watery stool) in >1/4 of defecations
- Abnormal stool passage (straining, urgency, or feeling of incomplete evacuation) in >1/4 of defecations
- Passage of mucus in >1/4 of defecations
- Bloating or feeling of abdominal distention >1/4 of days

Source: Reprinted with permission from Rome II: The Functional Gastrointestinal Disorders (2nd ed.), 2000, McLean, VA, DA Drossman, E Corazziari, NJ Talley, WG Thompson, & WE Whitehead (Eds), *www.romecriteria.org.*

outcome. A high prevalence of prior physical and sexual abuse has been reported in women with IBS compared with women with organic disorders. Psychiatric comorbidities such as anxiety, depression, and impaired psychosocial adjustment are more prevalent in patients with IBS than controls. Although these factors are etiologic, they are relevant to an understanding of the patient's adjustment to IBS and to the development of a treatment plan.

The hallmark of IBS is abdominal pain or discomfort associated with a change in the consistency or frequency of stools and relieved by defecation. The disorder is unique in that it has no structural, biochemical, or physiologic diagnostic markers. Instead the diagnosis of IBS has been enhanced and

Table 11.9.   Laboratory and diagnostic studies if patient has typical features of irritable bowel syndrome.

Age <50	Order complete blood count (CBC), electrolytes, liver function tests (LFTs), screen stool for occult blood, and consider sigmoidoscopy
Age >50	Order CBC, electrolytes, LFTs, and perform a colonoscopy or air-contrast barium enema with sigmoidoscopy

Table 11.10.   Atypical findings for irritable bowel syndrome that may suggest alternative or coexisting disease and require additional studies.

Anemia	Rectal bleeding	Nocturnal symptoms of pain and abnormal bowel function
Fever	Severe constipation	Family history of gastrointestinal cancer, inflammatory bowel disease, or celiac disease
Persistent diarrhea	Weight loss	New onset of symptoms in patients 50+ years of age

simplified through the use of symptom-based criteria with the Rome II criteria as the most recent standard. (Table 11.8) The combination of these criteria and a complete history and physical examination increase diagnostic accuracy allowing for a more conservative work-up. Table 11.9 outlines recommended laboratory and diagnostic studies.

Abdominal pain or discomfort is usually poorly localized and may be migratory in nature. Other symptoms include altered stool form, altered stool passage, and passage of mucus. Symptoms can occur in clusters or individually, in addition to exhibiting variable frequency among patients. There are atypical symptoms that may indicate a coexisting or alternative diagnosis (Table 11.10) and referral to a gastroenterologist should be considered.

The interplay of physiologic and psychosocial factors in IBS requires an integrated approach to treatment. The current management components of IBS are listed on Table 11.11. Education and reassurance are key to helping patients understand they have real symptoms but these are not life-threatening. It is important for patients to understand that IBS is a condition that can be managed, but not cured.

Medical management is directed at alleviating the most predominant symptoms (Table 11.12). Antispasmodics are the most frequently used

Table 11.11.   Current management components of irritable bowel syndrome.

Education
Reassurance
Dietary modification (e.g., reduction in alcohol, fat, and caffeine)
Fiber
Symptomatic treatment
Psychological/behavioral options
Realistic goals

Table 11.12. Current medical and psychological/behavioral treatment options.

Pain	Constipation	Diarrhea	Psychological
Antispasmodics	Fiber	Loperamide	Cognitive-behavioral therapy
a. Dicyclomine	Osmotic laxatives	Cholestyramine	Psychotherapy
b. Hyoscyamine sulfate	a. Magnesium sulfate	Alosetron (pending FDA reapproval with black box warning, 5-HT$_3$ receptor antagonist indicated for treatment of diarrhea predominant IBS in women)	Hypnosis
Tricyclic antidepressants (TCAs)	b. Lactulose		Relaxation training
a. Amitriptyline	c. PEG solution		Family or group therapy
b. Doxepin	Tegaserod		
Selective serotonin reuptake inhibitors (SSRIs)			
a. Fluoxetine			
b. Sertraline			
c. Paroxetine			
d. Citalopram			

medication. The anticholinergic effects of these medications relax smooth muscle. Tricyclic antidepressants and selective serotonin reuptake inhibitors are also used for symptomatic treatment of pain, but are reserved for patients with severe or refractory pain. Side effects of the antispasmodics and tricyclic antidepressants (TCAs) (dry mouth, drowsiness) can limit their use.

Fiber bulking agents are also useful for those patients with constipation. Osmotic laxatives may also be prescribed if fiber bulking agents are not helpful. Recently the FDA approved a selective partial $5\text{-}HT_4$ agonist, tegaserod, for the treatment of women with constipation-predominant IBS.

Antidiarrheals such as loperamide are typically prescribed for the diarrhea-predominant IBS patient. These agents slow intestinal transit and enhance intestinal water and ion absorption, thereby resulting in decreased stool frequency and improved stool consistency. Alosetron, a potent and selective $5\text{-}HT_3$ receptor antagonist, is the only FDA-approved drug for treating diarrhea-predominant IBS. Alosetron was removed from the market in November 2000 due to reports of ischemic colitis and severe constipation, but has since been rereleased with a "black box" warning.

Psychological and behavioral options for IBS include cognitive-behavioral therapy, psychotherapy, hypnosis, relaxation training, and family or group therapy. A disadvantage of these techniques is that patients can be quite resistant to referral to a mental health specialist. As a result, the initial approach to a patient with IBS should involve dietary and pharmacologic measures. If these fail after an adequate trial, then referral to a psychologist or psychiatrist should be made.

Musculoskeletal Causes of Chronic Pelvic Pain

Musculoskeletal Dysfunction

The musculoskeletal system can often contribute to chronic pelvic pain. Dysfunction may develop as a response to an initial gynecologic problem or it may develop primarily. Surgical incisions can also contribute to musculoskeletal findings. Common problems include shortening and spasm of the psoas, shortening of the abdominal muscles, and/or a general abnormal posture including increased lumbar lordosis and an anterior tilt of the pelvis. As pain increases, patients develop splinting and cessation of physical activities such as exercise.

Regardless of which came first, if left untreated, this musculoskeletal dysfunction may induce tissue damage that results in the development of trigger points. Myofascial trigger points such as those located within the abdominal wall may be injected with a variety of local anesthetics as described earlier. Although both diagnostic and therapeutic, this type of therapy may not yield long-term results unless it is used in conjunction with physical therapy. Physical therapy is an integral treatment to successful management of musculoskeletal abnormalities. NSAIDs and muscle relaxants may also be useful.

Psychiatric Causes of Chronic Pelvic Pain

Addressing both the somatic and psychological aspects of chronic pelvic pain is a fundamental approach to its diagnosis and treatment. Even when there is a clear etiology to the pain, it is important to understand that pain responses are affective and behavioral and therefore have a psychological component. Depression accompanies chronic pain up to 50% of the time, and depressed patients typically report a lower tolerance of pain as well as decreased functioning due to pain.

Psychological assessment early in the patient's evaluation includes depression screening, psychological history, and sexual history. Early evaluation allows identification of areas that require intervention, for example, depression, anxiety, or substance abuse. In addition, ascertaining the effect the patient's pain has had on the dynamics within her family and work life can identify social support, coping mechanisms, and the patient's role in the family (e.g., "sick role").

Medication such as antidepressants and anxiolytics should also be used when appropriate to treat depression and anxiety disorders. Treatment of these conditions can help the patient's ability to function and cope with chronic pain. Psychotherapy and counseling have been shown to be effective adjuncts in the treatment of chronic pelvic pain. In addition, biofeedback, relaxation techniques, hypnosis, meditation, and behavioral modifications have been shown to be effective treatments for chronic pain. Addressing and treating the psychological component of chronic pain will allow patients to understand the impact of stress on their condition and learn to manage their pain in order to maintain functional lives.

Conclusion

The patient with chronic pelvic pain presents a diagnostic challenge to the clinician. The causes are varied and can be multifactorial. A careful and detailed clinical history and physical examination can provide a starting point for creation of a list of possible differential diagnoses. The need for laboratory and diagnostic studies, if any, should be tailored to the individual patient's symptomatology and differential diagnoses. A single diagnosis is often unlikely. Clinicians should resist the tendency to pursue only one treatment modality, whether it is medical or surgical, without consideration of treatment of other components that may be contributing to the pain process. A collaborative approach to the patient that utilizes the expertise of other health care professionals such as psychologists, urologists, gastroenterologists, and physical therapists can lead to a coordinated treatment plan with maximal benefit to the patient. Expectations for the patient should be set early in the treatment process. Many causes of chronic pelvic pain are not curable but are manageable and management can provide patients with significant improvement in their quality of life. Keeping this advice in mind can make caring for the complicated chronic pain patient a rewarding rather than frustrating experience.

Suggested Reading

Blackwell RE, Olive DL, ed. *Chronic Pelvic Pain: Evaluation & Management.* New York: Springer-Verlag; 1998.

Howard FM, Perry CP, et al., ed. *Pelvic Pain: Diagnosis & Management.* Philadelphia: Lippincott Williams & Wilkins; 2000.

Margoles MS, Weiner R, ed. *Chronic Pain: Assessment, Diagnosis, and Management.* Washington DC: CRC Press; 1999.

Steege JF, et al., ed. *Chronic Pelvic Pain: An Integrated Approach.* Philadelphia: W.B. Saunders Company; 1998.

Turk DC, Melzack R, ed. *Handbook of Pain Assessment.* New York: The Guilford Press; 1992.

12

Contraception Update

Amitasrigowri S. Murthy and Bryna Harwood

Introduction

A discussion of contraceptive options would not be complete without reviewing the population that needs contraception. In the United States, 48% of the 6.3 million pregnancies that occur annually are unplanned. Approximately 50% of these unplanned pregnancies occur among the small percentage of women at risk for pregnancy who do not use contraception. There are approximately 60 million women in the United States who are in their reproductive years (ages 15–44). Of these women, 30% do not need contraception (they are heterosexually abstinent, pregnant, postpartum, or are attempting to get pregnant), 65% are using some sort of contraception, and 5% are not using but are still in need of contraception. Of the women who practice contraception, two-thirds use a method of reversible contraception, such as oral contraceptives or condoms. Among women who use the condom as their primary method of contraception, one-third report not using it with every act of intercourse. These women tend to mainly use the male condom; less than 1% report using the female condom as their primary method of barrier contraception. Condom use tends to decline as women age; only 16% of women aged 35–39 years used a condom at all. Twenty-eight percent of couples using contraception rely on tubal sterilization and 11% on male sterilization. As women and male partners age, they increasingly begin to rely on female methods of contraception, with over 44% of women aged 35–39 years relying on female contraceptive methods. Female sterilization is the most commonly used method in women who are over the age of 34 years, have been previously married, or have an income below 150% of the poverty level.

In 1995, the National Survey of Family Growth collected information on contraceptive use and compared it to similar information collected from 1988 and 1982. The proportion of reproductive aged women using contraceptives increased from 56% in 1982 to over 64% in 1995. More women were using a contraceptive with first intercourse as compared to women surveyed in 1980. Between 1982 and 1995, the proportion of sexually active women not using a contraceptive method declined by over 30%, while the proportion of women relying on condoms increased by 5% among women in all age groups. Use of the diaphragm and the intrauterine device (IUD) declined significantly, to 2% for diaphragm users and to less than 1% for IUD users. With these changes in contraceptive use, i.e., increased use but decreased reliance on the most reliable methods, unplanned pregnancy rates have increased to 50% in the United States. About half of these pregnancies are electively terminated. Any attempt to decrease the number of unplanned pregnancies and elective terminations must not only increase the use of contraception, but also the use of highly effective contraception. This requires that physicians counsel patients adequately about available methods of contraception and review their efficacy, mechanism of action, and proper use.

Counseling begins the moment the physician walks in the door. Asking the patient what her needs are, determining her goals, and ascertaining her risk of acquiring sexually transmitted diseases are as important as explaining what her choices are and the advantages and disadvantages of using each method. As with any other drug, prescribing contraception requires counseling—instruction on its use, expected side effects, and expected rates of efficacy. Unlike most medications, success with contraception is measurable only with the absence of a clinical outcome—that is prevention of pregnancy, which makes compliance with treatment more difficult to maintain and problems with a contraceptive method more difficult to solve. Compliance with contraception is increasingly successful when patients are counseled on all its aspects. Therefore, counseling patients appropriately will help them use more effective methods and be more compliant with the method and help prevent unintended pregnancy and its consequences.

Hormonal Contraception

Combined Hormonal Contraceptives

Oral Formulations (Table 12.1)

From the time the first oral contraceptive (OC) was introduced, the use of OCs has accelerated, becoming one of the most prescribed medications today. OCs, as they are now formulated and prescribed, are a safe and effective contraceptive option.

Table 12.1.   Key points of oral formulations.

Route	Dose schedule	Mechanism of action	Efficacy[a] (1 year)	Special clinical considerations
Oral	Daily	Inhibition of ovulation	95%	Hypertension, tobacco use, myocardial infarction, stroke

[a] True population rates are as low as 85%.

For someone new to prescribing OCs, the task of choosing a formulation may be daunting. All combined OCs available now contain 20–35 µg of ethinyl estradiol in combination with a progestin. The most common progestins in OCs are divided into two families: gonanes (norethindrone) and estranes (norgestrel, levonorgestrel, norethynodrel, desogestrel, norgestimate, and gestodene). All of these progestins are derived from testosterone. They vary in their bioavailability and metabolism. The most recent addition to the progestin family, drosperinone, is not derived from testosterone but rather from spironolactone. Its profile is much more similar to progesterone with antimineralocorticoid and antiandrogenic activity.

OCs act on the hypothalamus and inhibit gonadotropin secretion, thus inhibiting ovulation. This is the primary mechanism of action of all combined hormonal contraceptives. Exogenous estradiol exerts negative feedback at the level of the hypothalamus, thereby suppressing follicle-stimulating hormone (FSH) and the progestin similarly decreases luteinizing hormone (LH) secretion.

While the estrogen component improves bleeding and cycle control by stabilizing the endometrium, it is the progestin that provides most of the contraceptive and other clinical effects of OCs. It suppresses endometrial growth, thereby decreasing menstrual flow. It also promotes secretion and thickening of cervical mucus, which prevents ascent of sperm in the reproductive tract. Progestins also affect oviductal motility. These secondary actions may be important, if ovulation occurs.

Oral contraceptives are very effective, but require daily attention for their efficacy, which is the main drawback for this method. Failure with OC use can usually be attributed to missed pills or a prolonged period without an active drug (i.e., the placebo week is extended). In research studies with "perfect use" and compliance with the study protocol, ~1% of women become pregnant during the first year of use. However, in typical use, about 1 in 20 women become pregnant in the first year. Efficacy was also decreased in trials whose main population consisted of urban adolescents. They were much more likely to miss doses or to extend the placebo week past 7 days than older women. Therefore, adherence to the dosing schedule and the typical efficacy are important counseling points for OC use.

New Delivery Methods (Table 12.2)

Recently, there have been major advances in delivery systems of combined hormonal contraception. These new delivery systems do not require daily attention and this has improved compliance and ease of use. Now dosing of a combined hormonal contraceptive can occur monthly (injectable, vaginal ring) or weekly (transdermal patch).

The transdermal patch, (OrthoEvra®) is 4.5 cm^2 and beige in color. It releases daily 20 μg of ethinyl estradiol and 150 μg of norelgestromin, the active metabolite of norgestimate, at a steady rate. The patch is worn on the upper arm or trunk (excluding breast tissue) 1 week at a time for three consecutive weeks. The fourth week is "patch free" and allows for the withdrawal bleed to occur. After application of the patch, therapeutic levels are achieved within 2 days. The patch, like OCs, prevents pregnancy by inhibiting ovulation. In a direct comparison to an OC, the failure rate was the same (~1%) but compliance was better among patch users. A major drawback of this method is that it is not recommended in women who weigh over 198 pounds because of the high failure rate (approximately 10%) in that group.

Most side effects are similar to those of oral contraceptives; however, the patch has some unique side effects including complete or partial detachment and site reactions. Approximately 3–4% of patches will completely detach, which translates to one to two patches detaching in the first year of use per

Table 12.2. Key points of new delivery methods.

Route	Dose schedule	Mechanism of action	Efficacy[a] (1 year)	Special clinical considerations
Transdermal	Weekly	Suppression of ovulation	99%	Hypertension, tobacco use, myocardial infarction, stroke
Vaginal	Monthly	Suppression of ovulation	>99%	As above
Injectable	Monthly	Suppression of ovulation	>99%	As above

[a] In efficacy trials only.

woman on average. Site reactions are typically consistent with a mild contact dermatitis and can be easily treated with the use of topical corticosteroids.

The contraceptive vaginal ring first became available in the United States in 2001, marketed under the trade name NuvaRing®. It is a clear flexible ring made of ethylene vinylacetate, and is 2 in. (54 mm) in diameter and 1/8th in. (4 mm) thick. The ring is left in place in the vagina for 3 weeks and removed for 1 week to allow for a withdrawal bleed. Vaginal administration allows for a continuous release of the active hormones. The ring releases 15 µg of ethinyl estradiol and 120 µg of etonogestrel, the active metabolite of desogestrel, intravaginally daily. The ring does not need to be fitted or placed in a specific location; absorption will occur when the ring is in contact with the vaginal epithelium. Similar to OCs, the ring inhibits ovulation to prevent pregnancy. Unlike OCs, the pregnancy rate in the first year of ring use is much lower, 0.65 per 100 women-years as reported in clinical trials. Reported side effects are similar to those associated with oral contraceptives except for irregular breakthrough bleeding, which occurs less frequently compared to an OC. Another common side effect is that of increased vaginal discharge without odor or irritation, due to the local hormonal effects of the ring. This is not vaginitis and patients should be counseled to expect increased discharge not related to infection. Expulsion occurs rarely, in only about 2% of Nuva-Ring® users in the first year of use. Removal of the ring during intercourse is not required but women may do so and continue to rely on the efficacy of the ring as long as it is replaced within 3 hours. In fact, partners usually do not notice the ring when in place during intercourse.

Lunelle™, the combined injectable hormonal contraceptive, is an intramuscular injection of a suspension containing 25 mg medroxyprogesterone acetate and 5 mg estradiol cypionate, given every 28–30 days. This method is highly effective; the 1-year failure rate for typical use is approximately 0.1%. Estradiol is the active metabolite of estradiol cypionate and provides a regular bleeding pattern unlike the progesterone alone injection. After Lunelle™ administration, ovulation is inhibited for 40 days, providing a week of "forgiveness" if a dose is missed. If a patient presents by day 35, her next dose may be given and her contraception will be continuous. The withdrawal bleed, unlike most cyclic methods, usually occurs about 2 weeks after the injection, when the estrogen withdrawal occurs. Compared to OCs, Lunelle™ is associated with increased number of days of irregular bleeding or spotting. Otherwise the side effects are similar to oral contraceptives. Unfortunately, due to manufacturing concerns, Lunelle™ has been pulled from sale in the United States.

Side Effects

Side effects with combined hormonal contraceptives can be divided into those commonly caused by the estrogen component and those caused by the progestin component. Estrogen-related side effects include nausea, fluid retention, mastalgia, hypertension, and leukorrhea. On the other hand, those attributed to progestins include mood swings or depression, increased appetite, fatigue, and irregular bleeding. Side effects are cited as the most common reason for discontinuation of oral contraceptives. Fully one-third of women using OCs discontinue use due to side effects. Of these women, one-third cite breakthrough bleeding as the most bothersome. Breakthrough bleeding is usually associated with a recently started or an inconsistent dosing schedule. If irregular bleeding occurs in the first few cycles of use, reassurance that this is normal is usually sufficient. Breakthrough bleeding after three cycles should prompt consideration for an evaluation for other causes of bleeding (i.e., cervical infection), and possibly a change of OC formulation with a different class of progestin. Side effects of the patch and vaginal ring are similar to those of the combined oral contraceptive pill, except as mentioned previously.

Other side effects most commonly listed as bothersome include nausea and weight gain. Teenagers especially list weight gain as an important factor in their decision to continue use of the pill. Over a 2-year period a woman in the United States without exogenous hormones will gain, on average, 1 kg per year. The same trend is seen with OCs, except with the use of drosperinone (Yasmin®), which is not associated with a net change in weight in the first 12 months of use. Similarly, other combined hormonal regimens have not been associated with significant weight gain in studies. Patients should be counseled about weight control and their concerns should be addressed.

Combined hormonal contraceptives are associated with many metabolic changes that are not usually clinically significant. Most oral formulations cause a slight and reversible increase in blood pressure. Glucose metabolism is also affected by OCs but without any clinical significance, and OCs can be safely used in women with diabetes mellitus. OCs also affect the ratio of high-density lipoprotein (HDL) to low-density lipoprotein (LDL) and increase triglyceride levels. These effects are not usually clinically significant but can be avoided by a non-oral formulation (i.e., contraceptive ring or patch). The increased risk of gallstones is due to the effect of oral contraceptives on bile solubility. Exogenous estrogen causes a thrombophilic state due to increased fibrin formation and platelet aggregation. This leads to rare but clinically significant events and unfortunately the new delivery methods do not eliminate this risk.

It is important to counsel patients that use of combined hormonal contraceptives does not prevent sexually transmitted diseases, including HIV; in order to prevent transmission of these infections, hormonal contraceptives must be used in conjunction with a barrier method (e.g., microbicide or condoms).

Contraindications

There are a few absolute contraindications to the use of combined hormonal contraceptives. These include known thrombophlebitis or thromboembolic disorders, impaired liver function or known hepatic adenoma, undiagnosed abnormal vaginal bleeding, pregnancy known or suspected, and tobacco use in women over the age of 35 years. While the use of combined contraceptives increases the risk of a venous thromboembolism (VTE), it is important to remember that this risk is half the risk of VTE in pregnancy. This increased risk of VTE is associated with the dose of estrogen; the risk is greater in 50-µg pills than in lower doses. The progestin component does not increase the risk of VTE; but epidemiologic studies found an association between desogestrel or gestodene and an increased risk of VTE, as compared to other progestins. These studies, however, were confounded by several factors unrelated to the type of progestin. Current labels on combined oral contraceptives mention an increased risk with desogestrel-containing products; however, neither the Food and Drug Administration (FDA) nor the American College of Obstetricians and Gynecologists (ACOG) recommends that patients on these pills change to a different formulation. Certain inherited mutations, such as Factor V Leiden and protein S or protein C abnormalities, are associated with an increased risk of VTE. However, routine screening for these mutations in asymptomatic patients without a significant personal or family history of VTE is not recommended because these are rare and the risk of a fatal event in the presence of one of these mutations is also extremely low. If patients are routinely screened and those with such inherited mutations are not offered estrogen-containing contraceptives, more than 500,000 women would need to be screened to prevent one death from pulmonary embolism; these women would be denied effective contraception, increasing their risk of unintended pregnancy and its health consequences, including VTE. Currently there are no guidelines that recommend screening for these genetic mutations. Decisions on whether to start oral contraceptives should still be based on clinical judgment after taking a thorough history and adequate counseling about contraceptive options.

The FDA, along with the makers of the contraceptive patch released a report revealing their concerns that the patch exposes users to about 60% more estrogen overall than an OC containing 35-micrograms of ethinyl estradiol. What is unknown is what exactly the clinical effect of this increased exposure to estrogen is on VTE risk. The one study, recently published, that evaluated patch users as compared to OC users for non-fatal VTE found no difference in the number of VTE events between patch and OC users. Interim results from another study, submitted to the FDA but not yet published, suggest a twofold increase in the risk of development of a thrombus. VTE is a rare event in hormonal contraceptive users; the risk of VTE increases from 1/10,000 in non-pregnant, non-contraceptive users to 3 to 5/10,000 in combined hormonal contraceptive users. As the investigation is still ongoing, currently, there are no recommendations to change use patterns or prescribing patterns of the patch. Certainly women considering the contraceptive patch should be counseled about the increased estrogen exposure and the unknown effect and VTE, and women who have other risks for VTE (tobacco use, obesity, older age) should be counseled about their increased risk of VTE. Although the same study demonstrates less estrogen exposure for ring users compared to OC users or patch users, there are no recommendations about increased or decreased VTE risk for ring users. Counseling for ring users should be the same as for any combined hormonal contraceptive.

Nonsmoking women under the age of 35 years who use combined hormonal methods have no increased risk of myocardial infarction or stroke. However, there is an increased risk of developing chronic medical disorders like hypertension or coronary artery disease as age increases. For patients with chronic hypertension, the relative risk of myocardial infarction and stroke is increased. Women at risk for cardiovascular events include women who are over 35 years who also smoke more than 15 cigarettes per day, women with uncontrolled chronic medical disorders like hypertension, diabetes, and hyperlipidemia, and women with migraines with neurologic foci. Women over the age of 35 years and who smoke are at increased risk of having a cardiac event, while those women with migraine headaches with neurologic symptoms are at increased risk of stroke. This risk of vascular events increases dramatically with the use of tobacco. As women age, the risk of developing chronic disease, as well as the risk of having complications related to these diseases, increases. For example, for women under the age of 35 years with hypertension and who are nonsmokers, the risk of having a cardiac event is no higher than for age-matched controls. This is in contrast to those women who have hypertension and are over the age of 35 years who are at increased risk.

Women with diabetes can use OCs safely with no fear of impairing carbohydrate metabolism. Nor does OC use accelerate the development of diabetic complications such as vascular disease or retinopathy. Use of OCs does not precipitate the development of non-insulin-dependent diabetes, nor does past use increase risk. However, women at risk of cardiovascular events due to diabetic complications may not be candidates for combined hormonal contraception.

Women who experience migraine headaches with neurologic symptoms and who use OCs are at a 34-fold increased risk of stroke compared to women who do not use combination hormonal contraception. Although the absolute risk of a cerebrovascular event is extremely low, the consequences can be devastating, therefore, OC use is not recommended for women in this setting.

Women with hyperlipidemia can use OCs safely as well, as long as the formulation has less than 35 μg of estrogen and the hyperlipidemia is controlled. The estrogen component will increase removal of LDL cholesterol, while encouraging increases in HDL cholesterol; however, it will also increase triglyceride levels. This increase is mild and in the setting of a higher HDL level and lower LDL level, the mild elevation will not increase the risk of atherosclerosis.

Benefits of Combined Hormonal Contraceptive Use

There are many noncontraceptive benefits associated with combined hormonal contraceptive use. OCs have been used to treat menstrually related pelvic pain including dysmenorrhea and mittelschmertz (mid-cycle pain), to decrease menstrual blood loss, and to increase menstrual cycle regularity. Current formulations treat symptoms such as hirsutism, acne, or other androgen-related seborrheic dermatoses. Drosperinone is the only progestin available in the United States that has antimineralocorticoid activity.

There are preventive noncontraceptive benefits of OC use as well. OC use decreases the risk of developing certain gynecologic cancers. There is a decreased risk of developing epithelial ovarian cancer; this risk decreases after 1 year of use and the risk exponentially decreases with prolonged use of an oral contraceptive (over 10 years). The risk of developing endometrial cancer is also decreased with OC use; OC use for 1 year decreases the lifetime risk by about 20% and this protection is prolonged (up to 30 years after the last OC use). Risk of death from colorectal cancer is decreased significantly as well with OC use.

Breast disease and OC use is a highly controversial topic; however, recent data should be able to reassure patients and clinicians. With continued OC use, there is a reduction in all benign breast disease. The consensus opinion is that OC use does not cause breast cancer. However, there is a slightly increased risk of being diagnosed with breast cancer. This is likely due to two factors. First there is a detection bias in those women who use OCs, because of more regular annual screening in OC users compared with women not using OCs. And second, the exogenous hormones may promote the growth of a preexisting nidus of cancerous cells. This increased risk disappears by the time a woman reaches the age of 55 years. In OC users who have breast cancer diagnosed, the lesion is more likely to be localized, supporting the assertion of a detection bias of growth promotion. For women with a strong family history of breast cancer, many recent cohort studies have shown that OCs do not increase their risk of developing breast cancer. These studies also looked at women with a personal history of benign breast disease and found no increased risk of breast cancer with OC use. Similarly, OCs do not increase the risk of breast cancer in women with risk factors of a strong family history or benign breast disease compared to women without these risk factors.

Progestin-Only Methods

Progestin-only methods of contraception include progestin-only-containing pills and depot medroxyprogesterone acetate. Unlike combined hormonal contraceptives, the main method of action of progestin-only methods is not by inhibition of ovulation or by prevention of mid-cycle LH surge. The primary actions are (1) thickening of cervical mucus, thereby impeding sperm entry, (2) impairing tubal motility to slow the passage of the ovum, and (3) thinning the endometrium. The first of these, thickening of cervical mucus, is responsible for the early onset of contraceptive action (within 3 days) and provides significant contraceptive efficacy. The third mechanism, thinning of the endometrium, is responsible for the irregular and unpredictable bleeding pattern of these methods.

Table 12.3. Key points of progestin-only pills ("mini pills").

Route	Dose schedule	Mechanism of action	Efficacy (1 year)	Special clinical considerations
Oral	Daily	Ovulation suppression, cervical mucus thickening	95%	Strict adherence to timing of dose

Progestin-Only Pills ("Mini Pills") (Table 12.3)

Progestin-only oral contraception (POP) is sometimes called "mini pills" due to the absence of estrogen, but this is a misnomer—as the progestin dose is not significantly reduced. POPs do not reliably inhibit the LH surge, and it is the thickened cervical mucus that provides reliable contraception. Therefore, the tablets must be strictly taken at the same time every day. Taking a dose three or more hours late reduces the contraceptive efficacy and a back-up method of contraception should be used. However, unlike combined hormonal formulations, contraceptive efficacy can be reestablished in 72 hours due to the thickened cervical mucus. For these same reasons, there is a no placebo week and POPs are taken continuously. The probability of pregnancy is about 5% during the first year of use.

Bleeding can be irregular when using POPs and is often due to endometrial atrophy. Amenorrhea can occur after some months of use but is not common. Users of POPs may still ovulate and have more irregular bleeding if pills are not taken on time.

Long-Acting Hormonal Contraception (Table 12.4)

Depot medroxyprogesterone acetate (DMPA) is a long-acting injectable contraceptive. It is the only long-acting progestin-only contraception currently available in the United States that does not require a provider visit to discon-

Table 12.4. Key points of long-acting hormonal contraception.

Route	Dose schedule	Mechanism of action	Efficacy (1 year)	Special clinical considerations
Injectable	Every 3 months	Suppression of ovulation	>99%	Bone effects

tinue. Structurally similar to endogenous progesterone, it is given as an aqueous suspension of microcrystals of 17-acetoxy-6-methylprogesterone in a dose of 150 mg by intramuscular injection every 12 weeks. Labeling states that each injection is effective for up to 13 weeks, giving a 1-week period of forgiveness. DMPA is very effective, with a first year typical use failure rate of approximately 0.3% and has a high rate of acceptance among users. Approximately 70% of women will continue using DMPA after the first year. Current developments include approval of a subcutaneous injection of DMPA. This new option would improve ease of use and help improve compliance by making administration of the method totally patient controlled—much like self-subcutaneous injection of insulin for diabetics. Contraceptive efficacy of the lower dose subcutaneous DMPA is comparable to that of intramuscular DMPA and the side effect profile is similar.

Side Effects

Common side effects include irregular bleeding, directly due to the progestin effect on the endometrial lining. Many patients will develop amenorrhea with continued use of DMPA; up to 90% of women will be amenorrheic by the end of the first year. Two studies demonstrate that adequate counseling about the possible changes in their bleeding pattern helped reduce 12 month DMPA discontinuation rates from 42% to 11%.

Other side effects of concern, particularly with DMPA, include mood changes and weight change. DMPA was associated with a worsening of depressive symptoms in women already diagnosed with a mood disorder. However, two well-controlled studies found no causal relationship between the use of DMPA and depressive symptoms. In fact, in one of the largest prospective trials that included pre- and post-treatment evaluations of mood, women continuing on DMPA had lower depressive symptom scores at 1 year than did women who did not continue. Therefore, DMPA use is not contraindicated in patients with a psychiatric diagnosis.

A causal relationship between weight change and use of DMPA has not been found either. A clinical trial was performed where the effect of DMPA on energy expenditure, food intake, and weight was examined. In this randomized, placebo-controlled trial, 20 women were monitored for their body weight, food intake, and energy expenditure. After this, they were randomized to either receive DMPA or a saline placebo. After treatment, there was no significant difference in body weight over time between the two groups. Weight gain while using DMPA is not necessarily an inevitable side effect of the medication.

For lactating mothers, current labeling suggests waiting a period of 6 weeks before initiating DMPA. This recommendation is not supported by the literature. There is no known harmful effect of DMPA use on infant growth and development and there are no contraindications to starting DMPA immediately postpartum. Progestin-only contraceptives may actually increase the quality and duration of lactation. If a mother chooses to wait, then DMPA should be initiated 2 weeks postpartum (after lactation is established) because ovulation can occur as early as 3 weeks postpartum.

The other clinical concern about DMPA use relates to its effects on bone mineral density. While DMPA users are known to have similar peak estradiol levels in the midfollicular phase as cycling women, these levels may decrease over time and affect bone homeostasis. Some studies associate DMPA use with bone loss, but in these studies the bone loss was small and transient, deferring any clinical concern for decades. Furthermore, these studies do not show that the fracture risk is higher in DMPA users. Other studies show no association between bone loss and use of DMPA, but these are retrospective studies and the independent effect of DMPA use is difficult to discern. Therefore the relationship between use of DMPA and bone loss is controversial but a causal relationship has not been demonstrated, nor has a relationship been demonstrated with duration of therapy. No study has associated use of DMPA with any long-term increased risks due to decrease in bone density.

Recently, the FDA released a black box warning regarding prolonged use of DMPA and its effects on skeletal health. Specifically, the concern regarded the loss of bone mineral density (BMD) with prolonged use of DMPA and the possibility that this bone loss was not fully reversible once DMPA was discontinued. Contrary to this warning, multiple studies performed in both adolescents and in former users of DMPA reveal that not only is there no difference in BMD in former users of DMPA as compared to never users of DMPA, but also that this loss of BMD is temporary. The loss of BMD with DMPA use is less than that which occurs during lactation. Following discontinuation of DMPA, BMD in former users of DMPA was found to return to levels similar to or even higher than BMD in never users of DMPA. Given the transient nature of the changes of BMD noted with DMPA use, clinicians should feel comfortable prescribing DMPA to any woman in need of an effective method of contraception without worrying about its effects on skeletal health.

Benefits

As with combined oral contraceptives, there are many noncontraceptive benefits associated with the use of DMPA. These include a significant reduction in risk of endometrial cancer and a possible reduction in ovarian cancer risk. For women with seizure disorders, DMPA is highly effective; first, efficacy is not affected by use of anticonvulsant drugs and second, frequency of seizures actually decreases. Women with sickle cell disease may experience fewer crises while on DMPA. Women with pelvic pain due to endometriosis experience symptom improvement on DMPA.

DMPA and other long-acting contraceptives are thought to be responsible for the drop in the number of teenage pregnancies, abortions, and births. DMPA is one of the few methods that is not user or coital dependent and a single injection provides protection for up to 13 weeks.

Tables 12.5 and 12.6 list instructions for initiating hormonal contraception and for when doses are missed or late.

Table 12.5.   **Instructions for initiating hormonal contraceptives.**[a]

	Start day of cycle	Back-up method required?
Combined oral contraceptives	Day 1	None needed
	Sunday start[b]	For 7 days
	"Quick Start"[c]	For 7 days
Contraceptive vaginal ring	Cycle days 1–5	None
Contraceptive patch	Cycle days 1–7	None
Progestin-only pills	Cycle day 1	None needed
	Sunday start	For 2 days
	"Quick Start"	For 2 days
Progestin-only injectable (DMPA)	Cycle days 1–7	None

[a] Patients may switch directly from one hormonal method to another.
[b] Sunday start is defined as starting method on the first Sunday after cycle day 1.
[c] "Quick Start" is defined as starting method on any day of the menstrual cycle after day 1.

Intrauterine Contraception

Two intrauterine contraceptives are currently available in the United States, a copper-containing IUD and a levonorgestrel-releasing IUD (Table 12.7). While both IUDs have been in use for decades, the newer hormonal IUD was approved for use in the United States in 2000. Each one has a different mechanism of action and insertion technique. Intrauterine contraception is one of the most cost-effective methods of contraception, provided that the IUD is used for at least 2 years. The initial costs of the device are high (despite low manufacture costs), mainly due to the fact that there are few competitive products and that insertion requires special training, but there are no continuing costs associated with the IUD.

Copper Intrauterine Device (CuT380A or Paragard®)

The copper IUD available in the United States is a T-shaped device that is made of a radiopaque polyethylene, wrapped with 380 mm^3 of copper wire. It has two flexible arms that stay open in the uterus, to keep the copper coils against the fundus, but are able to flex for insertion and removal. The monofilament polyethylene string is threaded through the stem and knotted below a blunt ball at the base of the stem, creating a double string that protrudes through the cervix for removal and placement verification.

Table 12.6. Instructions for late or missed doses of hormonal contraception.

	Makeup dose required	EC recommended[a]	Backup recommended[a]	Restart
Combined oral contraceptives				
Missed one pill during cycle week 1	Take missed pill immediately	Yes	For 7 days	Continue current pill pack
Missed one pill in cycle week 2	Take missed pill immediately	No	No	Continue current pill pack
Missed one pill in cycle week 3	Take missed pill immediately	No	No	Start new pack
Missed 2 or more pills collectively in any cycle week	Take missed pills no more than 2 at once	Yes	For 7 days	Start new pack
Progestin-only pills				
If missed one or more pills by more than 3 hours	Take missed pill immediately	Yes	For 2 days	Continue current pill pack
Progestin-only injectable (DMPA) (depot medroxyprogesterone acetate)				

If given after cycle day 8	No	Yes	For 7 days	N/A
If patient late for repeat injection by more than 15 days	Give injection if urinary chorionic gonadotropin is negative	Yes	For 7 days	N/A
Contraceptive vaginal ring				
If ring removed for greater than 3 hours	Replace ring immediately	Yes	For 7 days	Continue cycle with ring
New ring inserted later than cycle day 5	No	Yes	For 7 days	N/A
Contraceptive patch				
If patch is detached for greater than 3 hours	Reapply immediately or place new patch	Yes	For 5 days	Start new patch, continue patch week, change on usual change day
Later than cycle day 7	No	Yes	For 7 days	Make new change date

[a] EC (Plan B®) should be given as soon as possible after unprotected intercourse when a lapse in contraceptive coverage has occurred.

Table 12.7.   Key points of comparison of intrauterine contraception available in the United States.

	Duration of use (years)	Mechanism of action	Average monthly blood loss	Pregnancy rate	Timing of insertion
Copper T380A (Paragard®)	10	Spermicidal	Increased	2% (10 years)	Cycle days 11–15
Levonorgestrel intrauterine system (Mirena®)	5	Increased cervical mucus viscosity	Decreased	1% (5 years)	Cycle days 1–7

The copper IUD is approved for use for 10 years; however, it is proven effective for contraception for up to 12 years. Its failure rate in the first year with typical use is 0.8%. The cumulative 10-year failure rate is about 2%, i.e., better than a traditional tubal ligation.

The mechanism of action of the copper-containing IUD is spermicidal. The copper ions inhibit sperm motility and enzyme activation, thus the sperm are unable to reach the tube and fertilize the ovum. In addition, there is evidence that a sterile inflammatory reaction within the endometrium phagocytizes the sperm. Its action prevents fertilization and therefore the copper IUD is not an abortifacient. The copper IUD increases menstrual blood loss by an average of over 30%, and also increases rates of dysmenorrhea. Both of these can be decreased by nonsteroidal antiinflammatory drug (NSAID) use. In addition, in the first 20 days after insertion, the risk of infection related to insertion increases slightly—about 1/1000 women will get pelvic inflammatory disease. The risk of uterine perforation is equally small and is related to insertion. The risk of expulsion is dependent on the timing of insertion. The risk of expulsion is increased if the copper IUD is inserted during menses or less than 6 weeks postpartum. However, this risk decreases over time; the longer the IUD is in place the lower the risk of expulsion. At the fifth year, the risk of expulsion is approximately 0.3%.

Levonorgestrel-Releasing Intrauterine System (Mirena®)

The levonorgestrel-releasing system was approved for marketing and general use in the United States in 2000. Although similar in shape and efficacy to the Paragard®, it differs in many ways. First, it is approved for use for 5 years and second, its main method of efficacy is hormonal and not spermicidal. In addition, there are differences in both its appearance and its string, as well as its insertion technique.

Contrary to the Paragard® IUD, the Mirena® has arms that are bent at forty-five degree angles. The strings are tied in a knot through a loop at the end of the stem and are different in color (brown) from those of the Paragard®. Insertion of the Mirena® differs widely from that of the Paragard® and clinicians require a review of its insertion technique. While the technique differs from that of the Paragard® insertion, complications are similar.

The reservoir has a stem containing 52 mg of levonorgestrel and is covered by a silicone membrane that is compounded with barium to make the stem radiopaque. This reservoir releases 20 µg per day of levonorgestrel; the serum level achieved is half that reached with Norplant® and one-quarter of that achieved with progestin-only pills. The levonorgestrel causes the cervical mucus to thicken, thereby impeding sperm entry into the uterine cavity. In addition, changes occur in the tubal fluid, which impair sperm migration. And lastly, the levonorgestrel does cause anovulation in a small percentage of cycles.

The Mirena's® main noncontraceptive benefit is the menstrual change that women experience after insertion. Although initially increasing the number of days of spotting after insertion, by the end of 1 year, 20% of users will develop amenorrhea. In most of the other users, menstrual blood loss is decreased by over 70%. Other advantages include a small protective effect against endometrial cancer, a decreased risk of ectopic pregnancy, and a decreased risk of pelvic inflammatory disease. Some physicians, in off-label use patterns, are using the Mirena® to deliver the progestin portion of hormone replacement therapy or to reduce the incidence of benign endometrial polyps in patients being treated with tamoxifen for breast cancer.

Barrier Methods of Contraception

Barrier methods of contraception are user-initiated and coital-dependent. There has been renewed interest in and increased use of barrier methods due to increased education and awareness of prevention of sexually transmitted diseases, including HIV. The most commonly used methods include cervical caps, diaphragms, spermicides and withdrawal, as well as male and female condoms. Barrier methods have some advantages as compared to longer acting or hormonal methods; they do not cause systemic side effects and do not alter bleeding patterns. They can also be used by a woman who needs contraception only intermittently and are immediately effective. When used correctly, barrier methods, particularly the diaphragm and cervical cap, decrease the incidence of cervical cancer by half. Barrier methods alone, however, are not nearly as effective as hormonal or intrauterine contraception at preventing pregnancy.

Condoms

The condom remains one of the most commonly used methods of reversible contraception in the United States (Table 12.8). Condom use has increased

Table 12.8.   Key points of condoms.

	Schedule	Mechanism of action	Efficacy	Special considerations
Male	With every act of intercourse	Act as barrier to sperm penetration	86% (1 year)	Decrease risk of STI
Female	As above	As above	~80% (1 year)	Cannot be used simultaneously

with increasing awareness of its role in preventing transmission of sexually transmitted diseases, especially among adolescents and men. Efficacy in condoms varies but among those using the condom as their primary method of contraception, the unintended pregnancy rate is about 14%. The varying rates of efficacy in condom use are usually attributed to inconsistent use. The rate of breakage and slippage of condoms is very small, as long as the condom is being used correctly. Condoms break less than 2% of the time during intercourse or withdrawal and slip off the penis during 5% of acts of intercourse. However, most studies do not differentiate between complete and partial slippage. The risk of pregnancy and transmission of infections differ between the two but the exact rates are unknown.

While there are several advantages to use of condoms, there are concerns expressed by users. These concerns include a decrease in male sensation and spontaneity and the possibility that they interfere with intercourse. All patients need to be counseled that for condoms to be effective they must be used during the entire act of vaginal intercourse. Male condoms provide very effective protection against most sexually transmitted infections, especially when placed on the penis before any genital contact.

Female condoms are differently designed to provide protection for the entire length of the vagina. They also partially shield the perineum. The female condom is a loose sheath and it has two rings; one lies inside at the closed end of the sheath and helps as an insertion mechanism and internal anchor. The second ring forms the external shield and remains on the perineum to provide protection to the labia and base of the penis during intercourse. The sheath is coated with a silicone-based lubricant that has no spermicide. It can be inserted up to 8 hours before intercourse. Female and male condoms should not be used simultaneously, as that can cause slippage or breakage. In studies, female condom use was found to be acceptable by a majority of users.

About 21% of women will experience an unintended pregnancy within the first year of use of the female condom. The polyurethane of the condom is impermeable and is presumed to provide protection from sexually transmitted infections similar to male condoms.

Diaphragms

There is only one diaphragm available for use in the United States. Diaphragms are dome-shaped rubber cups with a flexible rim and must be inserted before intercourse (Table 12.9). Once inserted correctly, the dome covers the cervix, the posterior rim rests in the posterior fornix, and the anterior rim fits behind the pubic bone. Diaphragms need to be fitted by a clinician for proper fit and size in the vagina. Spermicide is placed in the cup prior to insertion and held in place against the cervix. The diaphragm must be in place for at least 6 hours and provides contraception for up to 6 hours. If additional acts of intercourse occur within 6 hours, fresh spermicide should be applied vaginally (in front of the diaphragm) prior to each act. If the diaphragm is left in longer than 8 hours, then the entire device should be removed and spermicide reapplied to the cervical side of the cup before the next act of intercourse. Current developments to improve the diaphragm are under way. A diaphragm currently being studied for use, unlike currently available diaphragms, requires no fitting, has been designed to ease insertion, and relies on a suction fit to the vaginal tissue rather than a wedge fit behind the pubic bone.

Cervical Caps

The two cervical caps available for use in the United States include the Prentif cap® and the Femcap® (Table 12.10). Cervical caps, unlike diaphragms, fit snugly around the base of the cervix, close to the vaginal fornices. Like diaphragms, the concurrent use of a spermicide is required. The spermicide is

Table 12.9. Key points of diaphragms.

	Schedule	Mechanism of action	Efficacy	Special considerations
Diaphragm	Can be inserted up to 8 hours prior to intercourse	Barrier to sperm penetration	80% (1 year)	Only 56% continue use after 1 year. Must be used with spermicide. Should not be worn longer than 8 hours after intercourse

Table 12.10.   Key points of cervical caps.

	Schedule	Mechanism of action	Efficacy	Special considerations
Prentif® and FemCap®	Up to 6 hours prior to inter-course	Barrier to sperm penetr-ation	40% in parous women 20% in nulliparous women	Spermicide must be used. Cannot be worn longer than 48 hours. 42% continue use after 1 year
Lea's shield®	As above		20% at 1 year	Spermicide needs to be used. Does not require fitting

held in place against the cervix by the cap. Used correctly, the cervical cap provides continuous contraception for up to 48 hours. Additional applications of spermicide are not necessary for further acts of intercourse. The cervical cap should be worn for no less than 24 hours and not longer than 48 hours. As with diaphragms, these cervical caps require fitting around the cervix for ideal use.

Recently, the FDA approved a new cervical cap that does not require fitting. Lea's shield® is a cervical cap that comes in only one size. Like other cervical caps, it requires the use of a spermicide. Unique features of the Lea's shield include a valve that creates a seal between the device and the vaginal wall near the cervix and a loop over the dome for easy removal.

Spermicides

The efficacy of a spermicide depends upon correct and consistent use (Table 12.11). The spermicide needs to make contact with the cervix and should be placed correctly in the vagina no more than 1 hour before each act of inter-course. In studies, failure rates range widely from 5% to greater than 50% during the first year of use. Using spermicides in conjunction with a barrier method increases the efficacy. The advantage of a spermicide is that it can be purchased over the counter, and therefore does not require a visit to a clinician. They may also lower the risk of a sexually transmitted infection by 25%. Similar to barrier methods, spermicides can be stored for long periods of time if inter-course is occasional or unpredictable and can be used as a simple back-up method when hormonal methods are undependable (i.e., missed pills or anti-biotic use). Newer spermicides in development may protect against the HIV virus in addition to bacterial pathogens. Microbicides refer to a range of prod-ucts that prevent sexually transmitted infections, but are not necessarily sper-micidal and therefore do not necessarily provide contraception. Recent evidence

Table 12.11. Key points of spermicides.

	Schedule	Mechanism of action	Efficacy (1 year)	Special considerations
Spermicide	Insert prior to intercourse	Spermicidal	Ranges from 50% to 85%	Decrease risk of sexually transmitted infection, increase efficacy when combined with other barrier method

has emerged that nonoxynol-9, the most common spermicide, does not provide protection against the HIV virus *in vivo*. In addition, frequent use (over eight acts of sexual intercourse per day) can cause epithelial disruption of the vagina and vulva, and increase susceptibility to HIV.

The most common side effect of any spermicide is genital skin irritation, including the vagina, vulva, or penis. This is usually caused by mild local toxicity or allergy. In addition, spermicide can encourage selective colonization of the vagina with anaerobic bacteria and may explain the increased incidence of bacterial vaginosis in some women.

Emergency Contraception

Emergency contraception (EC) is contraception used after unprotected intercourse to prevent pregnancy. Currently, there are two FDA-approved methods available, although there are many off-label methods of EC. Plan B® (Table 12.12) is a progestin-only method of EC, marketed as Plan B®, and can be

Table 12.12. Key points of emergency contraception.

	Route	Dose schedule	Mechanism of action	Pregnancy rate	Special considerations
Plan B®	Oral	As soon after unprotected intercourse before 120 hours	Multiple	<1% in 24 hours	Advance prescription

used for up to 120 hours after unprotected intercourse. It is the most effective method with the fewest side effects available in the United States. The failure rate for Plan B® is about 1.1% when used within 72 hours of unprotected intercourse. The failure rate decreases further with early administration of Plan B. If Plan B is given within the first 24 hours after unprotected intercourse, the failure rate drops to 0.5%. The method continues to reduce the risk of pregnancy when administered up to 120 hours after unprotected intercourse. Side effects occur transiently (<10% of the time), are self-limited, and include nausea, vomiting, headache, mood changes, or change in next menses.

The mechanism of action of EC is not understood precisely. EC does not disrupt an established pregnancy implanted in the uterus. If EC is given before ovulation it may delay ovulation and disrupt normal follicular development. This is the main effect of EC. If given after ovulation, it may affect endometrial maturation and also it may cause thickening of cervical mucus, preventing sperm from entering the upper genital tract. EC can be given as an advance prescription to anyone who is at risk of pregnancy, to increase the likelihood it will be used if needed and to decrease the time interval to dosing. The advance provision of EC will not, however, decrease contraceptive use or increase risky behaviors, even in high-risk populations like adolescents.

Case Studies

Case 1. A 36-year-old G1P1 with well-controlled hypertension is on lisinopril. She is a nonsmoker and is in a monogamous relationship.

Choices for contraception include the following:

1. Combined hormonal contraception. Hypertension (HTN) is a WHO eligibility category 2 for OC use, a condition in which the advantages of using the method generally outweigh the risks of pregnancy with the condition. As long as the patient's hypertension is well controlled, her risk of adverse events, such as myocardial infarction and cerebral vascular accident, is no higher than if she did not use OCs. The risks would change if she smoked. At her age, her risk of an adverse event with use of combined hormonal contraception would be significantly increased. This is due to the increased risk of a thromboembolic event with tobacco use and age over 35 years. The risk of using combined hormonal contraception is still not greater than if she became pregnant, so effective contraception is indicated. Currently no data are available for the vaginal ring or the patch but recommendations for these methods are the same as OCs.

2. Progestin-only contraception. There is no increase in blood pressure with use of progestin-only methods. These would be recommended in patients with uncontrolled hypertension or those who are over the age of 35 years and are smokers.

3.   Intrauterine contraception. This is another excellent method that provides long-term contraception at no increased risk of complications from the patient's hypertension.

4.   Barrier methods. While barrier methods are also not contraindicated, their efficacy is lower than any other method available.

Case 2. A 35-year-old G3P2 has diabetes. Her diabetes is currently well controlled and the patient has normal renal function. She weighs over 220 pounds (BMI = 38).

Choices for contraception include the following:

1.   Combination hormonal contraception. This condition is listed as a category 3. This means a condition in which the risks of the method outweigh the advantages of the method. However, if this patient were to become pregnant, her course might be complicated. OCs have not been found to impair glucose metabolism or accelerate the incidence of vascular disease in diabetic women. Nor do oral contraceptives precipitate the occurrence of non-insulin-dependent diabetes. Despite the category 3 designation, OCs can be used in patients with well-controlled diabetes who have no evidence of untreated vascular complications like nephropathy or retinopathy. The patch and contraceptive vaginal ring can both be used in women with diabetes, as the recommendations remain the same. However, for this patient, the patch would be highly ineffective due to her weight.

2.   Progestin-only contraception. There is no evidence that these methods interfere with glucose metabolism or cause vascular complications and they can be safely used in diabetic women.

3.   Intrauterine contraception. The local action of the IUDs makes this an ideal method of contraception, without contraindications for this patient.

4.   Barrier methods. While barrier methods are also not contraindicated, their efficacy is lower than any other method available.

Case 3. A 26-year-old female has migraine headaches associated with neurologic symptoms on the left side of her face. These include mainly tingling and numbness. She has been using oral contraceptive for 5 years.

Choices for contraception include the following:

1.   Combination hormonal methods. Women using oral contraceptives who develop migraine headaches were noted to have a 6-fold increased risk of ischemic stroke in a large hospital-based case controlled study; this increases to over a 34-fold increased risk if the patient used OCs, had migraines, and smoked. Given the fact that this patient has migraine headaches associated with neurologic foci, combination hormonal methods are not an appropriate method of contraception.

2.   Progestin-only methods. Methods containing progestin alone are preferred because they provide effective hormonal contraception and do not increase the risk of stroke.

3.   Intrauterine contraception. Once again, this is highly effective contraception that avoids the increased risk of a thromboembolic event and is excellent for patients at risk of stroke.

4.   Barrier methods. While barrier methods are not contraindicated for use, their efficacy is lower than any other method available.

13

Coronary Heart Disease in Women: Diagnosis, Evaluation, and Preventive Therapy

Nanette K. Wenger

Background Information

Coronary heart disease, traditionally considered a problem predominantly for men, is currently the leading cause of mortality in adult women in the United States, responsible for about 250,000 deaths annually. The substantial age dependency of coronary heart disease in women is important in that one of eight or nine women aged 45 to 64 years has clinical manifestations of coronary heart disease, in contrast to one of three women older than 65 years. Despite these data, until very recently, most information used to guide preventive strategies, clinical recognition, and therapy of coronary heart disease in women was extrapolated from studies conducted predominantly or exclusively in middle-aged men.

The lifetime risk of mortality for menopausal women (and U.S. women today spend about one-third of their life in menopausal status) defines coronary heart disease as their major clinical problem, with a 31% mortality risk. This contrasts with less than a 3% mortality risk from hip fracture (as a surrogate for osteoporosis) and a less than 3% risk for breast cancer mortality. As the total U.S. population ages, more women survive to older age when coronary heart disease becomes clinically manifest. Coronary heart disease causes significant morbidity among women as well. Thirty-six percent of women aged 55–64 years with coronary heart disease are disabled by symptoms of their illness, with this percentage rising to more than 55% among women aged 75 years and older. This mandates intensive preventive efforts across their lifespan and appropriate diagnostic efforts in later life to minimize the current high rates of morbidity and mortality for women.

Based on 1990–1991 U.S. data, there were 0.8 million annual coronary heart disease-related hospitalizations for women, 3.9 million physician office visits, health care costs of $11 billion, and total economic costs of $22 billion, documenting coronary heart disease in women as an important challenge to our national public health.

Evaluation of Chest Pain Syndromes

Chest pain is the predominant initial and subsequent presentation of coronary heart disease in women, in contrast to myocardial infarction or sudden death as the predominant presentation for men. Additionally, more women than men are likely to have had antecedent stable angina prior to an initial myocardial infarction.

Therefore, a pivotal approach to the care of women with chest pain syndromes is to differentiate those due to coronary heart disease, which has a relatively unfavorable prognosis if untreated, from chest pain due to noncoronary causes, which often has a benign prognosis (Table 13.1). The clinical history alone is inadequate to do so, and objective confirmatory testing is required. Registry data from the Coronary Artery Surgery Study (CASS) document that among patients referred to coronary arteriography to evaluate chest pain syndromes, 50% of women, as compared with 17% of men, had minimal or no coronary atherosclerotic obstruction.

While the optimal timing and selection of noninvasive diagnostic procedures continue to evolve, substantial advances have occurred in the selection and utilization of these tests for women with chest pain.

The Exercise Electrocardiogram

Exercise testing remains the cornerstone of the noninvasive evaluation of myocardial ischemia. Owing to the lower pretest likelihood of coronary heart disease in women of young to middle age than for comparably aged men, an

Table 13.1.   Evaluation of chest pain in women: diagnostic testing.[a]

Test procedure	Data for women
Exercise ECG	Young women: low pretest likelihood → ↑ false-positive results
	Older women: many cannot exercise adequately, many have baseline ST abnormalities
Exercise radionuclide myocardial perfusion imaging	
Thallium-201	Gender-based criteria ↓ false-positive tests secondary to breast attenuation
Technetium 99 sestamibi	? ↑ value for women
Pharmacologic radionuclide perfusion studies	For women unable to exercise
	? ↑ side effects in women
Exercise radionuclide ventriculography	Cannot use ↓ exercise EF to suggest myocardial ischemia in women
Exercise/pharmacologic echocardiography	High sensitivity and specificity, even with single vessel disease
	Cannot always obtain adequate image
Ultrafast CT	Cannot quantify myocardium at risk
PET • under investigation	
MRI • ? ↑ diagnostic accuracy for women	No ionizing radiation
MRA • ↑ cost	No ionizing radiation

[a] ECG, electrocardiogram; EF, ejection fraction; CT, computed tomography; PET, positron emission tomography; MRI, magnetic resonance imaging; MRA, magnetic resonance angiography.

abnormal test is more likely to represent a false-positive result in these women. Some women in the older age group, who have a greater pretest likelihood of coronary heart disease, are unable to perform an adequate exercise-based test; their substantial prevalence of nonspecific repolarization abnormalities on the resting electrocardiogram (ECG) precludes exercise electrocardiographic studies. Further, older women more often have concomitant medical problems that may lead to false-positive exercise test results or limit their ability to exercise to adequate intensity. Thus, exercise ECG testing has been viewed by clinicians as a suboptimal diagnostic modality for women. Nonetheless, data from the CASS confirm that with a normal resting electrocardiogram and reasonable exercise tolerance, there is a comparable diagnostic value of exercise ECG testing by gender. A negative Duke Treadmill Score is described as better in excluding coronary heart disease for women than for men. Additionally, given the low pretest likelihood of coronary heart disease in young and middle-aged women, a normal exercise test result has powerful predictive value for excluding coronary heart disease, with this negative predictive value comparable to that for men.

The Task Force on Exercise Testing of the American College of Cardiology/American Heart Association suggests that because the exercise ECG for women is less specific than for men, an imaging study may often be a better initial choice. The average 57% sensitivity and 61% specificity of the exercise ECG in women contrasts with 78% and 86%, respectively, for imaging studies.

Exercise Radionuclide Myocardial Perfusion Imaging

Radionuclide-based exercise testing increases the sensitivity and specificity of the exercise test in both genders, with the predominant data available for thallium 201 perfusion imaging. Although earlier studies highlighted a large proportion of false-positive tests for women, resulting from breast attenuation artifact, contemporary gender-specific interpretation shows good predictive accuracy of exercise thallium scintigraphy for women. Technetium 99m sestamibi imaging, studied in populations of both genders, has shown good sensitivity and specificity of this test for women, with recent reports suggesting better results with technetium than with thallium perfusion imaging for women.

Women who have a normal myocardial perfusion imaging study have a low risk for future coronary events, with a risk as low as 0.6% described.

Exercise Radionuclide Ventriculography

There are gender differences in the response of the ventricular ejection fraction to exercise. Men achieve their exercise-related increase in cardiac output predominantly by an increase in ejection fraction, whereas in women and in elderly individuals of both genders this is accomplished predominantly by an increase in end-diastolic volume. Thus, lack of an increase in ejection fraction with exercise, highly suggestive of coronary heart disease in men, fails to provide diagnostic accuracy for women and is not recommended.

Pharmacologic Radionuclide Perfusion Studies

Limited data suggest that pharmacologic (persantine or adenosine) radionuclide perfusion studies, typically undertaken in patients unable to exercise, have comparable predictive accuracy for both genders, once correction is made for breast attenuation artifact.

Exercise and Pharmacologic Echocardiography

Although echocardiographic studies have involved small numbers of women, high sensitivity and specificity are reported even in the presence of single vessel disease, owing to the ability to detect focal wall motion abnormalities. Some reports describe exercise echocardiography as better than exercise ECG or exercise thallium testing for the identification of coronary heart disease in women. Detection of exercise-induced wall motion abnormalities independently predicted subsequent cardiac events in women and may be useful even with single and double vessel disease. However, adequate echocardiographic windows may limit the performance of these studies. Studies are lacking in populations of women with a low prevalence of coronary heart disease, such that the likelihood of false-positive studies remains uncertain.

Tests Under Investigation

The diagnostic value of electron beam ultrafast CT for detecting coronary calcification is currently under study. Women generally have similar age- and risk-adjusted coronary calcium scores as men. Nonetheless, this test is unlikely to provide adequate information regarding risk stratification, in that the extent of myocardium in jeopardy is not evaluated. Only limited data are available regarding positron emission tomography (PET) imaging, magnetic resonance imaging (MRI), and magnetic resonance angiography (MRA); however, available reports suggest that these may be gender-neutral tests, independent of body configuration, with substantial diagnostic value for women.

The emphasis to primary care physicians is the compelling need to evaluate chest pain syndromes suggestive of angina pectoris in women; objective confirmation of the presence and extent of myocardial ischemia is necessary for subsequent diagnostic and therapeutic decisions.

Clinical Characteristics and Therapies of Coronary Heart Disease in Women

Women with chest pain syndromes compatible with angina pectoris historically had far less aggressive diagnosis and management than did their male counterparts. Whereas two decades ago there was a 10-fold greater likelihood of men than women with abnormal noninvasive exercise-based tests being referred for coronary arteriography, there is currently almost comparable referral by gender. Coronary arteriography is a major determinant of access to revascularization procedures, with comparable gender revascularization described based on results of coronary arteriography; this is important in that the diagnosis of coronary heart disease entails a more adverse prognosis for women than for their male peers. Advances in diagnostic strategies may not yet be evident as improvements in clinical outcomes.

Women who present with angina pectoris tend to be older than men and to more frequently have associated hypertension, diabetes, and heart failure; as well, they were less likely to have had a prior myocardial infarction or prior myocardial revascularization.

The prevalence of chest pain appears similar in women and men with acute coronary syndromes, but women are more likely to have atypical symptoms as well. In the Euro Heart Survey Prospective Registry, more than 85% of women and men with acute coronary syndromes had typical angina pectoris at presentation, without clinically significant differences by sex. Women with acute coronary syndromes are more likely to have unstable angina than enzyme- or ECG-documented acute myocardial infarction. They also had greater delay in seeking emergency care than did men after the onset of symptoms. Studies of invasive versus conservative management for acute coronary syndromes identify that this decision should be based on objective risk stratification measures, rather than being influenced by the sex of the patient. Only in higher-risk women does the benefit of an invasive strategy seem to balance the early procedural risks.

Data from the National Registry for Myocardial Infarction (NRMI) identify that one-third of all myocardial infarctions in the United States occur in women. Women were older than men at presentation and had a longer time from symptom onset to arrival at hospital. They also had a greater mortality than men, even when matched for age, both with and without thrombolytic therapy. Women with myocardial infarction were less likely to undergo coronary arteriography, percutaneous coronary interventions and coronary artery bypass graft surgery (Table 13.2). The 1-year mortality following myocardial infarction is comparably increased, particularly early postinfarction mortality. A number of factors may be contributory. First is the frequent atypical presentation of myocardial infarction for women, who often describe shortness of breath and extreme fatigue, both with and without classic chest pain. Next is the decreased use of thrombolytic therapy for women with ST elevation acute myocardial infarction, in great part due to their late arrival at hospital, beyond the optimal time for such therapy. Additionally, because more women than men with myocardial infarction are incorrectly diagnosed at presentation, they are less likely to receive prompt life-saving medical management with heparin, β-blocking drugs, and aspirin therapy. Women are referred less frequently than men to rehabilitation following a coronary event, despite demonstrated comparable improvement in exercise capacity with exercise training; decreased application of risk reduction strategies may likewise have an adverse impact. Additionally, the prior less-frequent risk stratification following a coronary event may have limited referral for revascularization when appropriate. Women are more likely to have depression following myocardial infarction than their male peers, and this may also influence excess mortality rates.

Women who undergo coronary artery bypass graft surgery are older than their male counterparts and have more frequent comorbidity, particularly diabetes and hypertension. They have an almost doubled hospital mortality compared to men with such surgery, with women experiencing decreased graft

Table 13.2. Coronary heart disease in women: therapeutic strategies.

Intervention	Data for women vs. men
Antianginal drugs	Minimal gender-specific data
Lipid-lowering drugs	Comparable benefit
Angiotensin-converting enzyme inhibitors	Comparable benefit
Thrombolytic therapy	Comparable benefit
	↑ risk bleeding complications
Acute angioplasty (MI)	Comparable benefit
Aspirin	Similar secondary prevention benefit
Exercise rehabilitation	Current ↓ referral
	Comparable ↑ exercise capacity
Balloon angioplasty (PTCA)	Comparable procedural success, safety
	↓ symptom relief, ↑ mortality
Other transcatheter revascularization procedures	↓ procedural success, ↑ complications
Coronary artery bypass graft surgery	↓ operative mortality, complications
	Comparable long-term survival

Source: Adapted from Agency for Healthcare Research and Quality, Evidence Report/Technology Assessment Number 80 and 81, May 2003.

patency, less symptomatic relief, and more reoperation within the initial 5 years. Nonetheless, women who survive the hospital stay have 15-year survival rates comparable to those for men. Recent data suggest that the majority of excess mortality among women involves patients with diabetes or with urgent or emergency presentations. These features suggest a potential for improvement in outcomes. Off-pump compared with conventional coronary artery bypass graft surgery appears to reduce mortality, respiratory complications, and length of hospital stay for women.

Despite comparable procedural success rates and safety with percutaneous transluminal balloon coronary angioplasty (PTCA), women report less symptomatic relief and their long-term survival is less favorable, predominantly owing to older age at the time of the procedure. Recent data show that despite persistent high-risk characteristics for women undergoing percutaneous interventions, the procedural success rates and outcomes for women have improved over time. After controlling for other factors including older age, women did not have significantly greater likelihood of death or death and nonfatal myocardial infarction. Nonetheless, following percutaneous interventions, women continue to have more symptoms than men and these symptoms are associated with self-reported limitations in activity and quality of life.

Potential contributors to less successful revascularization outcomes for women include an excess of urgent or emergency procedures, the older age at which women undergo these procedures, and their substantially greater comorbidity, particularly diabetes and hypertension.

Coronary Preventive Interventions

Preventive interventions are the cornerstone of a primary care approach to coronary heart disease in women (Table 13.3). Lifestyle approaches including smoking cessation, regular exercise, a heart healthy diet, and weight management are recommended for all women. The contemporary emphasis is that the baseline level of cardiovascular risk of an individual woman should determine the intensity of coronary risk interventions.

Forty percent of all coronary events in women are fatal, and nearly two-thirds of all sudden deaths in women occur in those not previously

Table 13.3. Coronary risk reduction strategies.[a]

Component	Recommendations
Lifestyle interventions	
Smoking	Consistently encourage patient/family to stop smoking and avoid environmental tobacco.
Heart healthy diet	Consistently encourage healthy eating pattern including fruits, vegetables, grains, low- or nonfat dairy products, fish, legumes, protein sources low in saturated fat (poultry, lean meats, plant sources). Limit saturated fat intake <10% of calories and cholesterol <300 mg/day. Decrease transfatty acid intake.
Weight management	Consistently encourage weight maintenance/reduction through physical activity, decreased caloric intake, and formal behavioral programs to achieve BMI 18.5–24.9 kg/m² and waist circumference <35 in.
Physical activity	Consistently encourage at least 30 minutes of moderate intensity physical activity such as brisk walking on most days of the week.

Table 13.3. *Continued.*

Component	Recommendations
BP control	Lifestyle approaches to achieve optimal BP <120/80 mm Hg.
	Pharmacotherapy when BP ≥140/90 mm Hg or lower with BP-related target organ damage. Include thiazide diuretics in drug regimen unless contraindicated.

Major risk factor interventions

Lipid management	Lifestyle approach to achieve optimal levels: LDL <100 mg/dl, HDL >50 mg/dl, TG <150 mg/dl, non-HDL <130 mg/dl.
	With increased LDL or in high-risk women[b] decrease saturated fat intake <7% of calories, cholesterol <200 mg/day, decrease transfatty acid intake.
	High-risk women[b] LDL >100 mg/dl: initiate LDL lowering therapy, preferably with a statin simultaneously with lifestyle interventions. Initiate niacin or fibrate therapy with low HDL or elevated TG or non-HDL. Consider statin therapy in high-risk women with LDL <100 mg/dl.
	Intermediate risk women[c]: as above but with LDL ≥130 mg/dl. Niacin/fibrate therapy after LDL goal is reached.
	Lower risk women[d]: as above but with LDL ≥160 mg/dl with multiple risk factors or LDL ≥190 mg/dl with 0–1 risk factor. Niacin/fibrate therapy after LDL goal is reached.
Diabetes mellitus	Lifestyle and pharmacotherapy to achieve HbA$_{1C}$ >7% in diabetic women.

Preventive drug therapy

Aspirin	81–325 mg aspirin (or clopidogrel if aspirin intolerant) in high-risk women[b] unless contraindicated.

Continued.

Table 13.3. *Continued.*

Component	Recommendations
	Reasonable to use aspirin in intermediate-risk women[c] if BP is controlled and benefit outweighs risk of GI side effects.
	Do not routinely use aspirin for low-risk women.[d]
β-Blockers	Use indefinitely after MI or with chronic ischemic syndromes unless contraindicated.
ACE inhibitors	Use unless contraindicated in high-risk women.[b]
	Use ARBs in high risk-women[b] intolerant of ACE inhibitors.
Menopausal hormone therapy	Do NOT initiate or continue to prevent CVD in menopausal women.
Antioxidant drugs	Do NOT initiate or continue to prevent CVD.

[a] BP, blood pressure; BMI, body mass index; LDL, low-density lipoprotein; HDL, high-density lipoprotein; TG, triglyceride; GI, gastrointestinal; MI, myocardial infarction; ACE, angiotensin-converting enzyme; ARB, angiotensin receptor blocker; CVD, cardiovascular disease; CHD, coronary heart disease.

[b] High risk: CHD or risk equivalent. Global risk >20%.

[c] Intermediate risk: global risk 10–20%.

[d] Low risk: global risk <10%.

Source: Adapted with permission from Mosca L, Appel LJ, Benjamin EJ, et al. Evidence-Based Guidelines for Cardiovascular Disease Prevention in Women. Expert Panel/Writing Group, American Heart Association. *Circulation* 2004;109(5):672–93. Copyright 2004 Lippincott Williams & Wilkins.

known to have coronary heart disease. Although certainly not all sudden death events are coronary in etiology, a majority are likely to be so. Coronary risk factors appear to predict the occurrence of sudden cardiac death.

Coronary risk factors are highly prevalent among women in the United States. Based on 1991 data from the National Center for Health Statistics, one-third of U.S. women aged 20 to 74 years have hypertension, and one-quarter have hypercholesterolemia, are cigarette smokers, are overweight, or have a sedentary lifestyle (Table 13.4).

Coronary risk factors predominate among women with less favorable socioeconomic circumstances and lower educational levels, and commonly these coexist. As such, physicians who provide primary care for these women must appreciate the heightened need for coronary prevention. Although both cardiovascular and coronary mortality continue to decline in both genders, in recent years the decline for women has been less prominent than that for men. Further, the decline in coronary risk factors among women during the past two to three decades has been less pronounced than for men, partly related to targeting of risk reduction messages to populations of men.

Based on follow-up data from NHANES I, the relative risk of coronary heart disease by gender shows that hypertension imparts a comparable relative increase in risk, 1.5 for women and men; hypercholesterolemia imparts somewhat more risk for men, a 1.1 relative risk in women versus 1.4 in men; diabetes is a substantially higher contributor to the risk for women, with a relative risk of 2.4 versus 1.9 for men; overweight is slightly more important for women, 1.4 versus 1.3 for men; as is smoking, 1.8 for women versus 1.6 for men.

Cigarette Smoking

Of women in the United States aged 18 years and older, 23% still smoke cigarettes; this underestimates smoking prevalence among women in that teenaged girls are prominent among cigarette smokers. The current relatively comparable prevalence of cigarette smoking by gender relates to the far more effective smoking cessation among men in recent years. Among women, there is now a greater intensity of smoking as well as an earlier onset of smoking behavior. Further, smoking lowers the age of menopause by almost 2 years, with the longer time in menopausal status a potential added contributor to the smoking risk. Cigarette smoking accounts for about 60% of the coronary risk in middle-aged women. Smoking at least triples the risk for myocardial infarction, even for premenopausal women, and is an important contributor to sudden death in young women, mandating intensive efforts to effect smoking cessation. Data

Table 13.4. Prevalence of coronary risk factors—U.S. women—20–74 years of age.

1/3 Hypertension
1/4 Hypercholesterolemia
1/4 Cigarette smokers
1/4 Overweight
1/4 Sedentary lifestyle

Source: Adapted from 1991 data from the National Center for Health Statistics.

from the Nurses' Health Study suggest that within 2 years of smoking cessation, former smokers decrease their cardiovascular mortality risk by 24%. The benefit of smoking cessation does not decrease with older age, such that smoking cessation should be encouraged across the lifespan.

Hypertension

Fifty-one percent of white women and 79% of black women in the United States older than 45 years of age have hypertension; this percentage increases to more than 71% among women older than 65 years of age. The pattern of increase in blood pressure varies by gender. Whereas systolic blood pressure in men peaks in middle age, levels of systolic blood pressure in women continue to rise until beyond age 80 years, such that isolated systolic hypertension predominates in elderly women. After 65 years of age, more women than men have hypertension. Lifestyle modifications can prevent hypertension. Control of hypertension decreases both the risk of stroke and that of fatal and nonfatal coronary events and heart failure (Table 13.5). Goal levels of blood pressure treatment should be lower if multiple risk factors are present.

Cholesterol and Lipoproteins

The pattern of lipid levels also varies by gender, with hypercholesterolemia more prevalent in middle-aged and older women, being a particularly prominent problem in menopausal women. Across the life span, women have higher levels of high-density lipoprotein (HDL) cholesterol than do men, and this does not substantially change with menopausal status. At young to middle age, women have lower levels of low-density lipoprotein (LDL) cholesterol than do their male counterparts. Total cholesterol levels among women rise

Table 13.5. Classification of blood pressure for adults (aged 18 years and older).

Blood pressure	Systolic (mm Hg)		Diastolic classification (mm Hg)
Normal	<120	and	<80
Prehypertension	120–139	or	80–89
Stage 1 hypertension	140–159	or	90–99
Stage 2 hypertension	≥160	or	≥100

Source: Adapted from Chobanian A, Bakris G, Black H, et al. The Seventh Report of the Joint National Committee on Prevention, Detection, Evaluation, and Treatment of High Blood Pressure. The JNC 7 Report. *JAMA* 2003;289:2560–72.

progressively with aging, at least to age 70 years, because of a progressive increase in LDL cholesterol, which, in the menopausal years, exceeds the levels in comparably aged men. The combination of low HDL cholesterol and elevated triglyceride levels appears to impart greater risk for women than for men. Notably limited are primary prevention trials of lipid lowering in women in general and elderly women in particular. Nonetheless, the Adult Treatment Panel III of the National Cholesterol Education Program (NCEP) offers comparable recommendations for women and men. Five clinical trials of pharmacologic lipid lowering published between 1996 and 1998 showed that the overall reduction in major coronary events was similar in treated women and men, but a mortality benefit was not evident for women, likely owing to the small numbers of women studied. In the Heart Protection Study, 40 mg of simvastatin daily reduced coronary events by nearly one-third in both sexes, independent of age, diabetic status, and initial cholesterol level. A systematic review of the efficacy of lipid-lowering therapy to reduce coronary risk in women showed that this therapy reduced coronary mortality by 26%, nonfatal myocardial infarction by 36%, and major coronary events by 21%. Lipid lowering was not shown to reduce the rates of revascularization procedures or the risk of total mortality.

Glucose Intolerance and Diabetes Mellitus

Diabetes is a far more powerful risk factor for women than for men, essentially negating the gender-protective effect, even for premenopausal women. It remains unclear why diabetic women have a greater coronary risk than diabetic men, although diabetic women commonly have more and more severe coronary risk factors. Diabetes tends to cluster with hypertension, hyperlipidemia, and central obesity in the metabolic syndrome. Current recommendations are that diabetes mellitus be considered a coronary risk equivalent, such that concomitant coronary risk factors require more precise control in diabetic women.

In the Nurses' Health Study, maturity-onset diabetes was associated with a 3- to 7-fold increase in cardiovascular events, with this risk sizably augmented when associated with other coronary risk factors. The incidence of diabetes was reduced among women in the Nurses' Health Study who exercised regularly, suggesting that exercise was an important intervention for women with a strong family history for diabetes or women with gestational diabetes. Both lifestyle interventions and therapy with metformin can reduce the incidence of diabetes. Although diabetes is associated with a less favorable hospital and long-term prognosis following myocardial infarction for both genders, the adverse effect is accentuated among women, doubling their risk of recurrent myocardial infarction, and increasing 4-fold the risk of cardiac failure. Further, among patients undergoing myocardial revascularization, both coronary artery bypass grafting (CABG) and PTCA, the prevalence of diabetes is greater among women than among men, likely adding adversely to the prognosis.

Obesity and Body Fat Distribution

The prevalence of obesity in the United States is greatest among minority populations and those of lower socioeconomic and educational levels. National Center for Health Statistics data from 1998 indicated that 50% of black women and 30% of white women had body weight levels 20% or more greater than desirable. Framingham data define obesity as a significant independent predictor of cardiovascular disease, particularly among women; obesity is associated with elevated levels of total cholesterol, triglyceride, and LDL cholesterol, lowered levels of HDL cholesterol, as well as insulin resistance, hyperuricemia, and hypertension. Weight control, in a number of studies, improved the coronary risk profile. Recently reported 15-year follow-up data from the Nurses' Health Study showed that increased body weight was directly related to increased all-cause mortality, with the lowest mortality rate evident among women who weighed at least 15% less than the U.S. average, who never smoked, and who had stable weight since adulthood.

The pattern of body fat distribution is important because central obesity, i.e., a waist-to-hip ratio of 0.8 or greater, is associated with a substantial increase in coronary risk.

Exercise and Physical Fitness

Physical inactivity is a highly prevalent and independent risk factor for coronary heart disease in women. Whereas 25% of young women describe no leisure-time physical inactivity, this percentage increases to 50% in women of elderly age. Data from 1988 show that 6 of 10 U.S. women are sedentary, with a progressive trend to inactivity in recent years, most prominent in lower socioeconomic and educational groups. Objectively measured physical fitness is associated with a more favorable coronary risk profile, and this association is more powerful for women than for men. Primary care providers must encourage habitual physical activity for women. Habitual exercise is associated with a decreased coronary risk even in old age. In the Women's Health Initiative Observational Study, both walking and vigorous exercise were associated with substantial reductions in cardiovascular events in menopausal women. However, women appear to require more assistance and follow-up than men to induce the behavioral change of reversing a sedentary lifestyle.

Menopausal Hormone Therapy: Is There Evidence for Coronary Disease Prevention

Owing to the unfavorable outcomes of coronary events in women as compared to men and the older age of occurrence for coronary heart disease in women than men, interest was raised in the potential of menopausal hormone therapy to provide cardiac protection. This was buttressed by multiple biologically plausible benefits of estrogen use including a more favorable lipid profile, decreased LDL oxidation, a generally more favorable coagulation profile, decreased levels of homocysteine, decreased inflammatory response to athero-sclerosis and decreased vascular smooth muscle proliferation, and promotion of endothelium-dependent vasodilation, among others. Unfavorable effects were acknowledged including an increase in triglyceride concentration and in the inflammatory marker C-reactive protein with oral estrogen use. Addition-ally, a number of observational studies and metaanalyses of these studies uni-formly showed a 35–50% reduction in coronary risk, particularly among current estrogen users. Nonetheless, concern was raised with these observational data as selection bias, compliance bias, ascertainment bias, etc., may exaggerate benefits and underestimate risks of hormone use. To reinforce this concern, a recent reanalysis of the observational data just cited, where the studies were adjusted for socioeconomic status, educational level, and major coronary risk factors, failed to demonstrate cardiac protection with hormone therapy and thus to support the use of such therapy for the primary prevention of coronary and cardiovascular disease.

Pivotal randomized controlled clinical trial data further fail to support cardiac protection. The landmark Heart and Estrogen/progestin Replacement Study (HERS) compared the use of estrogen/progestin with placebo in women with documented coronary heart disease. There was no significant difference in the primary trial outcome of nonfatal myocardial infarction and coronary death. However, concern was raised by an excess number of coronary events in the hormone-treated group in the first year of treatment, with a trend to fewer events in subsequent years. Follow-up of 93% of surviving HERS participants in an observational study, HERS II, failed to provide evidence of reduction in the risk of coronary events, even after adjustment for potential confounding factors, including statin use. If coronary benefit had been demonstrated, limited harm might be acceptable; however, with lack of coronary benefit, potential harm, including a twofold increase in the risk of venous thromboembolism, predominantly in the initial years, and an almost 50% increase in the rate of gallbladder disease requiring surgery, raises substantial concerns. Based on the HERS data, this hormone regimen of conjugated equine estrogen plus medroxyprogesterone acetate should not be used to decrease the risk of cardiovascular events in women with coronary heart disease.

Primary prevention data derive from predominantly healthy meno-pausal women, aged 50–79 years, enrolled in the Women's Health Initiative (WHI) hormone trial. Approximately 17,000 women were randomly assigned to receive conjugated equine estrogen and medroxyprogesterone acetate daily versus placebo. As in HERS, this regimen was selected as the hormone prepa-ration most commonly used by U.S. women. The trial was halted prematurely at the recommendation of the Data Safety and Monitoring Board, after an average follow-up of 5.2 years, because of an increased risk of invasive breast cancer that exceeded the preset trial-stopping boundaries, combined with a lack of global risk benefit, again based on a preestablished global risk score. The parallel estrogen only versus placebo arm of WHI, for women who had a hysterectomy, is continuing. The harm in WHI included a 26% increased risk for invasive breast cancer; a 29% increase in the risk of coronary events, predominantly nonfatal myocardial infarction; a 41% increased stroke risk; and a doubled risk of venous thromboembolism. The benefits included a 37% decrease in colorectal cancer, a 33% decrease in hip fracture, and a 24% decrease in total fracture. Total mortality was not affected. Importantly, the risk for myocardial infarction began within the initial year of hormone therapy and that for stroke in the initial 2 years; myocardial infarction risk predominated in the younger women.

Although the majority of women in the WHI estrogen/progestin randomized trial had no adverse events, one adverse event can be anticipated for each 100 such women treated for 5 years. Importantly, the population risk, extrapolated to the 10 million menopausal women who are current hormone users, is substantial. The conclusion of WHI is that the global risk–benefit profile does not warrant recommendation of this therapy as a widespread preventive intervention for women. Data for estrogen only therapy are pending.

Further analysis of the estrogen/progestin versus placebo arm of the WHI randomized trial showed no clinically meaningful benefit in general health, vitality, mental health, depressive symptoms, or sexual satisfaction based on questionnaire data. As well, subset data on women older than age 65 years showed a doubled likelihood of developing dementia in hormone-treated women, although the absolute risk of dementia was low. Hormone therapy did not affect mild cognitive impairment. In another substudy, a small number of hormone-treated women had statistically significant and clinically important decrements in cognition compared with placebo-treated women.

Neither was hormone benefit demonstrated in the Women's Angiographic Vitamin and Estrogen (WAVE) trial, with potential for harm suggested, or in the WELL-HART (Women's Estrogen-progestin Lipid-Lowering Hormone Atherosclerosis Regression Trial), an angiographic study with a sizable percentage of women of racial or ethnic minorities.

The recommendation of the U.S. Preventive Services Task Force is that hormone therapy should not be used routinely for the prevention of chronic conditions in menopausal women.

The January 2003 labeling requirements of the U.S. Food and Drug Administration (FDA) for all estrogen and estrogen/progestin products require identification that they are not approved for heart disease prevention and that their use increases the risks of heart disease, heart attack, stroke, and breast cancer. The FDA advises women to discuss with their health care providers other approaches to reduce risk factors for coronary heart disease such as diet, smoking cessation, and blood pressure control. To these I would add exercise and lipid management, interventions documented to improve coronary heart disease outcomes.

Summary

Recent data highlight coronary heart disease as a major health problem for U.S. women. Also, women with established coronary heart disease have less favorable outcomes than do their male counterparts following both myocardial infarction and myocardial revascularization procedures. This warrants meticulous attention to the evaluation of chest pain syndromes, identifying those due to myocardial ischemia, and to the institution of the requisite medical and surgical therapies.

Preventive interventions are necessary and very beneficial. Primary care physicians should assess coronary risk status for women across the lifespan and institute appropriate preventive strategies.

Suggested Reading

Agency for Healthcare Research and Quality. Results of systematic review of research on diagnosis and treatment of coronary heart disease in women. Evidence Report/Technology Assessment Number 80. U.S. Department of Health and Human Services, Public Health Services. AHRQ Pub. No. 03-E034, May 2003.

Agency for Healthcare Research and Quality. Diagnosis and treatment of coronary heart disease in women: Systematic reviews of evidence on selected topics. Evidence Report/Technology Assessment Number 81. U.S. Department of Health and Human Services, Public Health Services. AHRQ Pub. No. 03-E036, May 2003.

American Diabetes Association. Implication of the Diabetes Control and Complications Trial. *Diabetes Care* 2003;26:S25.

American Heart Association. Heart Disease and Stroke Statistics—2003 Update. Dallas, TX: American Heart Association; 2002.

Chobanian A, Bakris G, Black H, et al. The Seventh Report of the Joint National Committee on Prevention, Detection, Evaluation, and Treatment of High Blood Pressure. The JNC 7 Report. *JAMA* 2003;289:2560–72.

Executive Summary of the Third Report of the National Cholesterol Education Program (NCEP) Expert Panel on Detection, Evaluation, and Treatment of High Blood Cholesterol in Adults (Adult Treatment Panel III). *JAMA* 2001;285:2486–97.

Grady D, Herrington D, Bittner V, et al. for the HERS Research Group. Cardiovascular disease outcomes during 6.8 years of hormone therapy: Heart and Estrogen/progestin Replacement Study follow-up (HERS II). *JAMA* 2002;288:49–57.

Mosca L, Appel LJ, Benjamin EJ, et al. Evidence-Based Guidelines for Cardiovascular Disease Prevention in Women. Expert Panel/Writing Group, American Heart Association. *Circulation* 2004;109(5):672–93.

Wenger NK, guest ed. Symposium: gender differences in cardiac imaging. *Am J Card Imag* 1996;10:42–88.

Wenger NK. Coronary heart disease: the female heart is vulnerable. *Prog Cardiovasc Dis* 2003;46:199–229.

Wenger NK. Menopausal hormone therapy. Is there evidence for cardiac protection? In *Contemporary Cardiology: Coronary Disease in Women: Evidence-Based Diagnosis and Treatment.* LJ Shaw, RF Redberg (eds). Totowa, NJ: Humana Press Inc.; 2003: pp 321–48.

Writing Group for the Women's Health Initiative Investigators. Risks and Benefits of Estrogen Plus Progestin in Healthy Postmenopausal Women. Principal results from the Women's Health Initiative Randomized Controlled Trial. *JAMA* 2002;288:321–33.

14

Dermatologic Disorders

Jeffrey P. Callen

Background Information
Approach to the Patient (Dermatologic Diagnosis)

Only with proper diagnosis can an appropriate approach to therapy and discussion of prognosis occur. Dermatologic diagnosis is based on history, physical examination, and laboratory evaluation. In addition, careful and complete documentation of cutaneous abnormalities is necessary.

Historical information should include the duration of the problem, the progression of the disease, whether there are any associated symptoms, and the type of previous therapy, including over-the-counter preparations. Often the physical examination is performed after a brief history, and then as a differential diagnosis is being formulated, a more in-depth history is added.

Physical examination of the skin should be complete. The examination involves visual inspection and palpation. Examination should also include the hair, nails, and mucous membranes. Findings are characterized by the type of lesions(s) present, the location of the process, the configuration, and the distribution. The examiner should assess for primary lesions, those related to the skin disease, and for secondary lesions, those related to secondary factors such as rubbing (lichenification), scratching (excoriations), infection (impetiginization), or loss of tissue (erosion, ulceration, or atrophy). The color of a lesion is also important, and at times subtle color differences are significant in the differential diagnosis.

Description of dermatologic lesions in objective terms is extremely useful in dermatologic diagnosis. Physicians in the late nineteenth and early twentieth centuries were superb clinicians and used careful description of cutaneous disease for diagnostic and classification purposes. These skills have often been undervalued in the age of advanced technology, but with a keen eye and careful description, the diagnosis—or at worst, a differential diagnosis—can be accurately made. To do this it is necessary to know how and to use proper terminology for lesions, configurations, and distributions (Table 14.1).

Dermatologic diagnosis can, in simplistic terms, be subdivided into growths and rashes. Growths can be further divided into those that affect the epidermis or the dermis and those that are pigmented. Rashes can be subdivided into those with epidermal involvement versus those with dermal involvement. An algorithmic approach to dermatologic diagnosis is presented in Figs. 14.1 and 14.2.

Table 14.1.   Definitions for cutaneous findings.

Lesion	Appearance
Macule	Flat with color (e.g., red, brown)
Patch	Flat with color and surface change (e.g., scale)
Papule	Elevated <0.5 cm in diameter
Plaque	Elevated >0.5 cm in diameter, but without depth
Nodule	Elevated and indurated, >0.5 cm in diameter and depth
Cyst	A nodule filled with fluid or semisolid content
Vesicle	A small blister, filled with visible clear fluid, <0.5 cm
Bullae	Same as vesicle, but >0.5 cm
Pustule	Same as vesicle except fluid is yellow
Wheal	Edematous plaque (hive)
Erosion	Partial loss of the epidermis
Ulcer	Wound with loss of all of the epidermis and part or all of the dermis
Descriptive terms	
Erythema	Blanchable redness due to dilated blood vessels
Purpura	Nonblanchable, deep red or purple color due to extravasated blood
Hyperpigmented	Increased pigment
Hypopigmented	Decreased pigment
Surface change	
Crust	Dried serum, pus, or blood on surface of skin (scab)
Scale	White or whitish flakes on surface of skin
Lichenification	Thickened skin with accentuated surface markings
Configurations/distributions	
Linear	In a line
Herpetiform	Grouped lesions
Annular	Active border
Dermatomal	Curvilinear following a dermatome
Photodistribution	Occurring on sun-exposed surfaces

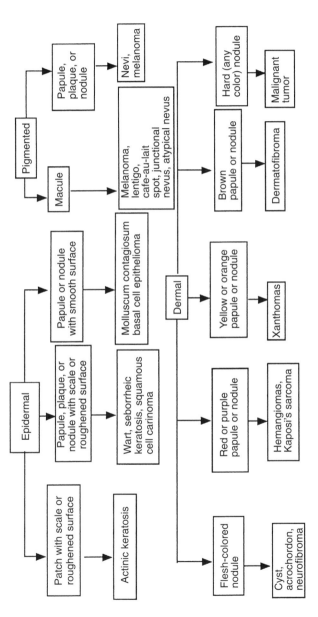

Fig. 14.1. Algorithm of growths.

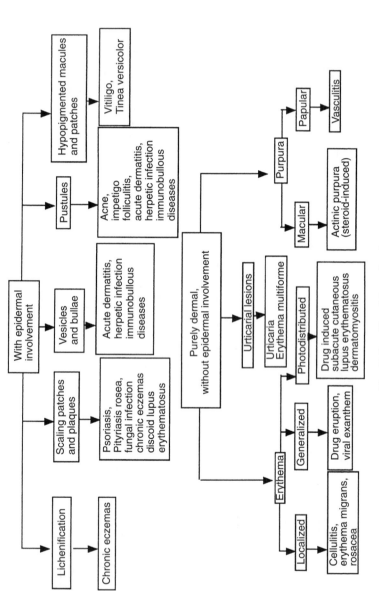

Fig. 14.2. Algorithm of rashes.

Laboratory evaluation in dermatologic diagnosis is invaluable in instances where diagnosis cannot be established by a history and clinical examination. The most frequent tests used are (1) microscopic analysis of skin scrapings for infectious agents, e.g., potassium hydroxide preparation for fungi, wet mount for scabies or pediculosis or Tzanck smear (for herpes virus infections), or (2) skin biopsy. Skin biopsy is an interpretive skill and is dependent on the proper selection of the site for biopsy and on the ability of the pathologist. While the procedure itself is quite simple, correct diagnosis is possible only when a representative lesion of appropriate age is sampled properly (by shave biopsy, elliptical incisional biopsy, or punch biopsy). Information about the clinical disease should be provided to the dermatopathologist rather than sending the specimen without any information or with information such as "rash" or "lesion." A clinical differential diagnosis is often useful in the examination of the specimen. It is important to be aware that the biopsy result is subjective rather than objective, and thus the "pathological" diagnosis must be interpreted in the context of the disease observed by the clinician (clinical–pathologic correlation). If the clinician is unequipped to provide the information to the pathologist or is unable to interpret the meaning of the pathologic diagnosis, a dermatologist should be consulted.

Common Tumors
Epidermal Tumors

These tumors are characterized by (1) a scaly patch, (2) a papule, plaque, or nodule with a scaly or roughened surface, or (3) a papule or nodule with a smooth surface. The most common epidermal tumor characterized by a scaly patch is the actinic (or solar) keratosis (AK) (Fig. 14.3; see color insert). There are most often multiple lesions, and they occur on exposed surfaces, particularly the head and neck, dorsal hands, extensor forearm, and anterior leg. These lesions are often better palpated than visualized, and they feel somewhat like sandpaper. Most authorities believe that somewhere between 0.25% and 20% of AKs will develop into a squamous cell carcinoma if left untreated. However, there are some lesions that may spontaneously disappear. AKs occur in the context of malignant lesions such as squamous cell carcinoma or basal cell carcinoma, and thus their recognition should lead to a careful inspection to rule out coexistent pathology. Treatment of AKs involves destructive methods (liquid nitrogen, curettage, and electrodesiccation, peels) or topical application of chemotherapeutic agents (diclofenac, fluorouracil, or imiquimod). Regular use of sunscreen with SPF of 15 or greater can reduce the appearance of new lesions as well as aid the process of spontaneous regression. Reexamination is necessary to follow patients and detect new AKs or other lesions.

Bowen's disease is a form of *in situ* squamous cell carcinoma and is also characterized by a persistent scaly patch. These lesions are at times mistaken for psoriasis or eczema, and thus when healing of such a lesion does not occur with appropriate therapy, a biopsy should be performed.

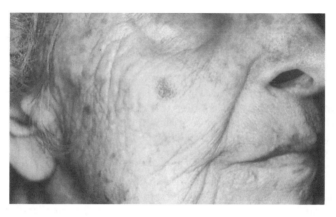

Fig. 14.3. Actinic keratosis: rough, scaly patch on the cheek. Note the background actinic damage, wrinkling, and solar lentigines. (See color insert.)

The most common papules, plaques, or nodules with a roughened or scaly surface are warts, seborrheic keratoses, or squamous cell carcinomas. Warts result from infection of the epidermis by various human papilloma viruses (HPV). The infecting agent varies by body site, and only a limited number are oncogenic. Warts commonly occur on the hands, the feet (plantar warts), or the genitalia (condyloma). Flat warts are a particular type that is commonly found on the legs of women. Shaving often enhances the spread of these lesions. Warts may be self-limiting, but treatment generally involves attempts at destruction.

Seborrheic keratoses (SKs) are benign epidermal tumors characterized most often by hyperpigmented verrucous plaques or nodules that appear to be "stuck on" the skin surface (Fig. 14.4; see color insert). They are generally of cosmetic concern, but lesions that are irritated, infected, or bleed can be treated by cryosurgical destruction or light curettage. SKs are acquired with their onset in persons 30 years or older, and they increase in size and number with age. Biopsy is indicated when the diagnosis is uncertain.

Squamous cell carcinomas tend to occur in sun-exposed skin of older patients. There is often a background of photodamage, and these patients frequently have AKs and lentigines accompanying the squamous cell carcinoma. Lesions are often flesh-colored, red, or tan with an adherent thick scale (Fig. 14.5; see color insert). As the lesion progresses, ulceration is possible. These lesions are locally invasive, but also there is some potential for metastases, particularly to local nodes. Various means of removal, destruction, or radiation therapy are effective.

The most common papules or nodules with a smooth surface that are found on the epidermis are molluscum contagiosum and basal cell carcinomas. Molluscum contagiosum are small, flesh-colored or pink papules with

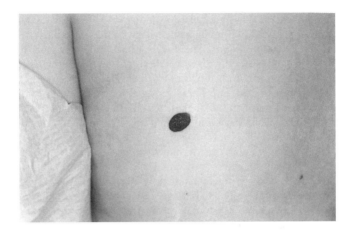

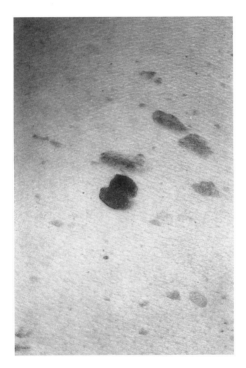

Fig. 14.4. Seborrheic keratosis. (top) Dark, sharply marginated, verrucous nodule on this patient's back. This lesion was regularly irritated by her bra, and it was therefore removed with curettage and destruction. (bottom) Multiple seborrheic keratoses. (See color insert.)

a central umbilication. They are caused by a pox virus. Molluscum contagiosum are common in children and in sexually active adults. In adults the lesions tend to occur in the groin area. The disease is self-limiting, except in HIV-positive patients and patients with atopic dermatitis in which the lesions may become quite extensive. Individual lesions may be removed with a sharp curette or blade or treated with liquid nitrogen for destruction. Imiquimod has also been used successfully for these lesions and is particularly useful in patients with multiple lesions, or in whom destructive methods are not desirable, such as children.

Basal cell carcinoma is the most common cancer in humans. The lesions occur most often on sun-exposed surfaces in older adults. These tumors are generally slow-growing and rarely metastasize. They may become locally invasive if left untreated and have been reported to cause death on rare occasions. The lesion is most commonly characterized by a pearly (translucent) papule with prominent telangiectasia (Fig. 14.6; see color insert). The border may be rolled, and central ulceration is common in more mature lesions. There are several clinical variants including superficial basal cell epitheliomas, pigmented basal cell epitheliomas, and sclerosing basal cell epithelioma. The sclerosing basal cell epithelioma is an important lesion to recognize because

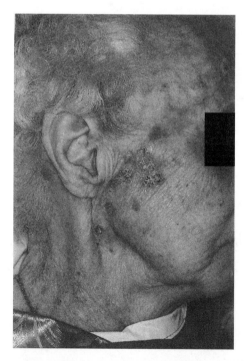

Fig. 14.5.   Squamous cell carcinoma. (See color insert.)

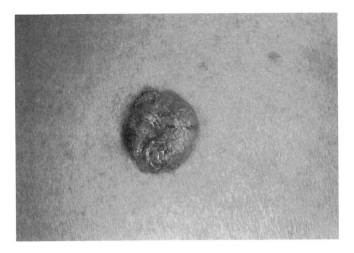

Fig. 14.6.   Basal cell epithelioma. (See color insert.)

invasion is much more aggressive. Surgical excision, destruction, and radiation therapy are effective methods of treatment of basal cell epitheliomas.

Dermal Tumors

Dermal growths represent proliferation of cellular elements in the dermis. They may be flesh-colored, red, purple, yellow, or brown papules, nodules, or tumors; or they may be hard nodules or tumors. Most dermal growths appear as nodules of the skin. If a nodule cannot be clinically diagnosed, an incisional or excisional biopsy should be performed.

Acrochordons (skin tags) are soft, pedunculated, skin-colored polypoid papules that are most common on intertriginous surfaces. They have a benign course, but can be removed if they bleed, become infected, are repeatedly irritated, or for cosmetic reasons.

Dermatofibromas are pea-sized nodules that may be slightly hyperpigmented. The lesion is firm and may be depressed or slightly elevated. On pinching the skin, they often will "dimple" or "button-hole." The cause is unknown, but they are often noted after minor trauma or an insect bite. The dermatofibroma is a benign lesion, but may be removed if it is continually irritated.

Sebaceous hyperplasia occurs on the face as small yellow or translucent papules. They occur in middle age and slowly increase in number and size. They need to be removed only when there is a question about whether they are basal cell epitheliomas.

The hypertrophic scar is a thickened, firm, flesh-colored, or reddish-brown growth in any area where trauma or a surgical incision occurs. The hypertrophic scar rarely overgrows the original injury and will spontaneously flatten or resolve over the course of several months or years.

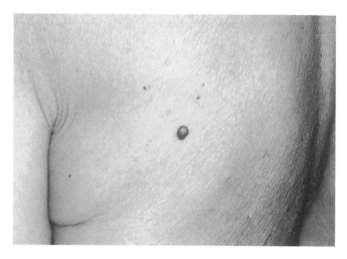

Fig. 14.7. Cherry angioma. (See color insert.)

In contrast, the keloid is an exuberant growth of collagen that may occur following injury or in some patients may occur spontaneously. Keloids are commonly treated with intralesional injections of triamcinolone acetonide. Other therapies include silicone gel dressing, excision, and radiation.

Chondrodermatitis nodularis helices are small, tender, flesh-colored to red nodules on the helix of the ear. Occasionally the surface has an adherent crust or scale. These lesions are possibly related to trauma and/or actinic damage. If there is a questionable malignancy, a biopsy should be performed, otherwise, they can be left alone, injected with corticosteroids, frozen with liquid nitrogen, excised, or destroyed.

The fibrous papule is a dome-shaped, translucent lesion most often noted on the nasal ala, but lesions can occur anywhere on the head or neck. They may be mistaken for intradermal nevi or basal cell epitheliomas. No treatment is necessary.

Cysts are nodules or tumors that have an epithelial lining. A miniature form of the epidermal inclusion cyst is known as a milium. These lesions are common on the face of women and are represented as small, white papules. No treatment is necessary unless the cyst becomes infected.

Syringomas are multiple, skin-colored to yellowish papules that usually occur on the lower eyelids and cheeks. They occur more commonly in people with Down's syndrome, but most patients with syringomas are otherwise healthy. No treatment is necessary for these lesions.

Cherry angiomas are common benign vascular tumors. They occur in adulthood and increase in number with age. They are manifest as small, bright red, smooth, dome-shaped papules, and are most common on the trunk (Fig. 14.7; see color insert). No treatment is needed unless the lesions bleed.

Another vascular tumor is the pyogenic granuloma. These are sessile or pedunculated growths that are usually solitary. They frequently bleed with minor trauma. There is often a history of trauma that precedes the onset of the lesion, and growth is often rapid. Pyogenic granulomas may be more frequent in pregnancy. Treatment with destructive methods, excision, or laser ablation is effective.

Pigmented Lesions

Melanomas are classified into at least four clinical types. The superficial spreading malignant melanoma, which has a horizontal growth, appears as an irregular, pigmented patch (Fig. 14.8; see color insert). The nodular melanoma, which has converted to a vertical growth, has a poorer prognosis. Lentigo maligna melanoma is an irregular pigmented patch on the face (Fig. 14.9; see color insert). This lesion is often large in diameter, but is superficial in depth. It may be preceded by a benign process, the lentigo maligna. The acral lentiginous melanoma occurs on acral areas.

Lesions that may be precursor pigmented lesions include congenital nevi, atypical nevi (Fig. 14.10; see color insert), and the lentigo maligna. The issue of whether these lesions should be removed is controversial. Large congenital nevi are difficult to remove, and it is these lesions that have the greatest risk. Atypical nevi (formerly dysplastic nevi) are not in themselves precursors, but their presence may represent the expression of a genetic process that predisposes to a greater risk of melanoma. Changing lesions should be removed. Photographic documentation is often useful in following patients with multiple atypical nevi.

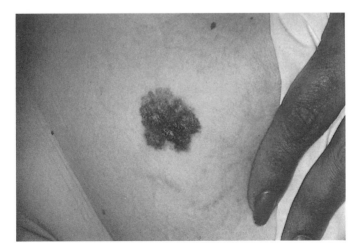

Fig. 14.8. Superficial spreading malignant melanoma. (See color insert.)

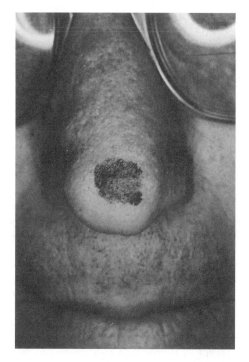

Fig. 14.9.   Lentigo malignant melanoma. (See color insert.)

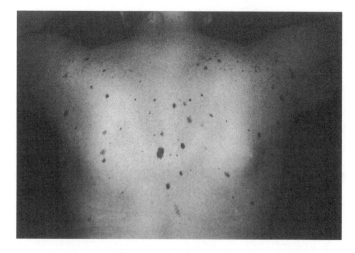

Fig. 14.10.   Atypical nevi—multiple. (See color insert.)

The common benign nevi are junctional, compound, or intradermal. These lesions appear in adolescence and early adult life and disappear with further aging beyond the fifth decade. The junctional nevus is a macular darkly pigmented lesion. Intradermal nevi are elevated tan or flesh-colored lesions, whereas compound nevi have both junctional and intradermal components. Less common nevi include the blue nevus, which is a benign dermatological collection of melanocytes, and the halo nevus, in which there is a depigmenation surrounding a junctional or compound nevus. A lentigo is a brown lesion, which is often sun-induced.

The most important issues are the recognition of melanoma and its differentiation from benign pigmented lesions. Melanoma is suspected when pigmented lesions exhibit *a*symmetry, *b*order irregularity, *c*olor variation, *d*iameter greater than 6 mm, and noted *e*nlargement. Not all melanomas will exhibit all features. Benign nevi do appear beginning in adolescence and ending in the third and fifth decades. Thus, not all lesions that are of recent onset are melanomas. When there is any question, an excisional biopsy should be performed. However, if the lesion is large, a representative area may be sampled without compromising the patient's prognosis.

Rashes

Epidermal Involvement

Scaly Patches and Plaques

Eruptions characterized by scaly patches and plaques may be acute or chronic. Common causes of eruptions include pityriasis rosea, secondary syphilis, seborrheic dermatitis, lichen planus, and superficial fungal infections. Common chronic eruptions include psoriasis, chronic eczemas, and discoid lupus erythematosus.

Pityriasis rosea is characterized by erythematous to fawn-colored plaques, most often distributed in a symmetric fashion on the trunk. There is often an initial round lesion, the so-called herald patch that precedes the development of multiple oral patches and plaques. The distribution takes on the appearance of a "Christmas" tree, as the lesions follow Blaschko's lines. Lesions develop over a period of 1 to 4 weeks. Pruritus may occur and can at times be intense. Diagnosis is confirmed on the basis of the clinical appearance, coupled with negative skin scrapings for fungal elements and a negative serologic test for syphilis. The course is self-limiting over a 4- to 8-week period, but ultraviolet B phototherapy may shorten the course and aid in relief of pruritus. One recent report has suggested that oral erythromycin shortens the course.

Secondary syphilis is an acute papulosquamous eruption that may simulate pityriasis rosea or lichen planus or seborrheic dermatitis. Mucosal involvement and involvement of the palms and soles are often clinically useful signs in distinguishing syphilis, but the diagnostic test is a positive STS

(VDRL, FTA, or other). Untreated secondary syphilis may self-resolve, thus serologic testing is indicated whenever syphilis is considered in the differential diagnosis.

Seborrheic dermatitis is often acute in its onset or exacerbation, but it is a chronic process. This disease is commonly characterized by a pruritic, scaly, erythematous scalp dermatitis. A "greasy" scale on an erythematous base of the eyebrows, the glabella area, the nasolabial folds, the midchest and the groin are common (Fig. 14.11; see color insert). When only the scalp is involved, seborrheic dermatitis may be difficult to differentiate from psoriasis. Scalp disease is treated with zinc or tar-based shampoos with or without a topical corticosteroid lotion. Cutaneous disease is treated with a low potency topical corticosteroid often combined with precipitated sulfa.

Lichen planus is a pruritic eruption characterized by flat-topped violaceous papules and plaques with a fine white scale. The scale may be reticulated, may be more noticeable when wet, and has been termed Wickham's striae. The lesions are commonly on the wrists and legs. Oral lesions occur in 25–50% of patients and more frequently appear as reticulated white patches along the bite line. Lichen planus-like disease may be drug-induced and therefore a careful analysis of drugs that patients might be taking is important. In addition, hepatitis C virus infection appears to be more common in patients with lichen planus, particularly those patients with severe erosive oral disease. Topical corticosteroids, oral antihistamines, and a short course of oral corticosteroids (2–3 weeks) are frequently effective. Recurrence, however, occurs in about 25% of the patients.

Superficial dermatophyte infections are common. Proper therapy depends on diagnosis, and thus when considering a fungal infection, skin

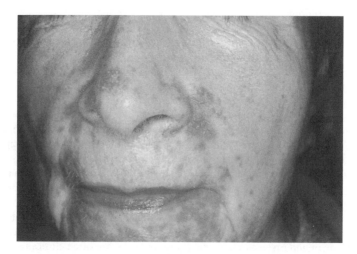

Fig. 14.11. Seborrheic dermatitis. (See color insert.)

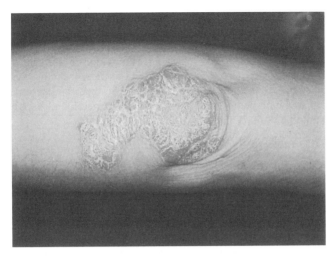

Fig. 14.12. Psoriasis. (See color insert.)

scrapings and/or culture should be performed. The scrapings are examined using potassium hydroxide, which is heated slightly to aid in scale dissolution.

Psoriasis is characterized by well-demarcated, erythematous plaques covered by a silvery white scale (Fig. 14.12; see color insert). It can occur at any time of life, but early adulthood is most common. Several stimuli are known to exacerbate psoriasis and include streptococcal infections, HIV infection, lithium therapy, systemic corticosteroid withdrawal, and antimalarial therapy. Psoriasis is most often distributed symmetrically on the extensor surfaces (elbows, knees) but also commonly affects the scalp, genitalia, and nails. The diagnosis is confirmed clinically, and disease of the scalp is differentiated from seborrhea, the nails from dermatophyte infection, and the genitalia from dermatophyte infection, candidal infection, or seborrhea. Localized disease is treated with topical corticosteroids, calcipotriol, tazarotene, tars, or intralesional injection of corticosteroids. Widespread disease is treated with phototherapy, methotrexate, oral retinoids, cyclosporin, or one of the newer biologic agents including etanercept, alefacept, efalizumab, adalimumab, and infliximab. The choice and administration of phototherapy or a systemic agent should occur only in the office of a physician familiar with the selection and safe use of these agents.

Chronic forms of eczema are characterized by thickened erythematous plaques with some scale. *Lichenification* is the term used to denote this thickening and signifies that the patient has rubbed or excoriated the lesion. Various forms of eczema exist, including atopic dermatitis and contact dermatitis. Pruritic eczematous eruptions can be due to infestation by scabies, and when considered appropriate, skin scrapings can aid in diagnosis. Patients with patterns of disease that suggest external factors should be carefully questioned and perhaps patch tested. Eczema responds to avoidance of irritants, clearing of any secondary infections, elimination of allergens if identified, topical corticosteroids, topical immunomodulators including tacrolimus and pimecrolimus, and oral antipruritics. Patients with widespread disease may be treated with phototherapy. Systemic corticosteroids, although widely used, should be avoided if at all possible.

Rashes Characterized by Vesicles and Bullae

Vesiculobullous disease can be divided into conditions that result in subcorneal vesicles, intraepidermal blisters of spongiotic, acantholytic, or ballooning degeneration variants or blisters at the epidermal basement membrane. Vesicles and bullae can eventually become pustules, and when they break, they become erosions. Thus when examining patients these diseases are considered when there are vesicles, bullae, pustules, or erosions. They may be acute or chronic. Acute vesiculobullous disorders include bullous impetigo, eczemas, superficial fungal infections, Stevens–Johnson syndrome (SJS), and herpes virus infections. Chronic vesiculobullous diseases include some eczemas, bullous pemphigoid, pemphigus, and other autoimmune blistering conditions.

Bullous impetigo is most often due to staphylococcal infection. It is characterized by flaccid blisters and erosions with a golden crust (Fig. 14.13; see color insert). It is more prevalent in warmer climates and in patients living under crowded conditions. Therapy with topical antibiotics or systemic antibiotics is curative. A search for a carrier state in patients or family members is advisable in patients with recurrent impetigo.

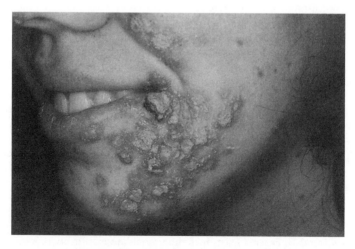

Fig. 14.13. Impetigo. (See color insert.)

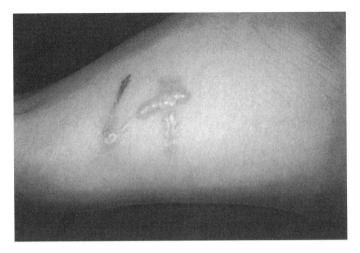

Fig. 14.14. Acute dermatitis due to contact with poison ivy (Rhus dermatitis). (See color insert.)

Acute eczemas are characterized by blistering. Acute exacerbations of hand eczema can cause subcorneal vesicles on the lateral aspects of the fingers. Acute contact dermatitis such as Rhus dermatitis is frequently manifested by blistering (Fig. 14.14; see color insert). Therapy depends on the severity of the reaction. In patients with moderate to severe disease, systemic corticosteroids should be administered in a tapering dose beginning with 0.5–1 mg/kg/day and tapered over 10–14 days.

Certain dermatophytes can cause a vesicular disease that mimics dermatitis. Potassium hydroxide preps or fungal cultures will confirm the diagnosis. Therapy with topical and possibly systemic antifungal agents is curative.

SJS or erythema multiforme major involves multiple mucosal surfaces with erosions and cutaneous vesiculation affecting less than 10% of the body. Individuals with greater than 30% body surface vesiculation are termed toxic epidermal necrolysis (TEN). SJS is rarely fatal whereas 30% of patients with TEN die. Therapy is drug withdrawal with supportive measures. Recent data from open-label trials suggest that the early administration of intravenous immune globulin (0.75 gm/kg for 4 days) results in cessation of disease progression and improved survival.

Herpes simplex virus (HSV) may occur on any body surface. Those on the face are frequently due to HSV type I, while those on the genitalia or buttocks are most often due to HSV type II. The process is marked by recurrent eruptions with vesicles, pustules, and eventually erosions. Several patterns exist. Herpetic whitlow is an infection of the fingers and is more common in dentists, dental hygienists, and pulmonary technicians. Eczema herpeticum is a widespread infection that occurs in patients with chronic eczema. HSV infections are more prevalent and more severe in patients infected by the HIV virus.

The varicella-zoster virus is responsible for chicken pox in its primary stage and herpes zoster (shingles) as a manifestation of recurrence. Herpes zoster often begins with unilateral pain that is followed within several days by grouped vesicles in a dermatomal distribution (Fig. 14.15; see color insert). The incidence of herpes zoster appears to be rising, and it occurs more frequently in HIV-infected individuals. Herpes zoster was the initial event leading to serologic testing and discovery of HIV. It is controversial whether all herpes zoster patients should be serologically tested for HIV, but I inform the patient of the association and offer testing. The eruption is self-limiting, but pain may persist following resolution. The frequency of postherpetic neurology rises with age. Newer antiviral therapy with famciclovir or valaciclovir may limit the acute eruption and reduce the duration of postherpetic pain.

Bullous pemphigoid is the most common immunobullous disease. Its prevalence is unknown. Bullous pemphigoid is generally a disease of the elderly (over 60 years old). The disease is characterized by tense bullae on an erythematous base. Prodromal phases of generalized pruritus or urticarial lesions may occur. The diagnosis is confirmed by biopsy for both routine and immunofluorescence processing. Bullous pemphigoid can be associated with other autoimmune phenomena or disorders; however, malignancy is no more

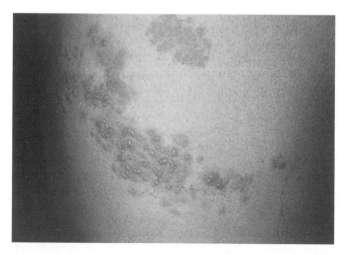

Fig. 14.15.   Herpes zoster: shingles. (See color insert.)

than in an age-matched population. Corticosteroids in low to moderate doses are usually effective. Steroid-sparing agents such as niacinamide, tetracycline, dapsone, or immunosuppressive drugs may be used in selected patients.

Rashes Characterized by Pustules

Pustules are due to infiltration of white blood cells into the skin. These can be follicular, as in acne vulgaris or folliculitis, or nonfollicular, as in impetigo or in later stages of blistering disorders.

Folliculitis refers to inflammation of the hair follicle. This may occur due to bacterial invasion of an irritated follicle or direct bacterial invasion. Tight-fitting clothing and poor hygiene are frequent causes of folliculitis. Cleansing with an antibacterial agent is often sufficient, while at times an oral antibiotic may be required.

Acne vulgaris is a disease of the follicles that is due to an abnormal keratinization that is at least in part hormonally triggered. In addition, bacteria that are part of the normal flora (propionbacterium acnes) act on excess sebum to cause inflammation. Almost all individuals will have acne at some point in their lives.

Therapy for acne is directed at affecting the pathophysiology of disease production. Topical application of a retinoid acts at the follicular level and alters keratinization. Benzoyl peroxides are topical antibacterial agents and may be combined with traditional, topical antibiotics. A new topical preparation, azeleic acid, may also affect keratinization. Oral antibiotics, tetracycline, erythromycin, doxycycline, or minocycline are utilized for inflammatory acne. These antibiotics are labeled by the FDA as possibly interacting with oral contraceptives; however, the prevalence of this "interaction" is unknown. In addition, vaginal candidiasis is more common with antibiotic use. Tetracycline and doxycycline are potential photosensitizers, and the patient should be cautioned about this aspect of the therapy. Oral isotretinoin is an extremely useful agent for patients with severe cystic acne. It is reserved for patients who fail to respond to less toxic therapies. Adequate birth control is necessary to prevent retinoid embryopathy.

Erosions

Erosions signify a loss of the epidermis. They are a "secondary" phenomena in patients with acute eczema or vesiculobullous diseases. They may be an early event in the patient with impetigo. Impetigo, characterized by superficial erosions and crusts, is due to staphylococcal or streptococcal infection. It is more prevalent in tropical environments and in overcrowded households. Antibiotics selected for effectiveness against the causative organisms are curative. Nonbullous impetigo due to certain streptococcal organisms can be complicated by acute glomerulonephritis and can lead to renal failure. It does not appear that the treatment of impetigo alters the risk for glomerulonephritis. However, preventive measures can lower the risk of impetigo.

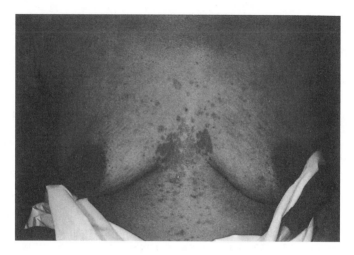

Fig. 14.16.   Tinea versicolor. (See color insert.)

Ulcers

Ulceration implies loss of the entire epidermis and some of the dermis. Healing will result in scarring. Ulcers are also considered to be a secondary phenomenon due to a preceding vasculopathy, a necrotic tumor, or eczematous process with external manipulation. Ulceration is most common on the leg and can generally be characterized as venous, arterial, or neuropathic. Separating these factors will lead to more effective therapy. Consideration of diseases that cause plugging or disruption of the small blood vessels such as vasculitis, paraprotein, or embolization should occur. Ulcers are usually cultured and biopsied to aid in their assessment.

Hypopigmented Macules and/or Patches

The most common cause of hypopigmented patches is tinea versicolor (TV). This disease can also result in hyperpigmented patches (Fig. 14.16; see color insert). The usual presentation of TV is asymptomatic, slightly scaly, hyperpigmented or hypopigmented patches on the upper trunk and upper extremities. The disease is often observed during summer months when tanning of the normal skin highlights the lesions of TV. A scraping for potassium hydroxide preparation is diagnostic. Treatment with a short course of an oral antifungal along with a prolonged course of a topical antifungal (imidazole or selenium sulfide) can control the process.

Vitiligo is an acquired loss of pigment. In this condition an immunologic aberration leads to dysfunction and possibly destruction of melanocytes. Periorifical and acral areas are often first affected. The lesions are asymptomatic, but sunburn can occur in the depigmented skin. Examination with a Wood's light will allow identification of otherwise unrecognized lesions. Diseases associated with autoantibodies are more common in vitiligo, but there is no agreement about the extent of evaluation of patients with vitiligo. Localized areas will occasionally repigment with potent topical corticosteroid or tacrolimus application. Extensive areas require narrow band UVB phototherapy, photochemotherapy (PUVA), or depigmentation. Vitiligo is a disease process, not merely a cosmetic problem.

Dermal Rashes (No Epidermal Involvement)

Erythema can be localized, facial, photodistributed, and generalized. Acute onset of localized erythema can occur in early lesions of contact dermatitis or can occur in cellulitis, a bacterial infection usually caused by β-hemolytic streptococci. Erysipelas is a superficial form of cellulitis that most often affects the face. Lesions of erysipelas are tender, erythematous, brawny, well-demarcated plaques. Fever is common. Systemic antibiotics are necessary for erysipelas and cellulitis.

Facial erythema is a common problem, for which clinical histopathologic and laboratory information must be combined to properly diagnose the patient. Photosensitivity diseases, including lupus erythematosus, polymorphous light eruption, dermatomyositis, and drug-induced phototoxicity, may present as facial erythema. Seborrheic dermatitis may have little scale and be confused with a facial erythema.

Rosacea is a common cause of facial erythema. It occurs in adults and is manifested as central facial erythema, telangiectasias, and inflammatory nodules and occasionally pustules (Fig. 14.17; see color insert). The red

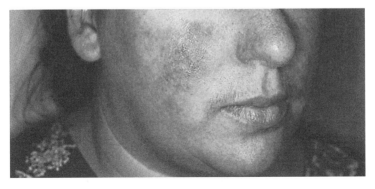

Fig. 14.17.   Rosacea. (See color insert.)

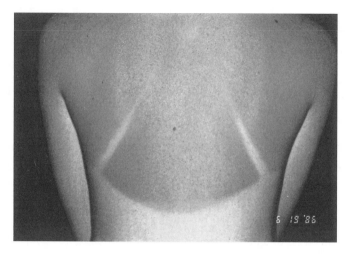

Fig. 14.18. Photosensitivity dermatitis: phototoxic reaction secondary to tetracycline. (See color insert.)

face that occurs in middle-aged women is often confused with lupus erythematosus. Since middle-aged women often have a positive antinuclear antibody (ANA), rosacea adds to this confusion. Biopsy for routine processing is helpful in the differential diagnosis. Rosacea is treated topically with low-potency topical corticosteroids combined with 1% precipitated sulfur, with topical metronidazole, or with topical azeleic acid, with or without oral antibiotics.

Photodistributed erythema is a special form of localized erythema. A photodistribution occurs with facial lesions, the sides of the neck, the upper chest and back, and exposed portions of the arms (Fig. 14.18; see color insert). The acral areas of the fingers are less affected than the proximal areas, and there is often sparing of the interdigital web spaces. The most common photosensitivity eruption is drug-induced phototoxicity. Commonly involved drugs include tetracyclines, thiazides, sulfonamides, and phenothiazines. Most photosensitivity is induced by UVA light, thus traditional sunscreens are often ineffective as a preventive measure. Photosensitivity is also a classic feature of systemic lupus erythematosus.

Generalized erythema is perhaps a misnomer since the entire skin surface will usually not be affected. Drug eruptions and viral exanthems are the most common causes of widespread, blanchable, confluent, erythematous macules.

Purpura—Macular and Palpable

Purpura represents extravasated red blood cells in the dermis. It can be macular or palpable. Macular purpura is most commonly caused by chronic actinic exposure or corticosteroid usage. Minor trauma induces these lesions. Macular purpura may also occur as a manifestation of capillaritis, a mild inflammatory reaction. Patients with capillaritis are generally well, and systemic involvement is extremely rare. In contrast, palpable purpura represents inflammation or occlusion of arterioles or postcapillary venules. Palpable purpura is representative of small vessel vasculitis (Fig. 14.19; see color insert). Embolic phenomena [subacute bacterial endocarditis (SBE), left atrial myxoma, cholesterol], infectious causes (Rocky Mountain spotted fever, gonococcemia, menigococcemia, SBE), and occlusive diseases (cryoglobulinemia or cryofibrinogemia) may simulate vasculitis. Vasculitis can affect any organ system but most commonly affects the joints, gastrointestinal tract, and kidneys. The major associations of vasculitis include infections, drugs, and rheumatologic disorders. Therapy of vasculitis depends upon the organ systems involved, but in severe cases high-dose corticosteroids with or without immunosuppressives are regularly instituted.

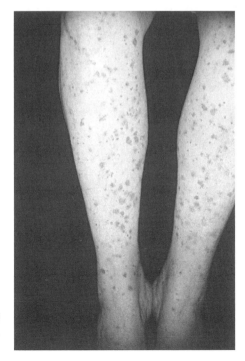

Fig. 14.19. Leukocytoclastic vasculitis due to ampicillin. (See color insert.)

Urticaria/Urticarial Lesions

Urticaria is characterized by pruritic erythematous or flesh-colored wheals (Fig. 14.20; see color insert). Angioedema is similar to urticaria but involves deeper dermal tissues and is most frequently observed on mucosal surfaces. Urticaria is an acute process in which the individual lesions resolve within hours of their appearance. When urticaria is of longer duration, the more appropriate term is urticarial. Urticaria may occur via immunologic (IgE dependent), non-immunologic (direct mast cell degranulation or indirect mast cell degranulation), or idiopathic mechanisms. Acute urticaria (less than 2 months duration) is often related to an ingestant (food or drug), whereas with chronic urticaria, the etiology is often not found. Urticarial lesions can occur in small vessel vasculitis. Therefore, in patients with individual lesions that persist more than 24 hours, a biopsy may aid in diagnosis.

Therapy of urticaria first involves a careful evaluation to identify a cause that can be treated or withdrawn. Then antihistaminic agents, both nonsedating as well as sedating, are used alone or in combination. Corticosteroids may give temporary relief but in this author's view should not be used. In patients whose conditions do not resolve, a restrictive diet may aid in the identification of triggering factor(s).

Erythema multiforme (EM) is characterized by erythematous macules or urticarial papules. The classic targetoid lesion is common, but not universal. Acute EM is most often due to drugs or infection. Recurrent EM has been closely linked to recurrent herpes simplex virus infection. Acute EM is self-limiting and only symptomatic therapy is needed. Recurrent EM can

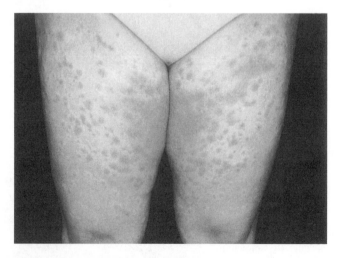

Fig. 14.20.   Urticaria: multiple erythematous plaques. (See color insert.)

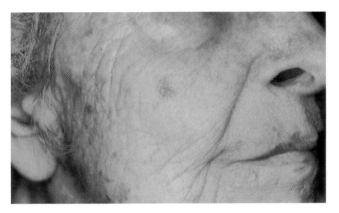

Fig. 14.3. Actinic keratosis: rough, scaly patch on the cheek. Note the background actinic damage, wrinkling, and solar lentigines.

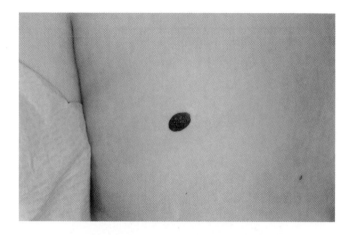

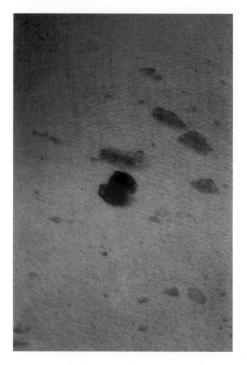

Fig. 14.4. Seborrheic keratosis. (top) Dark, sharply marginated, verrucous nodule on this patient's back. This lesion was regularly irritated by her bra, and it was therefore removed with curettage and destruction. (bottom) Multiple seborrheic keratoses.

Color Plate III

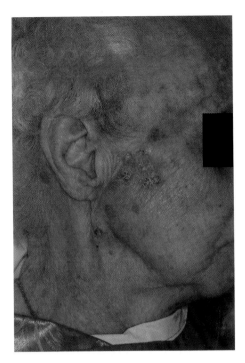

Fig. 14.5. Squamous cell carcinoma.

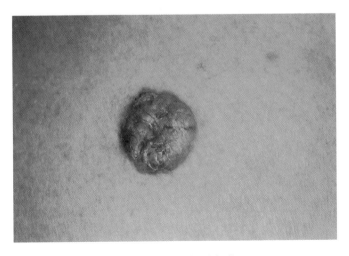

Fig. 14.6. Basal cell epithelioma.

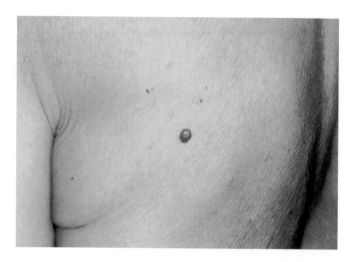

Fig. 14.7. Cherry angioma.

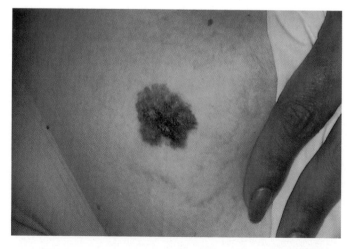

Fig. 14.8. Superficial spreading malignant melanoma.

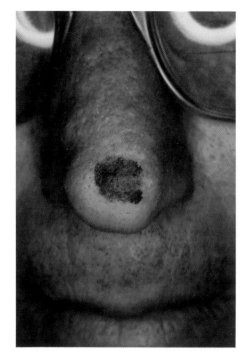

Fig. 14.9. Lentigo malignant melanoma.

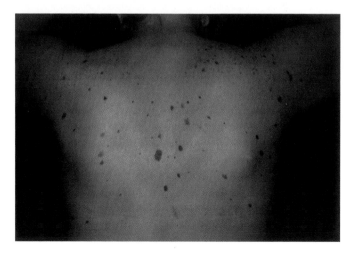

Fig. 14.10. Atypical nevi—multiple.

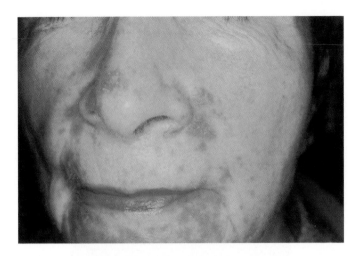

Fig. 14.11. Seborrheic dermatitis.

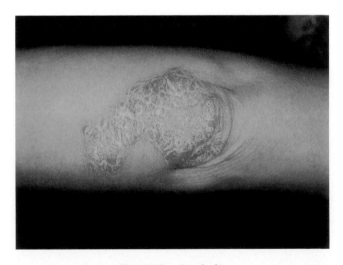

Fig. 14.12. Psoriasis.

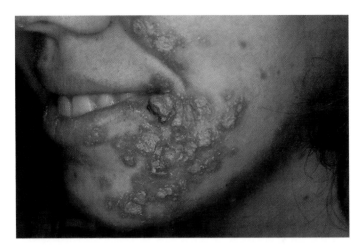

Fig. 14.13. Impetigo.

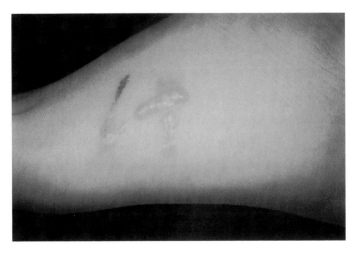

Fig. 14.14. Acute dermatitis due to contact with poison ivy (Rhus dermatitis).

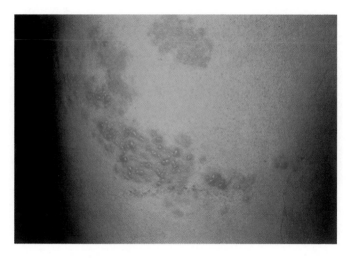

Fig. 14.15. Herpes zoster: shingles.

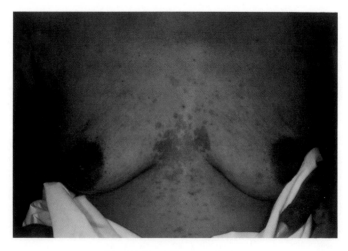

Fig. 14.16. Tinea versicolor.

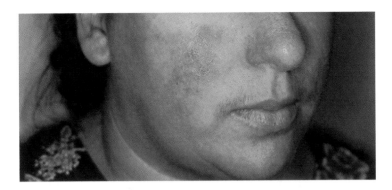

Fig. 14.17.   Rosacea.

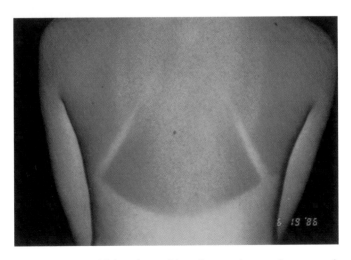

Fig. 14.18.   Photosensitivity dermatitis: phototoxic reaction secondary to tetracycline.

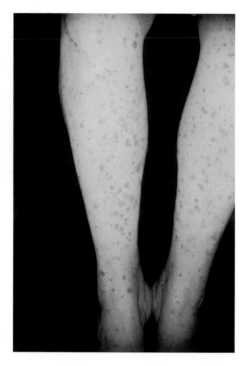

Fig. 14.19. Leukocytoclastic vasculitis due to ampicillin.

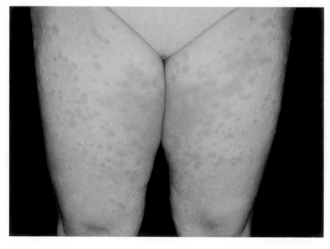

Fig. 14.20. Urticaria: multiple erythematous plaques.

be effectively suppressed with chronic antiviral therapy (valaciclovir, acyclovir, or famciclovir).

Pruritus Without Rash

Pruritus (itching) is a common cutaneous symptom. It occurs as a feature of many inflammatory conditions. However, pruritus may also occur without cutaneous changes. In this case a careful evaluation may lead to the recognition of a treatable process. Some causes of pruritus include hepatobiliary disease, thyroid abnormalities, diabetes mellitus, hematologic disorders, malignancies (particularly Hodgkin's disease), renal failure, parasitic infestation, HIV infections, psychiatric disease, and senescence. Before blaming psychiatric mechanisms or senescence, an evaluation should eliminate other possibilities.

Suggested Reading

Callen JP, ed. *Current Practice of Dermatology.* Philadelphia: Current Medicine; 1995.

Callen JP, Greer KE, Paller A, Swinyer L. *Color Atlas of Dermatology: A Morphological Approach*, 2nd ed. Philadelphia: W.B. Saunders Co; 2000.

15

Diabetes Mellitus

Sri Prakash L. Mokshagundam and Vasti L. Broadstone

Background Information

Diabetes mellitus is a complex of syndromes characterized by hyperglycemia and abnormal glucose metabolism. Persistent hyperglycemia leads to a variety of specific microvascular diseases involving the eye, kidney, and the peripheral nerves. In addition, diabetes mellitus is associated with an increased risk of macrovascular disease of the coronary, cerebral, and peripheral vasculature. It is estimated that approximately 6% of the U.S. population (approximately 14 million people) have been diagnosed with diabetes mellitus. An equal number of individuals probably have undiagnosed diabetes mellitus. Diabetes mellitus has a major economic and health impact. In 1992 the direct cost of treating individuals with diabetes mellitus was $85 billion, and the total cost of caring for these individuals was $105 billion. Thus, one in seven health care dollars was spent on treatment of individuals with diabetes mellitus. Individuals with diabetes mellitus are two to three times more likely to be hospitalized and two to four times more likely to have cardiovascular disease than the rest of the population. They also have the highest incidence of blindness, chronic renal failure, and nontraumatic foot amputation. Early diagnosis and appropriate management of diabetes mellitus can prevent or delay the development of complications.

Diagnosis

Diabetes mellitus is diagnosed by the measurement of blood glucose either in the fasting state or after an oral glucose load. Most patients with type 1 diabetes mellitus initially present with either the symptoms of hyperglycemia (polyuria and polydypsia) or with diabetic ketoacidosis. Some patients with type 2 diabetes mellitus also present with symptoms of hyperglycemia, but most are asymptomatic at the time of initial diagnosis. They are diagnosed while being evaluated for other medical problems or during screening for diabetes mellitus. In the absence of any symptoms of diabetes mellitus, screening for the disease is recommended in subjects with the following risk factors: (1) family history of diabetes mellitus, (2) obesity, (3) certain ethnic groups, e.g., Pima Indians, South Asians, etc., (4) previously identified impaired glucose tolerance, (5) aged 40 years and older, (6) hypertension and hyperlipidemia, and (7) history of gestational diabetes mellitus. Screening for diabetes mellitus is not recommended for the general population. The screening test of choice is the fasting plasma glucose level. Measurement of glycosylated hemoglobin (HbA_{1c}) is useful in the management of subjects with diabetes mellitus but is not recommended for making the diagnosis. The criteria used to make the diagnosis are given in Table 15.1.

Table 15.1.   Criteria for the diagnosis of diabetes mellitus.

A. Nonpregnant adult
    Oral glucose tolerance with 75-g glucose load
    1. Fasting plasma glucose >125 mg/dl on two or more occasions
    2. Plasma glucose level >200 mg/dl 2 hours after 75 g of oral glucose ingestion
    3. Random or postprandial plasma glucose >200 mg/dl on two or more occasions and in the presence of one or more symptoms of diabetes mellitus

B. Gestational diabetes mellitus
    Oral glucose tolerance test with 100 g of glucose performed at approximately 28 weeks of gestation, with samples drawn at 0, 1, 2, and 3 hours should reveal two or more of the following plasma glucose values:
    Fasting >95 mg/dl
    1 hour >180 mg/dl
    2 hour >155 mg/dl
    3 hour >140 mg/dl

Classification

Diabetes mellitus is a syndrome with heterogeneous clinical presentation. The clinical features, possible etiology, and need for insulin treatment are important criteria used to classify diabetes mellitus. The major classes of diabetes mellitus are outlined in Table 15.2. Most often the classification of individuals with diabetes mellitus is straightforward and based on clinical features. However, there can be some overlap of the clinical features, and additional tests may be needed in some patients. More than 90% of these subjects have type 2 diabetes mellitus. They are usually obese and have varying levels of insulin resistance and impaired insulin secretion. Measurement of plasma C-peptide can be useful. Plasma C-peptide is very low in subjects with type 1 diabetes mellitus, while it is high or normal in subjects with type 2 diabetes mellitus. Patients with type 2 diabetes mellitus can be managed without insulin, at least in the initial stages. However, some patients with type 2 diabetes mellitus need insulin to maintain fairly normal blood glucose, either from the onset of the disease

Table 15.2.   Classification of abnormal glucose tolerance.

Type	Characteristics
1. Type 1	Onset <40 years of age, insulinopenic, islet cell antibody positive, prone to ketoacidosis if untreated, requires insulin to control blood glucose and prevent ketosis.
2. Type 2	Onset >30 years of age, obese, insulin resistant, not prone to ketoacidosis, can be treated with diet or oral hypoglycemic agents
3. Gestational diabetes mellitus	Diabetes mellitus diagnosed for the first time during pregnancy, resolves after delivery, high risk of noninsulin-dependent diabetes mellitus later
4. Secondary diabetes mellitus	Diabetes is due to a separate identifiable disease; decreased insulin secretion or insulin resistance may be present
5. Impaired glucose tolerance	Obese, no risk of microvascular disease, increased risk of macrovascular disease, increased risk of developing diabetes mellitus
6. Maturity onset diabetes of the young (MODY)	Onset <30 years of age, strong family history, autosomal dominant inheritance, islet cell antibodies absent, no risk of ketoacidosis, defective insulin secretion, can be treated with oral hypoglycemic agents

or after an initial period of good response to therapy with oral hypoglycemic agents. Such patients are referred to as having insulin-requiring diabetes mellitus (IRDM). It is important to recognize that these patients do not develop diabetic ketoacidosis, a feature that distinguishes them from patients with type 1 diabetes mellitus. Type 1 diabetes mellitus is an autoimmune disorder and approximately 90% have circulating islet cell antibodies in the first few years of the disease. When the diagnosis is unclear after initial clinical evaluation, measurement of islet cell antibodies can be helpful in clarifying the nature of the disease. A small number of patients with diabetes mellitus have an identifiable cause (disease) that is responsible for the diabetes mellitus. These diseases can cause diabetes mellitus either due to impaired insulin secretion, insulin resistance, or both. It is important to look for clinical features that may suggest this diagnosis and initiate appropriate laboratory evaluation when needed.

Initial Evaluation of the Patient with Diabetes Mellitus

The initial evaluation of patients with diabetes mellitus should be comprehensive and aimed at determining its type and severity, the adequacy of any previous therapy, the presence of micro- or macrovascular complications, the presence of possible underlying causes or risk factors, and the need for diabetes education and nutritional counseling. The following information should be obtained:

History: Hypoglycemic or hyperglycemic symptoms, exercise and dietary habits, symptoms of long-term complications, history of cardiovascular disease/risk factors, and family history of diabetes and of complications of diabetes.

Physical examination: Anthropometric data (weight, height, waist–hip ratio), blood pressure (supine and standing), peripheral pulse, foot examination, complete neurologic examination, cardiovascular examination, and ophthalmoscopic examination.

Laboratory tests: Glycohemoglobin, serum lipids, serum creatinine, urinalysis, EKG (in type 2 diabetes mellitus), and 24-hour urine collection for measurement of microalbuminuria (5 years after onset in type 1 diabetes mellitus).

Management

The primary goal of management of diabetes mellitus is the prevention of acute and long-term complications of the disease. Microvascular complications (retinopathy, nephropathy, neuropathy) have been shown to be related to the level of blood glucose, as reflected by hemoglobin A_{1c} levels. In both type 1 (Diabetes Control and Complications Trial—DCCT) and type 2 diabetes mellitus

Table 15.3. Glycemic targets for subjects with diabetes mellitus.

	Goal	Action suggested
Preprandial glucose (mg/dl)	80–120	<80; >140
Bedtime glucose (mg/dl)	100–140	<100; >160
Hemoglobin A$_{1c}$ (%)	<7	>8

(United Kingdom Prospective Diabetes Study—UKPDS) intervention studies have clearly demonstrated the reduction in incidence and progression of microvascular complications by intensive treatment regimens. Macrovascular complications are related to several risk factors including fasting and postprandial blood glucose, glycemic spikes after a meal, lipid profile, blood pressure, lack of physical activity, obesity, cigarette smoking, abnormal platelet function, depression, and insulin resistance. While large epidemiologic studies have clearly demonstrated the association between elevated blood glucose and macrovascular disease, large randomized clinical trials that demonstrate the effect of intensive treatment on macrovascular disease incidence have not yet been published. Several studies have shown the benefits of blood pressure and lipid reduction in diabetes mellitus. It is important to define glycemic targets to enable the patient to achieve the best result (Table 15.3). Hypoglycemia is a major limiting factor to achieving glycemic targets. In subjects who have severe or frequent hypoglycemic episodes, the goals of treatment have to be modified. Optimal management of diabetes mellitus requires a team approach including the patient, physician, nutritionist, and diabetes educator (Table 15.4). In addition, other health professionals such as podiatrist, exercise physiologist, behavior therapist, ophthalmologist, cardiologist, and so forth need to be included whenever necessary.

The major components of management of diabetes mellitus are diet, exercise, and the use of hypoglycemic agents (insulin and oral hypoglycemic agents).

Diabetes Education

This is a key component of prevention of diabetes-related complications. In addition to improving glycemic control, diabetes education provides useful information to the subjects with diabetes about the rationale for treatment. In a chronic asymptomatic disease understanding the long-term consequences will be a major factor in improving adherence to diet, exercise, and medication recommendations. Education will also be extremely useful in instituting lifestyle changes to reduce coronary artery disease (CAD) risk and to ensure proper foot care.

Table 15.4.   General guidelines for diabetes management.[a,b]

1. Establish a diagnosis of DM
   A. FBG ≥140 mg/dl × 2, or
   B. Classical signs and symptoms of DM and random BG ≥ 200 mg/dl, or
   C. By OGTT (BG at 120 minutes ≥200 mg/dl)
      Do not perform OGTT if diagnosis of DM is already established.
   D. Classify DM as to type 1, type 2, etc.
2. Inform patient of diagnosis of diabetes and refer to diabetes education classes (to learn signs and symptoms of complication, BG monitoring, diabetic medications, sick days, etc.).
3. Place patient on diet with appropriate caloric, sodium, and lipid restrictions.
4. Establish cardiovascular risk factors.
5. Establish status of kidney function (serum creatinine, 24-hour urine albumin).
6. Evaluate for presence of neuropathy (refer to neurologist if symptomatic).
7. Establish extent of fundoscopic lesion (refer to ophthalmologist/ optometrist).
8. Check feet and toenails at each visit.
9. Use finger stick BG for daily diabetic control and urine check only for ketones (in type 1 diabetes mellitus).
10. Follow chronic glycemic control by HgA$_{1c}$ every 2 to 3 months (every 6 months in elderly) in the office.

[a] In addition to the above specific management procedures, it is understood that all patients who are seen for diabetes evaluation and have not been seen by other physicians for general health evaluation should have a complete history and physical examination and the following laboratory tests: complete blood count with differential, chemistry profile, lipid profile, urinalysis, thyroid function tests, and electrocardiogram (if indicated).
[b] DM, diabetes mellitus; FBG, fasting blood glucose; OGTT, oral glucose tolerance test.
Source: From Kitabchi A, Ghawji M. Diabetes in the nonpregnant patient. *Prim Care Update Ob/Gyn* 1994;1(2):86–94. Reproduced with permission from Elsevier.

Diet

Nutrition therapy plays a major role in the management of diabetes mellitus. The aims of nutrition therapy are to maintain near-normal blood glucose, maintain or attain ideal body weight (Table 15.5), achieve optimal serum lipid level, prevent and treat acute and long-term complications of diabetes mellitus, and improve the overall health of the individual with diabetes mellitus. These goals can be met only through an individualized approach to dietary recommendations. Ensuring compliance with dietary recommendations requires sensitivity to personal lifestyle and to cultural, ethnic, and financial considerations.

Exercise

Exercise is usually recommended for patients with diabetes mellitus. While the overall effect of exercise is beneficial to most patients, the effect of exercise on metabolism is complex. Hence an exercise program that is applicable to all patients with diabetes mellitus cannot be prescribed. The major benefits and risks of exercise are outlined in Table 15.6. Before prescribing an exercise regimen particular attention should be given to the degree of glycemic control, the presence of proliferative retinopathy and cardiovascular disease, and the frequency and awareness of hypoglycemic symptoms. If necessary, the assistance of an exercise physiologist must be sought.

Table 15.5. Simple formula to calculate ideal body weight (IBW) and caloric requirement for women.

Estimating desirable weight for women

Medium build	Allow 100 pounds for first 5 feet of height, plus 5 pounds for each additional inch
Small build	Subtract 10%
Large build	Add 10%

Caloric need for maintenance of IBW for adults can be estimated by using a food nomogram, or by adding basal calories and calories needed for activity, using the following:

Basal calories:	IBW (lb) $\times$ 10
Sedentary:	IBW (lb) $\times$ 10 + 30%
Moderate:	IBW (lb) $\times$ 10 + 50%
Strenuous:	IBW (lb) $\times$ 10 + 100%

Source: From Kitabchi A, Ghawji M. Diabetes in the nonpregnant patient. *Prim Care Update Ob/Gyn* 1994;1(2):86–94. Reproduced with permission from Elsevier.

Table 15.6. Benefits and risks of exercise in diabetes mellitus.

Benefits	Risks
1. Improved blood glucose control in type 2 diabetes mellitus	1. Hypoglycemia
	2. Hyperglycemia and ketosis
2. Increased cardiovascular fitness	3. Retinal hemorrhage (if proliferative retinopathy is present)
3. Improved serum lipids	
4. Improved feeling of well-being	4. Silent ischemia/cardiovascular event

Self-Monitoring of Blood Glucose

The ability to measure blood glucose at home has been a key factor in developing insulin regimens that achieve good metabolic control. Because of the expense and effort involved in this process, it is important that patients clearly understand the goals and reasons for performing self-monitoring of blood glucose (SMBG). In addition, the patient must be willing and capable of performing SMBG accurately and be committed to constructively modifying treatment plans based on the results of SMBG. A wide array of SMBG devices is available. Cost, ease of use, and accuracy are important considerations in prescribing a device. SMBG should be considered for all patients on intensive insulin regimens and by patients with gestational diabetes. SMBG is also useful in the detection and treatment of hypoglycemia and in determining the effect of diet and exercise on blood glucose in individual patients.

Insulin Therapy

Type 1 Diabetes Mellitus

All patients with type 1 diabetes mellitus are treated with insulin. Following the initial diagnosis of type 1 diabetes mellitus, there may be a period of 6 months to 1 year during which insulin requirements may decrease or may be unnecessary ("honeymoon period"), but all patients will eventually need daily insulin therapy. Several insulin regimens have been used, but the Diabetes Control and Complications Trial (DCCT) clearly demonstrated that intensive insulin therapy regimens (multiple daily injections of short- and intermediate/long-acting insulin 3–4 times daily/or insulin pump) provide better metabolic control and decrease the incidence of long-term complications. The dose of insulin selected for initiation of insulin therapy is based on the observation that the basal insulin requirement is 0.5–1 U/kg body weight/day and that 1 unit of regular insulin is needed to maintain the blood glucose level at premeal levels for every 12 g of carbohydrate (or 100 kcal) in the diet. Also, 1 unit of regular insulin will reduce the blood glucose level by 50–75 mg/dl. However, there is significant individual variation in the response to insulin and meals. Thus the dose has to be adjusted based on blood glucose monitoring in individual patients. It is important to make sure that the patient understands the principles of treatment and that trained professionals be available 24 hours a day to assist patients in making needed adjustments, especially at the time of initiation of treatment.

See Table 15.7 for the different insulin preparations.

Initiation of insulin therapy in type 1 diabetes mellitus:

1. *Conventional therapy:* A mixture of intermediate-acting (NPH or Lente) insulin is administered before breakfast and before dinner. Initiate with 0.5–1 U/kg/day: two-thirds as NPH (or Lente) and one-third as regular insulin; two-thirds before breakfast and one-third before dinner.

2. *Intensive insulin therapy:* (a) Mixture of NPH (or Lente) and short-acting insulin (preferably Lis-Pro or Insulin Aspart) before breakfast, short-acting insulin before dinner, and NPH (or Lente) insulin before bedtime. (b) Short-acting insulin before meals and NPH (or Lente) insulin before bedtime. Initiate with a total daily insulin of 0.5 U/kg/day divided into four equal doses and additional insulin before each meal calculated at 1 U/every 12 g of carbohydrate (or 1 U/every 100 kcal). (c) Glargine at bedtime and Lis-Pro/Ins-Aspart before each meal, with approximately 50% of the insulin dose being given as Glargine and the remaining as short-acting

Table 15.7. Insulin preparations.

Insulin	Onset	Peak/duration	Comment
Regular insulin (Humulin or Novolin R)	1 hour	2–4/6–8 hours	Short-acting insulin; now being replaced by Lis-Pro and insulin aspart; higher incidence of hypoglycemia
NPH/Lente insulin	2–4 hours	4–8/8–16 hours	Intermediate-acting insulin; bedtime or twice daily use
Ultralente	Variable	Variable (up to 24 hours)	Long-acting insulin but unpredictable; glargine is preferred as basal insulin
Lis-Pro (Humalog)	15–30 minutes	1–2/2–4 hours	Premeal insulin; can be used in insulin pump
Insulin Aspart (Novolog)	15–30 minutes	1–2/2–4 hours	Similar to Lis-Pro
Glargine (Lantus)	2 hours	None/24 hours	Currently preferred basal insulin

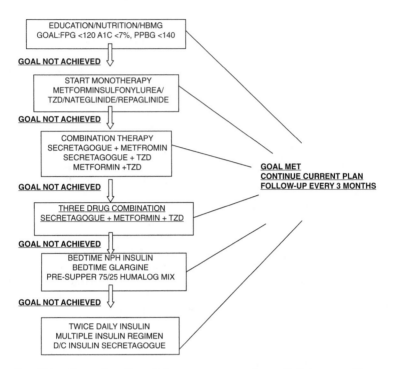

Fig. 15.1.   General outline of the management of type 2 diabetes mellitus.

insulin. (d) Continuous subcutaneous insulin infusion from an insulin pump with a basal background insulin dose and mealtime boluses. Initiate treatment with a basal rate of 0.6 U/hour and mealtime boluses based on the carbohydrate content of the meal. In addition, 1 U of regular insulin is administered for every 75 mg/dl blood glucose greater than 150 mg/dl at mealtime. These are only guidelines for initiating insulin therapy. Eventual doses will be based on the response to the insulin regimen.

Type 2 Diabetes Mellitus

Most patients with type 2 diabetes mellitus are initially treated with diet, with or without an oral hypoglycemic agent (Fig. 15.1). Some patients fail to respond to this regimen and will need insulin therapy. In addition, a significant number of patients who initially respond to diet and oral hypoglycemic agents will eventually fail to respond to the regimen and will require insulin therapy. Since there is some concern that the use of large amounts of insulin could predispose patients to cardiovascular disease, it is important to emphasize diet and exercise in individuals who are candidates for insulin therapy. The lowest dose of insulin that controls blood glucose should be used. Weight loss and exercise can decrease insulin requirements by decreasing insulin resistance. The following regimen may be used in patients with type 2 diabetes mellitus:

1. **_Single injection regimen:_** Once daily injection of intermediate (NPH/Lente) or long-acting (Ultralente) insulin. However, in most cases, single injection therapy is inadequate to normalize HbA_{1c}. It is probably most useful in newly diagnosed patients.

2. **_Combination therapy:_** Daytime sulfonylurea/bedtime NPH insulin. This is more effective in patients who (a) have had diabetes for less than 10–15 years, (b) are overweight, (c) developed diabetes after age 35 years, and (d) have fasting blood glucose less than 250 mg/dl.

3. **_Split-mixed regimen:_** This is the most widely used regimen of insulin administration in type 2 diabetes mellitus. A combination of NPH (or Lente) and regular insulin is administered before breakfast and before dinner. The total daily insulin dose is approximately 1 U/kg/day. This dose can be split equally between the prebreakfast and predinner doses.

4. **_Multiple insulin injections and insulin pump:_** Some patients with type 2 diabetes mellitus behave like patients with type 1 diabetes mellitus in their insulin needs. However, there is not enough experience in this insulin regimen in type 2 diabetes mellitus to make clear recommendations.

Oral Agents

Several oral hypoglycemic agents are currently available for the treatment of type 2 diabetes mellitus. A summary of the clinical use of these agents is given in Table 15.8. Since different classes of drugs act by different mechanisms it is possible to use combinations of oral hypoglycemic agents as well as combinations of oral hypoglycemic agents and insulin.

Sulfonylureas

The sulfonylureas are the most widely used oral hypoglycemic agents in the United States. Their main mechanism of action is to increase insulin secretion, although they are also known to decrease insulin resistance. A number of sulfonylureas are available and can be broadly classified as first- and second-generation agents. The second-generation sulfonylureas are more potent. Use of an improved delivery system has made it possible to administer glipizide once a day. Glimepiride is a newer sulfonylurea that has some effects that are different from other sulfonylureas.

Biguanides

The biguanide metformin has been available in the United States since 1995. It has several mechanisms of action. It improves peripheral and hepatic insulin action, and its use is associated with lower circulating insulin levels. It can also inhibit glucose absorption. When used alone it does not cause hypoglycemia. In addition to improving blood glucose it has a favorable effect on plasma lipids and can promote weight loss.

Table 15.8.   Oral agents for type 2 diabetes mellitus.

Drug	Daily dose	Duration of action	Comment
Sulfonylureas			
Glyburide	1.25–20 mg	12–24 hours	Increase insulin
(Diabeta)	1.5–12 mg	12–24 hours	secretion
Micronized	2.5–40 mg	12–24 hours	Hypoglycemia is a
glyburide	2.5–20 mg	24 hours	concern
(Glynase)			
Glipizide	1–8 mg	24 hours	
(Glucotrol)			
Glipizide GITS			
(Glucotrol XL)			
Glimepiride			
(Amaryl)			
Repaglinide	1.5–16 mg	4–6 hours	Increase insulin
(Prandin)			secretion; shorter acting than sulfonylureas; premeal dosing
Nateglinide	120 mg	2–4 hours	Increase in first-phase insulin secretion; excellent for postmeal glucose control; premeal dosing
(Starlix)			
Acarbose	300 mg	3–4 hours	Inhibit carbohydrate absorption
(Precose)			Limited by GI side effects
Metformin	500–2500 mg	12–24 hours	Major effect on hepatic glucose production; cannot be used in presence of renal disease, congestive heart failure
(Glucophage/ Glucophage XR)			

Table 15.8. *Continued.*

Drug	Daily dose	Duration of action	Comment
Rosiglitazone (Avandia)	2–8 mg (1–2/day)	12–24 hours	Weight gain, fluid retention, and cost are limiting factors; increase insulin sensitivity; high cost
Pioglitazone (Actos)	15–45 mg (1/day)	24 hours	

The most important side effect is lactic acidosis. The drug should not be used in the presence of liver disease, renal insufficiency, significant peripheral vascular disease, and in situations where there is increased risk of lactic acidosis. It should be discontinued during hospitalization of acute illness and prior to procedures using radiocontrast material. Gastrointestinal side effects are a more common but less dangerous side effect. The drug can be used alone or in combination with a sulfonylurea.

α-Glucosidase Inhibitors

Acarbose (Precose) and miglitol (Glyset) are approved for use in the United States. They inhibit the absorption of carbohydrates by inhibiting the intestinal digestion of complex carbohydrates. The effect on HbA_{1c} levels is modest (approximately 0.5–1.0%). Gastrointestinal side effects limit the use of these agents.

Thiazolidinediones (Glitazones)

There are currently two agents in this class for clinical use—pioglitazone (Actos) and rosiglitazone (Avandia). These drugs increase sensitivity to insulin in the skeletal muscle and other peripheral tissues. They can be used alone or in combination with sulfonylureas, metformin, or insulin. In addition to reducing blood glucose levels, this class of drugs has been shown to have effects that might prove useful in the management of type 2 diabetes mellitus. These include improvement in lipid profile (lower triglycerides and higher HDL cholesterol), hypertension, coagulation pathway, inflammatory pathway, and endothelial function. In addition, they have been postulated to improve the function of β cells. The nonhypoglycemic effects of these drugs have been postulated to decrease the risk of heart disease in subjects with type 2 diabetes mellitus. However, this has not yet been demonstrated in prospective clinical trials. Their main side effects are liver toxicity, weight gain, and fluid retention. Liver toxicity can been minimized by screening individuals with liver function tests before initiating treatment and periodically (every 2–4 months) thereafter.

Follow-up Evaluation of Patients with Diabetes Mellitus

The follow-up evaluation of patients with diabetes should include evaluation of diabetes control, the presence of diabetes complications, and continuing education needs. Most diabetics have to be evaluated three to four times a year. More frequent visits are necessary during initiation of treatment or with major changes in management. A thorough history of the patient's degree of blood glucose control, symptoms of hypo- or hyperglycemia, and symptoms of possible diabetes complications should be meticulously obtained. Education and nutritional counseling should continue. The suggested ongoing evaluations are outlined in Table 15.9. A general scheme for the evaluation, prevention, and treatment of diabetes-related complications is shown in Table 15.10. In addition, appropriate referrals should be made whenever clinical features warrant.

Immunization Recommendations

Table 15.9.   Recommended assessment and management goals for CVD risk factors in diabetes.

Parameter	Frequency	Goal
HbA_{1c}	3–4 months	<7% (<6.5%)[a]
Fasting blood glucose	2–7 times a week[b]	80–120 mg/dl
Postprandial blood glucose	2–7 times a week[b]	<140 mg/dl[a]
LDL cholesterol	Annual; 3–4 months, if abnormal	<100 mg/dl
HDL cholesterol	Annual; 3–4 months, if abnormal	>45 mg/dl
Triglyceride	Annual; 3–4 months, if abnormal	<200 mg/dl
Systolic blood pressure	Each visit	<130 mm Hg
Diastolic blood pressure	Each visit	<85 mm Hg
Microalbuminuria	Annual	Normal or no progression
Eye examination	Annual	Normal or no progression
Neurologic examination	Annual	Normal or no progression

[a] Recommended by AACE/ACE.
[b] No clear recommendation (need to individualize).

Table 15.10.   Complications of diabetes mellitus.

Complication	Screening	Prevention	Management
Nephropathy	Urine Microalbumin	Glycemic control Blood pressure control (ARB/ACE inhibitors)	ARB/ACE inhibitors Dialysis Renal transplant
Retinopathy	Dilated fundus exam	Glycemic control Blood pressure control	Laser Rx Vitrectomy
Neuropathy	Clinical history Clinical exam– monofilament test Tests of autonomic function	Glycemic control	Pain management— tricyclics, gabapentin, topiramate Preventive foot care Specialist referral for autonomic neuropathy
Cardiovascular disease	Risk factor screening EKG/stress test—as needed	Glycemic control Aspirin Diet and exercise Risk factors modification— blood pressure, lipids	Aggressive control of blood pressure, lipids Specialist referral for evaluation and management of heart disease

[a] ARB, angiotensin receptor blocker; ACE, angiotensin-converting enzyme.

The American Diabetes Association currently recommends immunization against influenza and pneumococcal pneumonia in subjects with diabetes mellitus. Although there are no controlled studies to demonstrate the effectiveness of these procedures in subjects with diabetes mellitus, the recommendations are based on the following facts. (1) Subjects with diabetes mellitus are at higher risk for complications, hospitalizations, and death from influenza and pneumococcal disease. (2) Subjects with diabetes mellitus can mount an effective response to vaccination. (3) The intervention is low cost and has low risk. Immunization for influenza is recommended on a yearly basis. Immunization for pneumococcal disease is recommended in all subjects with diabetes mellitus. Subjects >64 years who have been immunized when they were <65 years old should receive a one-time revaccination if the last immunization was >5 years ago. Subjects with nephropathy, chronic renal insufficiency, and postorgan transplantation are also candidates for revaccination.

Gestational Diabetes

Pregnant women who are at high risk for gestational diabetes should be screened for gestational diabetes mellitus between week 24 and 26 of pregnancy by measuring blood glucose 1 hour after a 50-g oral glucose load. If the blood glucose level is greater than 140 mg/dl, a full glucose tolerance test with a 100-g glucose load should be performed. The criteria for the diagnosis of gestational diabetes are given in Table 15.1. While in the past all pregnant women were screened for gestational diabetes mellitus, currently only "high-risk" individuals are screened. High-risk individuals include those with age >25 years, obesity, family history of diabetes mellitus, previous history of gestational diabetes mellitus, previous child weighing >9 pounds at birth, and those from high-risk ethnic groups (African-Americans, Latino/Hispanic, Asian, Native American). Gestational diabetes is associated with an increased risk of congenital malformations, macrosomia, and perinatal morbidity and mortality. It is essential to maintain strict control of blood glucose throughout the pregnancy. Oral hypoglycemic agents are contraindicated during pregnancy. All patients should monitor their blood glucose in the fasting state, 2 hours after each meal and at bedtime. The fasting blood glucose level should be less than 105 mg/dl, and the 2 hour postprandial blood glucose should be less than 120 mg/dl. If diet alone fails to control the blood glucose level within this range, insulin therapy should be initiated within a week. An intensive insulin regimen with multiple insulin injections is preferred. Early morning urine should be checked for ketones. If ketonuria is present and the blood glucose is not high, it may be necessary to increase the bedtime snack and, if necessary, to increase the insulin dose in the evening. The care of the patient with gestational diabetes mellitus requires excellent coordination among the diabetes team, the obstetrician, and the primary care provider. Blood glucose levels usually normalize immediately after delivery. A follow-up oral glucose tolerance test should be performed 6 weeks after delivery. There is a high rate of recurrence of gestational diabetes during subsequent pregnancies and an increased lifetime risk of developing noninsulin-dependent diabetes mellitus.

Suggested Reading

Ahmann AJ, Riddle MC. Current oral agents for type 2 diabetes. Many options, but which to choose when? *Postgrad Med* 2002;111(5):32–4, 37–40, 43–6.

American Diabetes Association. Implications of the Diabetes Control and Complications Trial. *Diabetes* 1993;42:1555–8.

American Diabetes Association. Implications of the United Kingdom Prospective Diabetes Study. *Diabetes Care* 2003;26(Suppl 1):S28–S32.

American Diabetes Association. Standards of medical care for patients with diabetes mellitus. *Diabetes Care* 2003;26(Suppl 1):S33–S50.

American Diabetes Association. Gestational diabetes mellitus. *Diabetes Care* 2003;26(Suppl 1):S103–S105.

Chan JL, Abrahamson MJ. Pharmacological management of type 2 diabetes mellitus: rationale for rational use of insulin. *Mayo Clin Proc* 2003; 78(4):459–67.

DeWitt DE, Hirsch IB. Outpatient insulin therapy in type 1 and type 2 diabetes mellitus: scientific review. *JAMA* 2003;289(17):2254–64.

Diabetes Control and Complications Trial (DCCT). *N Engl J Med* 1993; 329:683–9.

Diamant M, Heine RJ. Thiazolidinediones in type 2 diabetes mellitus: current clinical evidence. *Drugs* 2003;63(13):1373–405.

Edelman SV, Henry RR. Insulin therapy for normalizing glycosylated hemoglobin in type II diabetes: applications, benefits, and risks. *Diabetes Rev* 1995;3:308–34.

Expert Committee on the Diagnosis and Classification of Diabetes Mellitus. Report of the Expert Committee on the Diagnosis and Classification of Diabetes Mellitus. *Diabetes Care* 2003;26(Suppl 1):S4–S20.

Hirsch IL, Paauw DS, Brunzell J. Inpatient management of adults with diabetes. *Diabetes Care* 1995;18:870–8.

Inzucchi SE. Oral antihyperglycemic therapy for type 2 diabetes: scientific review. *JAMA* 2002;287(3):360–72.

Kitabchi A, Ghawji M. Diabetes in the nonpregnant patient. *Prim Care Update Ob/Gyn* 1994;1(2):86–94.

Lebovitz HE. Treating hyperglycemia in type 2 diabetes: new goals and strategies. *Cleve Clin J Med* 2002;69(10):809–20.

Petrie J, Small M, Connell J. "Glitazones," a prospect for non-insulin-dependent diabetes. *Lancet* 1997;349:70.

Santiago JV. Lessons from the Diabetes Control and Complications Trial. *Diabetes* 1993;42:1549–54.

Tsui EYL, Zinman B. Exercise and diabetes: new insights and therapeutic goals. *Endocrinologist* 1995;5:263–71.

Turner RC. The U.K. Prospective Diabetes Study. A review. *Diabetes Care* 1998;21(Suppl 3):C358.

16

Gastrointestinal Disorders

Roger P. Smith

Background Information

Our primary focus will not be on topics such as acute disease, appendicitis, hernias, massive bleeding, or hematemesis. The diagnosis and management of these entities are either obvious or outside the scope of routine office care. We will, instead, concentrate on gallbladder disease, and conditions affecting the stomach, small and large bowel, colon, and rectum.

Gallbladder Disease

Gallbladder disease may occur at any age, but 70% of patients are over 40 years. Age per se represents one of the major risk factors in the development of cholelithiasis. Specific additional factors are addressed in Table 16.1 The disease rate is three times higher in women. The effects of pregnancy, estrogen (both natural and pharmacologic), and other unique female factors have been studied; however, the exact reason for this sex difference is unknown. Obesity is also a recognized risk factor. A patient who is 15–20 pounds overweight has a two-fold increase in the risk of cholelithiasis, while a 50–75 pound excess in weight increases this risk sixfold. Medical conditions such as cirrhosis, diabetes, and Crohn's disease also increase the risk of cholelithiasis. Certain geographic and genetic factors also may play a role. A family history of cholelithiasis in siblings or children results in a twofold increase in risk.

Table 16.1.   Risk factors for cholelithiasis.

- Age >40
- Sex (female:male = 3:1)
- Pregnancy
- Oral contraceptives
- Oral estrogen replacement
- Obesity
- Diet and medications
- Cirrhosis
- Diabetes
- Crohn's disease
- Family history

Pregnancy, oral contraceptives, and estrogen replacement have been implicated in increasing the risk of gallstones. During pregnancy, bile secretion roughly doubles, while the rate of gallbladder emptying decreases. Three to four percent of pregnant patients will have symptomatic gallstones. Parity plays a role in the development of gallstones with 75% of affected patients having had one or more pregnancies. Oral contraceptives are thought to accelerate the course of cholelithiasis, rather than increasing the rate.

Upper Gastrointestinal Complaints

The most common upper gastrointestinal complaints are familiar to everyone: upper abdominal pain, nausea, vomiting, dyspepsia, heartburn, and "gas." For the gynecologist, esophageal reflux, gastroenteritis and chronic gastritis, peptic ulcer disease, and duodenitis are the most common upper gastrointestinal problems encountered.

Gastroesophageal Reflux

The reflux of gastric acid to the sensitive esophagus causes heartburn, the cardinal manifestation of gastroesophageal reflux disease (GERD). The most common etiology is the decrease in tone of the lower esophageal sphincter pressure. Symptoms are most common after large meals, consuming certain foods, and upon assuming the recumbent position. Prolonged exposure of acid to the esophagus may lead to stricture formation and dysphagia. Nocturnal aspiration may occur and be mistaken for asthma.

Peptic Ulcer Disease

Peptic ulcer disease is the result of disruption of host factors in the stomach or duodenum in the presence of acid and pepsin. Patients may have multiple abnormalities that lead to ulcer formation. Little evidence supports a strong genetic basis for the disease in the majority of patients. Up to 40% of patients have an increased secretion rate of acid; however, larger groups of patients have normal rates of secretion. Breakdown of the mucosal barrier is probably the most important factor in peptic ulcer disease. Definite factors that contribute to disruption of the mucosa include (1) infection with *Helicobacter pylori*, (2) cigarette smoking, and (3) nonsteroidal antiinflammatory drugs (NSAIDs). Many etiologies such as alcohol use, stress, and adrenocorticosteroids are now thought to be less important.

Helicobacter pylori infection has been isolated in 95% of patients with duodenal ulcers and 70% with gastric ulcers. The influence of *H. pylori* in peptic ulcer disease is now well established. *H. pylori* is associated with inflammation that disrupts the mucosal barrier and allows for the disruptive action of acid and pepsin. Cigarette smoking is associated with increased acid formation and alteration in blood flow, and interferes with prostaglandin production. NSAIDs have a direct effect on disruption of the mucosal barrier and range from superficial lesions to deep ulceration. Recently introduced cyclo-oxygenase-2 (COX-2) inhibitors are less prone to cause gastrointestinal side effects but at the doses required for the treatment of gynecologic conditions such as dysmenorrhea, a clear superiority has yet to be established.

Small Bowel Disease

Problems associated with the small bowel specifically are an infrequent source of complaints seen in gynecologic practice. Lactase insufficiency, leading to lactose intolerance, is perhaps the most common. Lactase deficiency occurs in 5–15% of whites but in 60–90% of American Indians, black Americans, and Asians. Symptoms of lactase insufficiency are generally not seen until adulthood. Patients with this deficiency are intolerant of milk products, experiencing bloating, cramps, and diarrhea. The diagnosis may be suspected by history and confirmed by a hydrogen breath test. (Hydrogen increases abnormally in response to a lactose challenge.) Treatment consists of dietary avoidance of lactose or the addition of lactase at meals.

Large Bowel and Colon Disease

Spanning the small and large bowel are diseases such as enteritis and irritable bowel syndrome. So-called regional enteritis may affect both the terminal small bowel and the colon. Irritable bowel syndrome appears to involve an abnormality of motility that includes the small bowel. Functional gastrointestinal symptoms are identified in up to 20% of women and 70% of irritable bowel syndrome sufferers are women. Both entities may bring patients to the gynecologist's office with complaints of abdominal or pelvic pain, abdominal "distention," altered bowel habits, and mucous in the stool. Diarrhea is a common complaint with many of these entities leading to a long list of possible causes (see Table 16.2).

Table 16.2.   Common causes of diarrhea.

- Iatrogenic (dietary—tea, coffee, etc.)
- Infectious enteritis
- Inflammatory bowel disease
  Regional enteritis
  Ulcerative colitis
  Crohn's disease
- Irritable bowel syndrome
- Lactose intolerance
- Laxative abuse
- Drug induced (antacids, antibiotics, colchicine)
- Diverticular disease
- Malabsorption (lactose insufficiency)
- Metabolic (diabetes, hyperthyroidism)
- Mechanical (impaction)
- Neoplastic

Irritable Bowel Syndrome

The irritable bowel syndrome (IBS), the most common clinical entity seen in clinical practice, has a 2:1 female/male ratio. It accounts for up to 50% of patient visits to gastroenterologists. Colonic wall motility is altered in these patients with evidence suggesting altered colonic wall sensitivity. Patients with IBS have altered motor reactivity to various stimuli, including meals, psychological stress, and balloon distention of the rectosigmoid, resulting in altered transit time, pain, constipation, and diarrhea. Studies using rectosigmoid balloon distention have shown that IBS patients have a significantly lower threshold for visceral pain than do healthy controls. Parallel studies do not demonstrate a similar hypersensitivity to peripheral stimuli. Because 5-hydroxytryptamine (5-HT) receptors may inhibit the activation of pain pathways in the peripheral nervous system, researchers have examined the role of 5-HT in IBS. Most affected patients are young to middle age. A high prevalence of psychopathology has been reported among IBS sufferers. These patients tend to have more somatizational disorders, stress, anxiety disorders, depression, hysteria, and hypochondriasis. The coexistence of these factors should be investigated and complicate both the diagnosis and treatment.

There are three common clinical variants: (1) "spastic colitis" characterized by chronic abdominal pain and constipation; (2) intermittent diarrhea, which is usually painless; and (3) a combination of both with alternating diarrhea and constipation. Symptoms are generally worse 1–1.5 hours postprandial, with 50% of patients experiencing pain that lasts for hours or days. Episodes of pain may last for weeks in up to 20% of patients. The pain is generally worse with high fat meals, stress, depression, or menstruation. Symptoms are often better after a bowel movement.

Inflammatory Bowel Disease

Inflammatory bowel disease includes both Crohn's disease and ulcerative colitis. In both of these conditions, the intensity and type of symptoms encountered depend on the extent and severity of the bowel involvement. The pain experienced may come from either the viscera itself or from inflammatory processes at extraintestinal sites. In many cases, the symptoms reported may be difficult to separate from other conditions such as irritable bowel syndrome. Symptoms may be either chronic or intermittent. Abdominal pain is more common in Crohn's disease than in ulcerative colitis, but may occur in either.

Ulcerative Colitis

Ulcerative colitis involves an inflammatory process limited to the mucosa of the large bowel and is found primarily in the descending colon and rectum, though the entire colon may be involved. Most sufferers are between the ages of 20 and 50 years. Acute pain and diarrhea are the most common complaints of these patients. The pain encountered is generally mild to moderate. The pain is frequently relieved by bowel movement, but many report the sensation of incomplete evacuation. Most patients experience voluminous, watery diarrhea with occasional blood. Ulcerative colitis may be differentiated from IBS by the frequent presence of fever or bloody stools. Symptoms, combined with sigmoidoscopy, barium enema, or rectal biopsy, will establish the diagnosis.

Crohn's Disease

The inflammatory process in Crohn's disease is transmural and involves both the large and small bowel in 50% of cases. Bowel thickening, stenosis, and internal fistula formation are common with most cases presenting between the ages of 15 and 30 years. Approximately 80–85% of patients with Crohn's disease experience abdominal pain associated with diarrhea and fever, often lasting for days or weeks. The pain described is frequently mid-abdominal or right lower quadrant in location, though generalized pain is often present. Patients may present to their gynecologist with complaints of dyspareunia, vulvar or perineal fissures or fistulas, or occasionally with vulvar granulomas. As with ulcerative colitis, suspicion, symptoms and imaging (upper gastrointestinal X-ray with small bowel follow-through), and colonoscopy will establish the diagnosis.

Diverticular Disease

Diverticular disease is common, occurring in approximately 40% of patients over the age of 60 years, but only about 20% of these patients have symptoms.

Those who do may have significant morbidity including diverticulitis, bleeding, perforation, and pericolonic abscesses. While the symptoms experienced by many patients (pain and diarrhea) are similar to those of patients with IBS, these patients do not have the psychopathology or the exacerbations with stress seen in IBS. Diverticulosis is itself asymptomatic. Only when inflammation, perforation, or other problems occur do symptoms ("diverticulitis") appear.

Colon Cancer and the Gynecologist

Colorectal cancer is the second most common cancer in the United States. An estimated 152,200 new cases occurred in the year 2002, with 77,900 of them in women. The annual mortality is estimated to be 57,100 (29,100 women). Most cases develop in patients 50 years or older, but about 8% are discovered prior to age 40 years.

High fiber diets have become popular in this country largely due to an associated decrease in the incidence of colorectal cancer. (Studies of African tribes on high fiber diets indicate a reduced occurrence of bowel cancers.) High fiber diets are thought to decrease stool transit time and therefore limit bowel wall contact with potential carcinogens in fecal material. This theory is limited by the lack of correlation between diverticular disease (found frequently in patients with low fiber diets) and colorectal cancer. Recent evidence from the National Women's Health Initiative study suggests that estrogen replacement therapy may be associated with a significant reduction in the incidence of colon cancer, but the final role this may play is still being investigated. Studies have also associated the use of some NSAIDs with a reduction in colon polyps, a risk factor for colon cancer, but here again the final answers have not been established.

Hemorrhoids are an anatomic fact of life. Few escape an occasional flare-up of hemorrhoidal symptoms. Either internal or external hemorrhoids may provide symptoms. External hemorrhoids tend to present with irritation, itching, bleeding, and fecal soiling while internal hemorrhoids most often cause blood with bowel movements or on wiping. Either type may undergo thrombosis. A history of rectal bleeding should not be ascribed to hemorrhoids without direct visualization of the bleeding or ruling out other potentially more ominous causes. Over-the-counter medications generally provide adequate relief when combined with strategies designed to avoid extremes of diarrhea or constipation.

Establishing the Diagnosis
Gallbladder Disease

The diagnosis of cholelithiasis is based on history, physical examination, and laboratory investigation. Classically, patients with cholelithiasis complain of fatty food intolerance, variable right upper quadrant pain with radiation to the back or scapula, nausea, or vomiting (Table 16.3). These symptoms frequently

Table 16.3.   Clinical characteristics of cholelithiasis.

Asymptomatic (60–70%)
   50% will become symptomatic
   20% will develop complications
Dyspepsia and fatty food intolerance (10–30%)
Biliary colic (5–10%)
   Due to obstruction
   Right upper quadrant to scapula pain
   Fever
   Nausea and vomiting
Jaundice (<5%)

---

will be evanescent, with variable symptom-free intervals. Fever is usually associated with cholangitis. Symptoms are often mistaken for "indigestion."

Laboratory evaluation is supportive, but often not diagnostic (Table 16.4). A complete blood count may indicate inflammation by leukocytosis. An elevated serum bilirubin may be useful in diagnosing obstruction and serum amylase may indicate the presence of pancreatitis. Determination of

Table 16.4.   Diagnosis of gallbladder disease.

History
Laboratory
   Complete blood count—for inflammation
   Serum bilirubin—for obstruction
   Serum amylase—for pancreatitis
   Serum alkaline phosphatase—indicates obstruction
   Serum aminotransferases (SGOT, SGPT)—metabolic function of liver
Imaging
   Ultrasonography ("gold standard")
   Computed tomography
   Magnetic resonance imaging
   Oral cholecystogram
   Plain X-ray
   Nucleotide imaging
   Endoscopic retrograde cholangiopancreatography
   IV cholangiography
   Transhepatic cholangiography

---

serum alkaline phosphatase may indicate obstruction. Alkaline phosphatase is often elevated during pregnancy, compromising the utility of this test in pregnant patients. Elevated serum amino transferase (SGOT or SGPT) can indicate altered metabolic function of liver cells in cases where obstruction causes damage.

The standard diagnostic tool is abdominal ultrasound and is 96% accurate in making the diagnosis of sludge or stone in the gallbladder. Ultrasonography has surpassed oral cholecystograms as the diagnostic test of choice. The false-negative rate with oral cholecystograms is high and 20% of patients have experienced nausea, vomiting, or diarrhea from the contrast agent. A flat plate of the abdomen will demonstrate only 20% of stones with enough calcium for accurate imaging.

Upper Gastrointestinal Complaints

Gastroesophageal Reflux

Formal evaluation (when indicated) is best accomplished by upper gastrointestinal endoscopy. The information gained will eliminate other potential causes of GERD, including esophageal motility disorders, erosive esophagitis and peptic ulcer disease (gastric or duodenal). A satisfactory working diagnosis may be established on purely clinical grounds and the results of a therapeutic trial with antacids, histamine blockers, or proton pump inhibitors.

Peptic Ulcer Disease

Common symptoms of peptic ulcer include nausea, vomiting, anorexia, fullness and bloating, and pain in the upper abdomen. Pain is described anywhere in the upper abdomen and may be cramping, gnawing, or burning. Pain may last only a few minutes, and response to meals is variable. A correlation between symptoms and demonstrated ulcers is poor and a high degree of suspicion is necessary to make the diagnosis. Physical examination is rarely helpful, unless a more serious complication such as perforation or obstruction is present. Diagnosis is established either by radiographic studies (which may miss as many as 20% of cases) or more reliably by endoscopy.

Large Bowel and Colon Disease

Irritable Bowel Syndrome

The diagnosis of IBS is made by careful history and exclusion of other pathology (Table 16.5). A travel history for exposure to possible bacterial or parasitic infections should be taken. A rectal examination should always be performed. If the history is suspicious for ulcerative colitis or inflammatory bowel disease (by the intensity of symptoms or the presence of bloody stools), the patient should be referred for a barium enema and sigmoidoscopy or colonoscopy.

Consensus in the specialty literature supports the position that taking a detailed history can prevent unnecessary investigation and referrals in patients with IBS. These observations suggest that of the four main symp-

Table 16.5.   Diagnoses to consider for patients with abdominal pain and bowel dysfunction.

Malabsorption: postgastrectomy syndrome, sprue, pancreatic insufficiency

Dietary factors: lactose intolerance, caffeine, alcohol, and fat-containing or gas-producing (e.g., cruciferous vegetables) foods

Infection: bacteria (e.g., *Campylobacter jejuni, Salmonella* spp.), common parasites like *Giardia lamblia*

Inflammatory bowel disease: Crohn's disease or ulcerative colitis, microscopic colitides (e.g., collagenous colitis or mast-cell disease—diagnosed by colonic biopsy)

Psychological disorders: panic disorder, depression, and somatization

Miscellaneous conditions: endometriosis, dysmenorrhea, endocrine tumors (e.g., carcinoid, Zollinger–Ellison syndrome, VIPoma), HIV disease and other associated infections

toms, the more that are present the more likely the diagnosis of IBS. In addition, they document that when mucus and feeling of incomplete evacuation were also present, the patient is most unlikely to have organic disease, requiring further investigation. The Rome II criteria are a simplification of the original diagnostic criteria for application to clinical practice (Table 16.6). These criteria define IBS as a functional bowel disorder that is characterized by the presence of symptoms for at least 12 weeks, not necessarily consecutive, during the preceding year. Furthermore, it presumes a lack of either a structural or biochemical explanation for the symptoms. By adding "onset" to relevant symptom features, the criteria elucidate how discomfort and pain are temporally related to a change in frequency and form of stool.

IBS is characterized by abdominal pain and discomfort, changes in stool frequency and consistency, urgency to defecate, bloating, and mucus in the stool. If a patient presents with chronic (≥ 12 weeks) bowel function disorders including abdominal pain as the dominant symptom with altered bowel function, a diagnosis of IBS is quite likely. Alternative or coexisting diagnoses

Table 16.6.   Rome II diagnostic criteria for irritable bowel syndrome.

At least 12 weeks, which need not be consecutive, in the preceding 12 months, of abdominal discomfort or pain that has two of three features:

Relieved with defecation

Onset associated with a change in frequency of stool

Onset associated with a change in form (appearance) of stool

Source: Reprinted with permission from Rome II: The Functional Gastrointestinal Disorders (2nd ed.), 2000 McLean, VA, DA Drossman, E Corazziari, NJ Talley, WG Thompson, & WE Whitehead (Eds), *www.romecriteria.org.*

are suggested by symptoms such as weight loss, rectal bleeding, or anemia (Table 16.7). Laboratory studies and a physical examination are performed to confirm the absence of organic disease. Sigmoidoscopy should be strongly considered.

Inflammatory Bowel Disease

The inflammatory process in Crohn's disease is transmural and involves both the large and small bowel in 50% of cases. This transmural character results in thickening and the possibility of internal fistula formation that may be detected on contrast enhanced radiographic studies and confirmed by sigmoidoscopy or colonoscopy with biopsy. Granulomas may be found in 15% of patients.

Ulcerative colitis is characterized by an inflammation limited to the mucosa of the large bowel and found primarily in the descending colon and rectum (though the entire colon may be involved). Sigmoidoscopy or colonoscopy may demonstrate superficial inflammation, with ulceration common. Hyperemia and hemorrhage are also common. The rectum is involved in 95% of cases but the inflammation extends proximal in a continuous manner, at times even involving the terminal ileum.

Colon Cancer Screening

Routine testing of stool with hemoccult (cards) is simple and inexpensive and should be a routine part of the pelvic and rectal examinations of patients over the age of 40 years (Table 16.8). Occult blood should never be assumed to be hemorrhoidal unless the source is visualized. Routine observation with flexible sigmoidoscopy has been advocated every 3–5 years, however, cost/benefit analysis has not supported its use at present. The family history may be an important screening tool to select patients who may benefit from further, more aggressive diagnostic workup.

Table 16.7.   Symptoms that suggest diagnoses beyond functional bowel disease.

Anemia
Fever
Persistent diarrhea
Rectal bleeding
Severe constipation
Weight loss
Nocturnal symptoms of pain and abnormal bowel function
Family history of gastrointestinal cancer, inflammatory bowel disease, or
    celiac disease
New onset of symptoms in patients 50+ years of age

Table 16.8.   Colon cancer screening.

Low risk
    Digital examination annually after age 40 years
    Stool guaiac annually after age 50 years
    Over age 50 years—flexible sigmoidoscopy annually then every 3–5 years
       (colonoscopy now preferred but sigmoidoscopy is acceptable)
High risk
    Begin at age 35 years
    Repeat every 3–5 years
       Colonoscopy or barium enema
       Flexible sigmoidoscopy

Clinical Intervention

Gallbladder Disease

Management of cholelithiasis depends on a number of factors, including patient and physician preference. Variables considered in therapeutic options include the severity and character of symptoms, stone composition and size, and availability of various treatment modalities.

Selected patients may be treated with watchful waiting. Dietary modifications aimed at reducing cholesterol and fatty food exposure may decrease the frequency and severity of recurrences. This will probably not alter the progression of symptoms over time because spontaneous reabsorption of existing gallstones is rare.

Depending on the size and character of the stones, oral therapy may be an option. Ursodeoxycholic acid increases the solubility of cholesterol in bile by promoting the formation of a lecithin-cholesterol liquid layer on the stone surface. Ursodeoxycholic acid therapy also causes a concomitant decrease in bile secretion and a decrease in the secretion and reabsorption of cholesterol. This agent has been very effective in decreasing the size of cholesterol gallstones over time without an adverse impact on serum lipids or cholesterol. The rate of stone dissolution (approximately 1 mm per month) limits its applicability to stones greater than 1.5–2 cm in size. Fortunately, the majority of gallstones fall below this size.

Reabsorption of cholesterol stones has been favorable with oral therapy, with resolution of symptoms in 2–3 months. Fifty percent of patients experience a recurrence of stones after cessation of therapy. Eighty-five percent of patients with recurrent stones are asymptomatic. Retreatment with oral therapy in the remaining patients is usually successful.

Surgery

For years, surgery was the definitive therapy for gallstones. Cholecystectomy ranked second only to endoscopy in the frequency of digestive system surgery. Surgical complications are common, with 0.7–1.2% mortality in asymptomatic patients, which rises to almost 5% in patients with acute cholangitis or pancreatitis. Risks of complications triple when associated with common duct exploration.

Lithotripsy

Lithotripsy mechanically disrupts the stone, but has no effect on reabsorption. Many physicians combine lithotripsy with oral therapy to hasten absorption and decrease the possibility of small fragments becoming a nidus for further stone growth. Success with this combined approach has been good.

Upper Gastrointestinal Complaints

Gastroesophageal Reflux

Empirical therapy is appropriate in patients with uncomplicated GERD (Table 16.9). Medications that contribute to reduced esophageal pressure, such as diazepam and calcium channel blockers, should be eliminated. NSAIDs, common in gynecologic practice, may contribute to direct damage to the esophageal mucosa. Cigarette smoking contributes to lowering esophageal pressure, delays esophageal acid clearance, and therefore increases the risk of prolonged acid exposure. Patients should not lie down for 2–3 hours after

Table 16.9.   Therapeutic options for heartburn.

- Lifestyle change
  Stop smoking
  Do not eat within 2–3 hours of bedtime
  Extra pillows/bed wedge
- Dietary change
  Reduce acidic liquids (e.g., orange juice)
  Reduce fatty foods and chocolate
  Avoid onions, garlic, peppermint, and liquors
- Antacids
- Histamine (H_2) antagonists
  Cimetidine, famotidine, nizatidine, ranitidine
- Proton pump inhibitors
  Esomeprazole magnesium, lansoprazole, omeprazole, pantoprazole
     sodium, rabeprazole sodium

Table 16.10.   Therapeutic options for dyspepsia and chronic gastritis.

- Lifestyle change
  Stress reduction
  Stop smoking
- Dietary change
  Slow, stress-free meals
  Balanced diet, moderate amounts
  Increased fiber
  Avoid irritants
- Medications
  Bethanechol, antiemetics, phenobarbital
- Antacids
- Histamine (H_2) antagonists
  Cimetidine, famotidine, nizatidine, ranitidine
- Proton pump inhibitors
  Esomeprazole magnesium, lansoprazole, omeprazole, pantoprazole
    sodium, rabeprazole sodium

consuming large meals. Placing the bed on 6–8 inch blocks or using a bed wedge has been shown to decrease acid exposure and is as effective as medication in healing reflux esophagitis. Diet should be modified by eliminating liquids with high acid content (such as orange juice). Fatty foods and chocolate decrease esophageal pressure and delay gastric emptying that contribute to symptoms. Substances found in onions, garlic, peppermint, and certain after-dinner liquors increase gas, belching, and lower esophageal pressure. These foods should be eliminated from the diet.

Before the widespread availability of H_2-antagonists and proton pump inhibitors, antacids were the preferred therapy. Due to the frequent dosage intervals required, compliance was a problem. Antacids often resulted in diarrhea, bloating, and constipation. Cimetadine, ranitidine, and famotidine are common medications that have become available without prescription. For those with resistant symptoms or when esophageal damage is suspected or documented, the use of proton pump inhibitors is more appropriate. The mechanism of action is the inhibition of the hydrogen potassium pump in gastric acid-producing cells. Due to a lack of long-term follow-up, the use of these drugs should be limited to 8–12 weeks. Referral of patients with this degree of disease severity is prudent.

Similar treatment strategies may be applied to those with chronic dyspepsia and gastritis as well (Table 16.10).

Peptic Ulcer Disease

Several therapies are effective in treating ulcers (Table 16.11), but ulcers usually require 12 weeks of therapy to completely heal. Treatment regimens with antisecretory agents include H_2-receptor antagonists (cimetidine, ranitidine, and famotidine), proton pump inhibitors (esomeprazole magnesium, lansoprazole, omeprazole, pantoprazole sodium, rabeprazole sodium), antimuscarinic drugs (rarely used due to side effects of blurred vision and dry mouth), and prostaglandins (misoprostol). As in esophageal reflux, antacids are rarely used due to frequent dosage schedules and side effects of diarrhea or constipation. Sucralfate is an aluminum hydroxide salt of sucrose octasulfate that is effective in duodenal ulcers. In patients with *H. pylori* infection, a combination of bismuth (Pepto-Bismol) and an antibiotic (metronidazole 250 mg q6 hours,

Table 16.11.   Therapeutic options for peptic ulcers.

- Lifestyle change
  Stress reduction
  Stop smoking
- Dietary change
  Slow, stress-free meals
  Balanced diet, moderate amounts
  Increased fiber
  Avoid irritants
- General medications
  Bethanechol, antiemetics, phenobarbital
- Proton pump inhibitors
  Esomeprazole magnesium, lansoprazole, omeprazole, pantoprazole
    sodium, rabeprazole sodium
- Bismuth/Antibiotic (2 week therapy)
  Metronidazole 250 mg q6h
  plus
  Tetracycline 500 mg q6h
  or
  Amoxicillin 500 mg q8h
- Antibiotic + acid suppression (4 week therapy)
  Clarithromycin (Bixin)
  plus
  Omeprazole (Prilosec)
  or
  Bismuth citrate (Tritec)

tetracycline 500 mg q6 hours, or amoxicillin 500 mg q8 hours) has been recommended for 2 weeks. A 4-week treatment with clarithromycin (Bixin) and either omeprazole (Prilosec) or ranitidine bismuth citrate (Tritec) is also an option.

Large Bowel and Colon Disease

Irritable Bowel Syndrome

Treatment of IBS is difficult due to the chronicity of the condition. Because many of these patients have hysterical, depressive, and bipolar personality disorders, psychological support is important. Bulk agents and increased dietary fiber in association with patient education may be helpful. Mild sedation with phenobarbital and tranquilizers may afford some relief, though long-term success is generally poor. In some studies, placebo response rates are as high as 80%.

Many of the pharmacological agents that are used for the treatment of IBS target only one symptom. Consequently, patients may need to take more than one medication to control their symptoms. Medications should be targeted toward the predominant symptom (e.g., pain, diarrhea, or constipation). Tricyclic antidepressants and selective serotonin reuptake inhibitors (SSRIs) are often prescribed for patients with severe or refractory pain.

Because of the role of $5\text{-}HT_3$ in the development of IBS, $5\text{-}HT_3$ receptor blocking agents would seem promising, but recently introduced agents have had to be withdrawn because of side effects or untoward outcomes. For many patients whose primary symptom is constipation, fiber is often recommended. If this is unsuccessful, osmotic laxatives may be prescribed. Stimulant laxatives (e.g., bisacodyl, phenolphthalein) enhance intestinal motility and stimulate accumulation of water and electrolytes in the colonic lumen. These agents are effective in relieving constipation associated with IBS. In some patients, laxatives can exacerbate abdominal pain and bloating, and should be used with caution when these symptoms are already present.

Inflammatory Bowel Disease

The management of both ulcerative colitis and Crohn's disease is complicated, long, and disappointing. Referral to a gastroenterologist is strongly suggested.

Case Studies

Case 1. A 34-year-old G3P3003 white woman presents with a 3-month history of crampy upper abdominal pain. She has also experienced burping, dysphagia, and occasional nausea, all of which seem to be worse after meals. What diagnoses would you consider and how would you proceed to evaluate this patient?

Based on this patient's symptoms, both esophageal reflux and cholelithiasis would be possible diagnoses. While we do not specifically have a history of fatty food intolerance or any high-risk factors, cholelithiasis is still possible because often the earliest symptoms of gallbladder disease are vague and nonspecific. More likely with the limited information we are given is esophageal reflux—GERD. Because it is reasonable to make this diagnosis on clinical grounds alone, a therapeutic trial may result in both consolidation of the diagnosis and relief of the symptoms. Initial therapy with antacids is acceptable, but the use of either an H_2 or proton pump inhibitor might be more expeditious.

Case 2. A 22-year-old G2P1001 woman returns to the office for a routine prenatal examination at 34 weeks of gestation. You have cared for her since her eighth week of pregnancy. Today she reports: "I have been having increasing problems with heartburn after I eat, difficulty swallowing, a sour taste in my mouth, and I have a persistent dry cough. I have tried to eat some peppermints to see if I can make it better and it only gets worse." She smokes 1 pack of cigarettes per day and drinks alcohol occasionally. Her blood pressure is 118/64 mm Hg. She weighs 56 kg (123 lb) and is 155 cm (5 ft 1 in.) tall. The uterus is palpable to 36 cm above the symphysis and fetal heart tones are normal. What is the most likely physiologic explanation for the symptoms this patient is experiencing?

While there is no doubt that (appropriate) uterine enlargement is present and there is a reasonable expectation that the patient's intraabdominal pressure is somewhat elevated, the most likely explanation of this patient's symptoms is a physiologic reduction in lower esophageal tone. The elevated hormones of pregnancy result in a physiologic relaxation of the lower esophagus. When this is combined with the reduced gastric emptying time typical of late pregnancy and the exacerbating effects of things like peppermint, alcohol, and smoking, this explanation is the most likely. If antacids are chosen, agents such as Gaviscon that form a layer high in the stomach or those that coat the lower esophagus may be more effective. Proton pump and H_2 inhibitors are generally pregnancy category B, and some may be used with caution for selected patients.

Suggested Reading

American Gastroenterological Association. Irritable bowel syndrome: a technical review for practice guideline development. *Gastroenterology* 1997; 112:2120–37.

American Gastroenterological Association Patient Care Committee. American Gastroenterological Association medical position statement: irritable bowel syndrome. *Gastroenterology* 1997;112:2118–9.

Bearcroft CP, Perrett D, Farthing MJG. Postprandial plasma 5-hydroxytryptamine in diarrhea predominant irritable bowel syndrome: a pilot study. *Gut* 1998;42:42–6.

Boston Collaborative Drug Surveillance Program. Surgically confirmed gall-bladder disease, venous thromboembolism, and breast tumors in relation to postmenopausal estrogen therapy. *N Engl J Med* 1974;290:15–9.

Drossman DA. Review article: an integrated approach to the irritable bowel syndrome. *Aliment Pharmacol Ther* 1999;13(suppl 2):3–14.

Everson GT, McKinley C, Kern F, Jr. Mechanisms of gallstone formation in women. *J Clin Invest* 1991;87:237–46.

Feldman M, Burton ME. Drug therapy: histamine$_2$-receptor antagonists—standard therapy for acid-peptic disease. *N Engl J Med* 1990;323:1672–80, 1749–55.

Humphrey PPA, Bountra C, Clayton N, Kozlowski K. Review article: the therapeutic potential of 5-HT3 receptor antagonists in the treatment of irritable bowel syndrome. *Aliment Pharmacol Ther* 1999;13(suppl 2): 31–8.

Ikard RW. Gallstones, cholecystitis and diabetes. *Surg Gynecol Obstet* 1990;171:528–32.

Katz PO. Gastroesophageal reflux disease—state of the art. *Rev Gastroenterol Disord* 2001;1:128–38.

Maclure KM, Hayes KC, Colditz GA, Stampfer MJ, Willett WC. Dietary predictors of symptom-associated gallstones in middle-aged women. *Am J Clin Nutr* 1990;52:916–22.

McSherry CK, Ferstenberg H, Calhoun WF, Lahman E, Virshup M. The natural history of diagnosed gallstone disease in symptomatic and asymp-tomatic patients. *Ann Surg* 1985;202:59–63.

Mitchell CM, Drossman DA. The irritable bowel syndrome: understanding and treating a biopsychosocial illness disorder. *Ann Behav Med* 1987; 9:13–8.

Paterson WG, Thompson WG, Vanner SJ, et al. Recommendations for the management of irritable bowel syndrome in family practice. *Can Med Assoc J* 1999;161:154–60.

Peterson WL. Current concepts: *Helicobacter pylori* and peptic ulcer disease. *N Engl J Med* 1991;324:1043–8.

Rapkin AJ, Mayer EA. Gastroenterologic causes of chronic pelvic pain. *Obstet Gynecol Clin N Am* 1993;20:663–84.

Sastic JW, Glassman CI. Gallbladder disease in young women. *Surg Obstet Gynecol* 1982;155:209–11.

Smith RP, Ellis JW. COX-1 and COX-2: understanding the differences. *OBG Manage* 2002;14(7):79.

Smith RP, Nolan TE. Gallbladder disease and women: etiology, diagnosis and therapy. *Female Patient* 1992;17:99–113.

Smith WL, Garavito RM, DeWitt DL. Prostaglandin endoperoxide H synthase (cyclooxygenase)-1 and -2. *J Biol Chem* 1996;271:33157.

Soll AH. Pathogenesis of peptic ulcer and implications for therapy. *N Engl J Med* 1990;322:909–16.

Thompson WG, Longstreth GF, Drossman DA, Heaton KW, Irvine EJ, Müller-Lissner SA. Functional bowel disorders and functional abdominal pain. *Gut* 1999;45(suppl 2):1143–7.

17

Headaches

Douglas W. Laube

Background Information

Headache as a Presenting Symptom

Headache is generally accepted as one of the 10 most common causes for visits to a physician's office. It can be the source of disability, lost time from work and school, as well as a significant expense item as a medical workup is initiated. The obstetrician-gynecologist as a primary care provider is faced with the task of differentiating common, benign conditions from more serious causes with appropriate therapy being a natural outgrowth of this initial determination. The majority of headaches are identified as either due to muscle contractions or migraine headaches with other etiologies being less common.

Community surveys suggest that up to 80% of women report headaches during any given month, with the prevalence of headaches declining with age. However, the frequency of visits to see physicians for the management of headaches increases with age.

As most headaches are self-limited, patients seek treatment primarily because of (1) severity, (2) recent onset, (3) chronicity, (4) failure of relief from over-the-counter analgesics, or (5) possible relationship to head injury or other medical problems. It is not uncommon for the patient to be seeking reassurance that organic pathology such as a brain tumor is not present.

As with other medical problems, the relationship between the physician and the patient is critical in diagnosis and treatment. The physician should develop a systematic yet sympathetic approach to diagnosing and managing these patients considering the possibility of underlying medical problems as well as the environmental issues that may be involved (i.e., social, emotional, and psychological factors). The ability to care for patients over time may prove critical in the success of any therapy. A physician should consider the following issues when evaluating a patient:

1. What are the environmental issues involved?
2. Is there an underlying etiology?
3. What medical tests should be ordered?
4. Is there drug-seeking behavior?

These and other issues should be part of the overall evaluation of any patient with headache.

Diagnosing Headaches

Headaches can be classified as primary or secondary with primary headaches defined as those not directly related to underlying disease and secondary headaches reflecting an underlying pathologic condition. Historically, physicians and medical students are admonished to "first rule out brain tumor" when a patient's principal symptom is headache. This is not sound advice because intracranial causes of headaches are rare as compared to extracranial causes. A general rule is not to search for something in the least likely place. A preferable approach is to seek the pain source in the most probable places and, having found it, quit looking. The method is familiar: take a thorough history and do a focused physical examination with the goal of being on the safe side and the inexpensive side of the skull (the outside). In the diagnosis of headache, sensitivities, specificity, and predictive value are in the following order: best for history; good for examination; and poor for chemical, electrical, and radiographic tests.

The diagnosis of headache is outlined in Table 17.1 by considering elements of the history and physical examination. Other headache characteristics are summarized in Table 17.2.

Diagnostic Tests

Tests have less to offer than generally supposed. Skull and sinus radiographs are seldom helpful in the absence of injury or suspicion of sepsis. The electroencephalogram (EEG) is great for seizure diagnosis but poor for headache diagnosis. The computerized tomographic (CT) head scan is grossly overused and seldom revealing with common headache symptomatology. CT and magnetic resonance imaging (MRI) tests are at their best when central nervous system symptoms or signs are part of the headache syndrome. Both are too expensive to use as diagnostic tests early in the workup of headache without specific symptomatology or neurologic findings.

Table 17.1. History and physical.

History	Physical
Past history	Focal neurologic
• Time and circumstance of onset?	• Pupils; reflexes
• Head injury? (within past 2 weeks)	
• Medications (including OCPs)	Fundoscopic examinations
• Spontaneous retinal venous	
Current History	Pulsations (SRVP) are *normal*;
• Frequency and duration	they are absent in papilledema
• Quality (pulsatile; valsalva)	
• Location (unilateral; bilateral;	Scalp vessels
front; back)	• Temporal arteries/pulsations
• Associated symptoms?	• Temporomandibular joints
• Other ailments? (depression)	• Neck rigidity
• Family history	
• Vocational history (noise; toxins;	
lights)	
• Previous R_x/self-R_x	

Classification of Headaches

Headache classification directs therapy and may be categorized into two major types. These are tension headaches, of which the most common is episodic tension headache and migraine. Migraine is further subdivided into migraine with aura (classic migraine) and migraine without aura (common migraine). Table 17.3 summarizes the major categories of headache.

Primary Headaches

Headaches can be classified as "primary" or "secondary." Primary headaches are defined as those not directly related to underlying disease while secondary headaches reflect an underlying pathologic condition. This latter includes conditions such as structural abnormalities, infection, inflammation, trauma, tumors, intracranial bleeding, drug abuse, environmental exposures, and psychosocial factors. Exclusion of these etiologies is critical as part of the evaluation of headaches and the presumptive treatment for a primary cause.

Table 17.2. Headache characteristics.

	Migraine	Tension	Cluster	Temporomandibular joint	Temporal arteritis	Tumor
Usual age at onset (years)	15 to 25	Variable	20–30	20–40	>60	Any
Childhood history	Common	15%	No	No	No	No
Family history	Yes	+/-	No	No	No	No
Sex distribution	F > M	F > M	M >> F	F > M	+/-	M = F
Aura	+Classic	No	No	No	No	No
Pain character	Throbbing	Aching	Stabbing	Aching	Ache	Ache
Pain distribution	+/- Unilateral	Diffuse	Retroorbital	Ear	Temporal	Variable
Pain duration	Hours to days	Hours to constant	20–40 minutes	Variable	Constant	Progressive
Associated symptoms	Nausea Photophobia Phonophobia	Depression	Horner's lacrimation coryza	Jaw click Tenderness	Malaise High ESR	Focality

Table 17.3.   Migraine and tension headache.

Migraine without aura (common migraine)
  A. At least five attacks
  B. Headache lasting 4–72 hours
  C. Headache has at least two of the following characteristics:
      1. Unilateral location
      2. Pulsating quality
      3. Moderate to severe intensity
      4. Aggravation by routine physical activity
  D. During headache at least one of the following:
      1. Nausea and/or vomiting
      2. Photophobia and phonophobia

Migraine with aura (classic migraine)
  A. At least two attacks
  B. At least three of the following four characteristics:
      1. One or more fully reversible aura symptoms indicating focal
          cerebral cortical or brainstem dysfunction
      2. At least one symptom develops gradually over more than 4
          minutes or two or more symptoms occur in succession
      3. No aura symptom lasts more than 60 minutes
      4. Headache follows aura with a free interval of less than 60
          minutes (it may also begin before or simultaneously with the
          aura)

Episodic tension headache
  A. At least 10 previous headache episodes
      Headache days <180/year (<15/month)
  B. Headache lasting from 30 minutes to 7 days
  C. At least two of the following pain characteristics:
      1. Pressing/tightening (nonpulsating) quality
      2. Mild or moderate intensity (may inhibit, but does not prohibit
          activities)
      3. Bilateral location
      4. No aggravation by routine physical activity
  D. Both of the following:
      1. No nausea or vomiting (anorexia may occur)
      2. Photophobia and phonophobia are absent, or one but not the
          other is present

Tension Headaches

The pain of tension headache is usually described as dull, aching, and constant and characteristically does not have pulsatile or throbbing components more likely associated with vascular headache. The distribution of tension headache is usually bilateral with the temporal and occipital regions being most commonly affected, thus giving it the so-called "hatband" distribution. Although tension headaches may become manifest at any time in life, they often begin in childhood and progress with varying frequency through adulthood. Typically, the pattern is not progressively more severe and often is associated with episodes of emotional stress. The key feature in the history is that tension headaches build as stress builds whereas vascular and most migraine syndromes start quickly after a stressful event. A tension headache can almost always be diagnosed clinically and therapy begun using simple analgesics once organic disease has been ruled out by history and a focused physical examination. Because depression may often be associated with chronic tension headaches, this disorder should be assessed with the expectation that headaches will improve as the depression is treated.

Headaches—Migraine or Not?

For the gynecologist, an appreciation of the need for management of menstrual migraine is obvious. This disorder can be treated successfully with relatively simple therapy the majority of the time. Menstrual migraine is defined (using the International Classification) as a migraine headache beginning between 1 day before menstruation and 4 days after the onset of menstrual flow. The most common day to develop headache is day 0 (the first day of bleeding). Because of the predictability of the onset of headache symptoms, this variant of migraine is amenable to a variety of therapies. Treatment for menstrual migraine is therefore usually effective when appropriate prophylactic medication is used prior to the onset or at the time of the onset of early symptoms. This "physiologic migraine diary" is used successfully in the majority of menstrual migraine sufferers after review of the headache history and appropriate counseling based on the timing of symptom onset.

Treatment of Migraine Headaches

Whether menstrually related or not, migraine headaches pose a significant problem to patients. Of the approximately 18 million women in the United States who do suffer from migraine, exacerbation at the time of menses is not uncommon. In addition to supportive counseling, validation of symptoms using a headache diary is critical. Nonmedical therapies as well as medical therapies have been described.

As the assumption underlying the onset of menstrual migraines is a drop in estrogen levels, prophylactic treatment can be rendered by using two

0.05-mg transdermal estrogen patches beginning the day before expected menstruation or one long-acting 0.1-mg (7-day) transdermal patch applied the day before expected menstruation. This effectively provides the patient with continuous estrogen levels throughout the cycle.

For the postmenopausal patient, continuation of estrogen on a regular, uncycled schedule is the obvious alternative. For patients who are already on a continuous estrogen preparation with intermittent cyclic progestins, additional 0.05-mg transdermal patches may be used after the progestin withdrawal and during menstruation. It is unclear why some post-menopausal women continue to have "menstrual migraines" despite being on continuous estrogen replacement. However, empiric treatment of this group of patients may include additional 0.05-mg transdermal patches through the time following progestin withdrawal and expected menstruation. Alternatively, the various prevention medications listed in Table 17.4 may also be applied depending on the patient's general health and cardiovascular status.

Triptans are a new class of vasoactive headache therapy developed over the past several years. These medications provide a fast-acting, effective therapy for migraine. They generally fall in the class of medications that function as serotonin agonists. They may be administered subcutaneously, sublingually, or orally. Generally, they are not used for prophylaxis, but for acute abortive therapy. A list of these is given in Table 17.5. These should be used cautiously in the older patient and may be contraindicated in patients who have ischemic heart disease.

For younger women on oral contraceptives who experience menstrual migraine in the pill-free interval, additional transdermal or oral estrogen may be indicated as a way to ameliorate the sudden drop of synthetic estrogens that occurs following the ingestion of the final active tablet. Even though these younger women have endogenous estrogen levels, their ovaries remain relatively inactive secondary to the effects of the oral contraceptive pill. Therefore, withdrawal of the contraceptive pill creates an artificial drop in relatively high estrogen levels. Management of vascular headaches generally falls into three categories: prophylactic therapy, abortive therapy, and emergency therapy. Prophylactic treatment of migraine is generally considered in patients who have predictable or frequent attacks. Two categories are included in this group. The first is the menstrual migraine sufferer and the second is the patient with more than three attacks per month. Other patients for whom prophylactic treatment should be considered are those who are refractory to abortive treatments and patients who have contraindications to the most effective abortive medications. An example of this group would be the older patient with ischemic heart disease or vascular insufficiency such that there are contraindications to the vasoactive drugs. Tables 17.4 and 17.5 list medications for prophylactic treatment and medications used as abortive therapy, respectively.

Table 17.4. Medications for prevention of migraines.

Drug	Daily oral dosage range	Comments
β-Blockers		
Propranolol	40–329 mg/day	Effective; side effects: drowsiness, nightmares, insomnia, depression, memory disturbances, decreased exercise tolerance
Atenolol	50–150 mg/day	
Nadolol	40–240 mg/day	
Timolo maleate	10–30 mg/day	
Calcium-channel blockers		
Verapamil	240–720 mg/day	Benefit may lag 3 to 4 weeks; side effects: hypotension, edema, headache, constipation
Nifedipine	30–180 mg/day	
Diltiazem	120–360 mg/day	
Antidepressants		
Nortriptyline	10–125 mg/day	
Amitriptyline	10–300 mg/day	
Fluoxetine	20–80 mg/day	
Serotonin antagonists		
Methylergonovine	0.2–0.4 mg, 4 times per day	
Methysergide	2–8 mg/day; continuous usage should not exceed 6 months at a time, with a drug-free interval of 4 weeks	

Table 17.5.   Medications for treatment of headache.

Drug	Route of administration	Dosage range
Simple analgesics ± caffeine		
Acetaminophen 250 mg and/250 mg; caffeine 65 mg	po[a]	Limit dose to 1 g stat, or Aspirin 4 g/day; avoid daily use
Combination analgesics ± butalbital		
Aspirin 325 mg or acetaminophen 325 mg; butalbital 50 mg; caffeine 40 mg	po	Limit dose to 1 or 2 stat, 4/attack, 24/month
Aspirin 650 mg or acetaminophen 325 mg; butalbital 50 mg	po	
Combination analgesics with narcotics		
Aspirin 325 mg; butalbital 50 mg; caffeine 40 mg; codeine phosphate 30 mg	po	Limit dose to 1 or 2 stat, 6/attack, and 16/month
Aspirin 325 mg; codeine 30 mg		
Acetaminophen 125, 300, or 325 mg; codeine 7.5, 15, 30, or 60 mg	po po	
Nonsteroidal antiinflammatory drugs commonly used		
Naproxen sodium 2.75 mg	po	Maximum initial dose 825 mg[b]
Ibuprofen 200, 300, 400, 600, or 800 mg	po	Maximum initial dose 800 mg[b]
Meclofenamate sodium 50 or 100 mg	po	Maximum initial dose 100 mg[b]

Continued.

Table 17.5. *Continued.*

Drug	Route of administration	Dosage range
Sympathomimetic agents		
Isometheptene, acetaminophen, dichloralphenazone	po	Dose: 2 stat, can repeat in 1 hour (limit: 3 times/week)
Ergotamine tartrate[c]		
Caffeine 100 mg; ergotamine tartrate 1 mg	po/rectally	Dose: up to 6 mg po or 2 suppositories stat. Limit monthly use to 8 events or 24 mg po, or to 12 suppositories
Dihydroergotamine mesylate[c]		
Dihydroergotamine mesylate 1 mg/ml ampule	Intramuscularly/ intravenously	Dose: up to 1 mg stat, 3 mg/day. Limit monthly use to 12 events or 18 ampules
Serotonin agonists[d]		
Sumatriptan	Subcutaneously (sc)/po	6 mg sc; can be repeated after 1 hour (limit: 2 injections/24 hours); 100 mg po; can be repeated after 1 hour (limit: 2 tablets/24 hours)
Eletriptan	po	20–40 mg to 80 mg maximum daily
Navatriptan	po	1–2.5 mg to 5 mg maximum daily

[a] Route po, per os.
[b] Up to maximum dose may be taken stat.
[c] Keep 3 days between dosing with ergotamine in patients with frequent or daily headache.
[d] For protracted migraines, serotonin agonists may be used.

Table 17.6.   Migraine triggers.

Dietary
Alcohol
Aspartame (NutraSweet)
Caffeine
Cheese
Chocolate
Monosodium glutamate
Nitrites, nitrates (hot dogs, fast foods)
Nuts

Hormonal
Menstruation
Oral contraceptives
Ovulation

Sensorial
Bright lights
Flickering lights
Odors

Medications
H_2 blockers
Danazol
OCPs

Other
Changes in diet, eating pattern (skipping meals, dieting), personal or work schedule, season, sleeping pattern, weather, stress

---

Additionally, common migraine triggers (Table 17.6) should be considered. This aspect of treatment is necessarily part of the counseling involved with prophylactic treatment of vascular headaches. Approximately 10–20% of patients will have sufficient amelioration of headaches by simple counseling techniques designed to identify the triggers and help the patient avoid these common dietary or situational triggers.

Summary

As a primary care physician for women, the obstetrician-gynecologist should be prepared to deal with a broad array of presenting symptoms. Of these, headache is quite common and differentiation between primary and secondary headaches is critical. Just as important is the differentiation among primary sources of migraine and nonmigraine headache.

Suggested Reading

Farkkila M, Olesen J, Daholf C, et al. Eletriptan for the treatment of migraine in patients with previous poor response or tolerance to oral sumatriptan. *Cephalalgia* 2003;23:413–71.

Granella F, Sances G, Zanferrari C, et al. Migraine without aura and reproductive life events: a clinical epidemiologic study in 1300 women. *Headache* 1993;33:385–9.

Headache Classification Committee of the International Headache Society. Classification and diagnostic criteria for headache disorders, cranial neuralgia, and facial pain. *Cephalalgia* 1988;8:1–96.

Silberstein SD. The role of sex hormones in headache. *Neurology* 1992; 42:37–42.

Silberstein SD. Migraine and other headache disorders. *Clin Update Women's Health Care* 2002;1(3).

Stewart WF, Lipton RB, Celentano DD, et al. Prevalence of migraine headache in the United States. *JAMA* 1992;267:64–9.

18

Nutrition, Obesity, and Eating Disorders

Bernadette McIntire and Joseph A. Lacy

Introduction

In 1947, the World Health Organization stated that health is a complete state of physical, mental, and social well-being and not merely the absence of disease. Yet today, despite living 6.4 years longer than men, women suffer poorer health outcomes and greater disability from disease.

The 10 leading causes of death in the United States for women of all ages and races result from diseases of the heart, malignant neoplasms, cerebrovascular disease, chronic obstructive pulmonary disease, pneumonia and influenza, diabetes, accidents, Alzheimer's disease, kidney disease, and septicemia. Nutrition is involved in the etiology or treatment of 50% of the 10 leading causes of death in women.

Women's health encompasses emotional, social, cultural, spiritual, and physical well-being. It is determined by their genes and by the social, political, and economic context of their lives.

Cardiovascular Disease

Risk factors in women include smoking, hypercholesterolemia, obesity and central adiposity, diabetes, hypertension, physical inactivity, and poor diet. Women who gain 20 pounds or more in early adulthood double their risk of heart disease. Because they have more risk factors, postmenopausal women have a two- to three-fold greater rate of heart disease than premenopausal women.

Nutrition is a major component in preventing cardiovascular disease through lifestyle change. Modest changes in dietary cholesterol have a small (if any) effect on plasma cholesterol levels. Dietary saturated fatty acids generally increase low-density lipoprotein (LDL) cholesterol, whereas monounsaturated fatty acids and polyunsaturated fatty acids lower LDL by increasing the liver's uptake of LDL. Dietary trans fatty acids increase the risk of developing cardiovascular disease. Trans fatty acids are found mainly in hydrogenated vegetable fats (stick margarines, shortenings, processed foods).

Fish and shellfish, rich in omega-3 fatty acids, provide beneficial effects in cardiovascular disease (see Table 18.1). Omega-3 fatty acids affect the ability to synthesize and clear very low-density lipoproteins and chylomicrons. Two to three fish meals per week are recommended.

Obesity, a major risk factor for heart attacks, heightens the inflammatory response. Overweight and obese people tend to have higher levels of high sensitivity C-reactive protein (hs-CRP). Smoking increases hs-CRP and exercise reduces it.

A high intake of whole grains, especially soluble fiber, reduces blood lipids and decreases the risk of heart disease. For 1–2 g of soluble fiber consumed daily, LDL is lowered by 1%. Optimally, 10–25 g of soluble fiber should be consumed per day (see Table 18.2).

Soy foods contain protein and isoflavone components that have special effects on reducing cardiovascular disease as follows:

- Soy protein favorably affects all blood lipid levels.
- Soy isoflavones are important antioxidants that prevent oxidation of LDL.
- Soy foods decrease the tendency to form blood clots.
- Soy isoflavones have health-promoting effects on blood vessels.

Table 18.1.   Fat content in fish.

Fish (6 ounces cooked)	Grams fat	Grams omega-3 fat
Salmon, Atlantic, farmed	21	3.7
Salmon, Atlantic, wild	14	3
Rainbow trout	12	2.0
Swordfish	9	1.4
Oysters	4	1.1
Flounder or sole	3	0.9

Table 18.2.   Soluble fiber in some foods.

Food	Grams soluble fiber
½ cup cooked oatmeal	1
1 cup Wheat Chex	1
1 cup collard greens, cooked	3.5
½ cup kidney beans	3
½ cup pinto beans	2
½ cooked brussels sprouts	3
1 medium apple with skin	1
I medium orange	2
½ cup prunes	3

- Soy protein intake is associated with a 9.3% reduction of serum cholesterol.
- Soy protein is associated with a 2.9% reduction in serum LDL.
- Soy protein is associated with a 10.5% reduction in serum triglycerides.

Chick peas and legumes are good sources of isoflavones. To obtain 25 g soy protein a day consume four (eight-ounce) cups soy milk or 12 ounces of tofu daily. To prevent cardiovascular disease:

- Achieve and maintain a desirable weight.
- Limit dietary fat (see Table 18.3).
- Limit animal sources rich in saturated fatty acids and cholesterol.
- Eat an abundance of fruits and vegetables, complex carbohydrates, and whole grains.
- Consume fish at least twice a week.
- Use vegetable oils rich in monounsaturated fatty acids (olive oil).

Table 18.3.   Dietary fat guidelines.

Daily calories	Maximum grams total fat
1200	40
1500	50
1800	60
2000	67
2400	80

Hypertension

Women with intact ovaries have lower blood pressure than age-matched men. Menopause abolishes the differences and women may develop a "male pattern" of hypertension. Premenopausal women tend to be more resistant to salt effect on blood pressure than men until menopause ensures there is loss of estrogen, at which point they become more sensitive to salt than men.

Here are five strategies to help lower blood pressure or to minimize its upward trend with aging:

1. Lose weight if overweight. Losing as few as 10 pounds can make a difference.
2. Cut sodium to less than 2400 mg a day.
3. Exercise for 1 hour of accumulated physical activity per day.
4. Women who drink alcohol should limit intake to one drink a day.
5. Try a lower salt DASH diet, which may lower blood pressure (see Table 18.4). Such a diet is low in total fat and saturated fat and high in fiber, potassium, calcium, and magnesium.

Table 18.4. Following the DASH Eating Plan.

Food Group	Daily Servings	Serving Sizes
Grains*	6–8	1 slice bread 1 oz dry cereal[†] ½ cup cooked rice, pasta, or cereal
Vegetables	4–5	1 cup raw leafy vegetables ½ cup cut-up raw or cooked vegetable ½ cup vegetable juice
Fruits	4–5	1 medium fruit ¼ cup dried fruit ½ cup fresh, frozen, or canned fruit ½ cup fruit juice
Fat-free or low-fat milk and milk products	2–3	1 cup milk or yogurt 1½ oz cheese
Lean meats, poultry, or fish	6 or less	1 oz cooked meats, poultry, or fish 1 egg[‡]
Nuts, seeds, and legumes	4–5 per week	⅓ cup or 1½ oz nuts 2 Tbsp peanut butter 2 Tbsp or ½ oz seeds ½ cup cooked legumes (dry beans and peas)
Fats and oils[§]	2–3	1 tsp soft margarine 1 tsp vegetable oil 1 Tbsp mayonnaise 2 Tbsp salad dressing
Sweets and added sugars	5 or less per week	1 Tbsp sugar 1 Tbsp jelly or jam ½ cup sorbet, gelatin 1 cup lemonade

* Whole grains are recommended for most grain servings as a good source of fiber and nutrients.
[†] Serving sizes vary between ½ cup and 1½ cups, depending on cereal type. Check the product's Nutrition Facts label.
Source: Your Guide to Lowering Your Blood Pressure with DASH. U.S. Department of Health and Human Services, National Institutes of Health, National Heart, Lung, and Blood Institute.

Weight Control

Today, 60% of adults in the United States are overweight or obese. Thirty-five percent of American adults are overweight, and an additional 26% are obese. Fat in our diet has fallen from 40% in 1990 to 34% today.

In 1960 3100 calories were consumed per person per day. That figure climbed to 3700 calories in 1990 according to the United States Department of Agriculture.

Body Mass Index

The body mass index (BMI) represents weight in kilograms divided by height in meters squared or BMI = kg/m^2 (see Table 18.5).

Obesity is defined as BMI greater than 30, while someone is considered to be overweight with a BMI greater than 25.

BMI does not work for

- Anyone less than 18 years old.
- Competitive athletes.
- Body builders.
- Pregnant or nursing women.
- Frail or sedentary elderly persons.

The following serious health hazards are associated with obesity:

- Coronary heart disease.
- Stroke.
- Hypertension.
- Hypercholesterolemia.
- Hypertriglyceridemia.
- Gallbladder disease.
- Obstructive sleep apnea.
- Degenerative joint disease.
- Gout.
- Certain cancers (breast, endometrial cancers).

Obesity is associated with poor pregnancy outcome, miscarriage, infertility, and polycystic ovarian syndrome. Not only does obesity increase the risk of several diseases, it also places a great psychological burden on women. Women who are obese may suffer from prejudice in society and experience a reduced quality of life.

Shape Up America! The antiobesity campaign launched by former United States Surgeon General C. Everett Koop, MD, advocates the ranges for body fat listed in Table 18.6. The basal metabolic rate tends to drop an estimated 2% every decade starting at the age of 30 years. The result is that after 30 years, a person needs fewer daily calories to remain at the same weight.

Table 18.5. Weight (pounds) by height and body mass index.[a]

BMI

Height	22	23	24	25	26	27	28	29	30	31	32	33	34	35	36	37	38	39	40
4'10"	105	110	115	119	124	129	134	139	143	148	153	158	163	167	173	177	182	186	191
4'11"	109	114	119	124	128	133	138	143	148	153	158	163	169	173	179	183	189	193	193
5'0"	113	118	123	128	133	138	143	148	153	159	164	169	175	179	185	189	195	200	204
5'1"	116	122	127	132	137	143	148	153	158	164	169	174	180	185	191	196	202	206	211
5'2"	120	126	131	136	142	147	153	158	164	169	175	180	186	191	197	202	209	213	218
5'3"	124	130	135	141	146	152	158	164	169	175	181	187	192	198	204	209	215	220	225
5'4"	128	134	140	145	151	157	163	169	174	180	187	193	199	204	210	215	222	227	232
5'5"	132	138	144	150	156	162	168	174	180	186	193	199	205	210	217	222	229	234	240
5'6"	136	142	149	155	161	167	173	180	186	192	199	205	211	217	224	229	236	241	247
5'7"	140	147	153	159	166	172	178	185	191	198	205	212	218	224	230	236	243	249	255
5'8"	145	151	158	164	171	177	184	191	197	204	211	218	224	230	237	243	250	256	262
5'9"	149	156	162	169	176	182	189	196	203	210	217	223	231	237	244	250	258	264	270
5'10"	153	160	167	174	181	188	195	202	207	216	223	230	237	244	251	258	265	272	278
5'11"	158	165	172	179	186	193	200	208	215	222	230	236	244	251	259	265	272	279	286
6'0"	162	169	177	184	191	199	206	214	221	228	236	243	251	259	266	273	281	287	294
6'1"	167	174	182	189	197	204	212	220	227	235	243	250	258	265	273	280	289	295	302
6'2"	171	179	187	194	202	210	218	226	233	241	250	257	265	272	281	288	297	303	311
6'3"	176	184	192	200	208	216	224	232	240	248	256	264	272	280	289	297	305	312	319
6'4"	181	189	197	205	213	222	230	238	246	254	263	271	280	288	296	304	313	320	328

[a]BMI: <18.5 = underweight; 18.5–24.9 = healthy weight; 25.0–29.0 = overweight; 30–39.9 = obesity; >40 = morbid obesity.
Source: Adapted from Clinical Guidelines of the Identification, Evaluation and Treatment of Overweight and Obesity in Adults, The Evidence Report, National Heart, Lung, and Blood Institute, in cooperation with the National Institute of Diabetes and Digestive

Table 18.6.   Healthy range of body fat for women, by age.

Age	Healthy range of body fat for women
18–39	21–32%
40–59	23–33%
60–79	24–35%

Estimating Energy Needs

Harris–Benedict Equation

Female: Basic Energy Expenditure (BEE) = 655 + [4.4 × WT (lb.)]
+ [4.3 × HT (in.)] – (4.7 × Age in Years) × Activity Factor
= calories per day

Activity factors:

Very light activity = 1.3 × BEE (driving, typing, sewing, ironing, and no regular exercise).

Light activity = 1.4 × BEE (carpentry, golf, sailing, and some regular exercise).

Moderate activity = 1.5 × BEE (includes walking/running 3.5–4 mph, skiing, tennis, and regular exercise three to four times per week, 30–40 minutes in duration).

Heavy activity = 2.0 × BEE (heavy manual digging, basketball, climbing, soccer, and regular exercise four times per week, 40 minutes or more in duration).

Alternative Method for Determining Women's Caloric Needs

Very light activity = 12 × body weight
Moderate activity = 15 × body weight
Heavy activity = 18 × body weight

Weight Loss Diets

Some weight loss diets are nutritionally balanced and follow recommendations for healthy eating; others are fad diets encouraging irrational and sometimes unsafe practices.

Sugar Busters

- Claims refined carbohydrates cause obesity by raising blood sugar.
- Foods to avoid: sugar, white flour, carrots, corn, and beets.
- Diet low in calcium. Restricts or avoids some healthful foods such as carrots, bananas.
- Menu's range from 7 to 44 g saturated fats.

Dr. Atkins

- Claims restricting carbohydrates enables the body to burn fat.
- Foods allowed: meats, eggs, cheese, butter, nuts, some starchy vegetables.
- Diet high in saturated fats; may cause bad breath and constipation; low in calcium and fiber.

The Zone

- Claims the correct ratio of carbohydrates to protein to fat is 40:30:30, which promotes weight loss and health.
- Foods allowed: low-fat protein (chicken, fish), fruits and vegetables, with a small amount of olive and canola oil.
- Low in whole grains and calcium. Includes healthy food choices.

Dean Ornish

- Can lose weight and feel satiety by eating fat-free healthful foods.
- Foods allowed: vegetables, fruits, whole grains, beans, egg whites, limited yogurt.
- Low in saturated fats; restricts seafood, poultry, and dairy products; low in calcium.

While high fat diets may promote short-term weight loss, the potential hazards for increasing the risk of atherosclerosis override the short-term benefits. Long-term use of the Atkins diet may increase cholesterol by 25% while long-term use of the Ornish diet would decrease it by 32%. A high-fiber, lower fat diet would have the greatest effect in decreasing serum cholesterol.

Higher protein intake may have a greater satiating effect than higher carbohydrate intake, but further research is required (Tables 18.7 and 18.8).

Surgery

Gastric bypass surgery has been shown to be the most effective approach in generating long-term weight loss in extremely heavy persons. More than 90% of patients experience significant (greater than 20–25%) weight loss, and between 50% and 80% maintain weight loss for over 5 years.

Prior to surgery, patients should be fully evaluated by a multidisciplinary team. Accepted indications for surgical weight loss therapy include having a BMI greater than 40, or a BMI 35–39 with one or more obesity-related disorders; and having previously unsuccessful nonsurgical attempts at long-term weight management.

Pharmacotherapy

Food and Drug Administration (FDA)-approved medications for the treatment of "clinically significant" obesity (BMI greater than 30 or BMI 27–29 with one or more obesity-related disorders) include Sibutramine and Orlistat. Sibutramine is a centrally acting serotonin and adrenergic reuptake inhibitor.

Table 18.7. Nutrient analysis of weight loss diets at 1600 kcal.

	Atkins	Protein Power	Sugar Busters	The Zone	ADA	High fiber	Ornish
% Carbohydrate	5	8	40	40	60	63	74
% Protein	35	35	28	28	20	16	18
% Fat	59	53	32	32	20	21	7
% Saturated fat	26.2	18.6	9.4	6.6	6.1	4.2	2.0
% Monounsaturated fat	8.6	12.2	7.4	9.3	6.2	8.9	2.8
% Polyunsaturated fat	23.5	23.7	14.4	11.5	7.4	4.0	1.9
Carbohydrate (g)	21.6	33.4	162.4	170.3	239.4	253.6	299.3
Protein (g)	145.6	148.8	113.0	119.5	81.5	66.5	73.8
Fat (g)	103.5	96.9	55.4	48.8	35.2	30.5	11.9
Saturated fat (g)	46.5	33.1	16.7	11.8	10.9	7.5	3.5
Monounsaturated fat (g)	15.3	21.7	13.1	16.6	11.1	15.9	5.0
Polyunsaturated fat (g)	41.7	42.7	25.6	20.4	13.2	7.1	3.4
Cholesterol (mg)	923.9	657.0	279.8	264.0	112.1	57.6	29.5
Dietary fiber (g)	4.0	10.6	23.8	18.1	22.3	28.5	49.1
Sugar (g)	7.8	13.2	68.0	66.6	90.2	79.8	101.3

Source: Health Advantages and Disadvantages of Weight—Reducing Diets: A Computer Analysis and Critical Review. Dr. James Anderson, Journal of the American College of Nutrition, Vol. 19, No. 5, 578–590 (2000).

Table 18.8. Sample menu plans.

Meal	Atkins	Protein Power	Sugar Busters	The Zone	ADA	High fiber	Ornish
Breakfast	Fried egg Sausage Butter Decaf coffee	Cottage cheese Berries Coffee	Orange juice Oatmeal Skim milk Coffee	Orange juice Oatmeal Skim milk Coffee	Bagel Oatmeal Skim milk Coffee	Low fat yogurt Oat muffin Strawberries Lite margarine	Bran cereal Nonfat yogurt Blueberries Orange juice Coffee
Lunch	Bacon cheeseburger (no bun) Small tossed salad with blue cheese dressing Seltzer water	Grilled chicken Green salad Olive oil Vinaigrette Black olives ½ apple Mineral water	Turkey Whole grain bread Mustard Lite mayo Lettuce Tomato Diet soda	Turkey Whole grain bread Mustard Lite mayo Lettuce Tomato Nuts	Chicken noodle soup Soft cheese Whole wheat roll Pear Light margarine	Vegetable juice Soy chili Pear	Whole wheat burrito with vegetarian red beans and 7 grain dirty rice Tomato salsa Chopped cilantro Tossed salad
Snack		Beef tenderloin Broccoli	Apple	Apple	Pretzels	Banana	Whole grain crackers

Dinner	Shrimp cocktail Mustard Mayo Clear consommé Steak Tossed salad Salad dressing Diet jello with heavy cream	Sauteed shrimp in olive oil Tomato and mozzarella salad Sauteed broccoli White wine Mineral water	Grilled pork tenderloin Brown rice Green beans	Grilled chicken Tossed salad Olive oil Vinaigrette Squash Margarine Coffee	Fresh tuna Eggplant Summer squash Dinner roll Margarine Angel food cake with strawberries	Garden salad Garbanzo beans Low fat dressing Chicken breast Green beans Potatoes Steamed tomatoes Blueberries Low fat yogurt Popcorn	Whole grain crackers Spinach Ravioli Creamed lentil soup with celery garlic crouton Tossed salad Peaches
Snack	Any meat	Nuts Peaches Mineral water	Nuts	Turkey Grapes Lite mayo	Popcorn Skim milk	Popcorn	Strawberry

Source: Health Advantages and Disadvantages of Weight—Reducing Diets: A Computer Analysis and Critical Review. Dr. James Anderson, Journal of the American College of Nutrition, Vol. 19, No. 5, 578–590 (2000).

It carries the potential complication of hypertension and increased heart rate. Orlistat (Xenical) is a pancreatic lipase inhibitor that inhibits absorption of up to 30% of dietary fat. Steatorrhea, bloating, distention, and anal leakage are potential complications, as well as possible fat-soluble vitamin deficiencies. Reported losses with these medications combined with a low calorie diet average 2–10 kg per year. If the medications are discontinued weight gain results.

Herbal preparations for weight loss do not have standardized amounts of active ingredients and have been reported to have harmful effects.

Leptin is a hormone secreted by fat cells in the body. Thought to maintain balance on appetite and thermogenesis, to date, data do not indicate that leptin is the much sought after magic bullet to lose weight.

PYY3-36 is a hormone that communicates to the brain that the stomach is full. It is released by cells in the digestive tract in response to luminal food. A complex array of genes links our stomach to our brain and more research is needed to clarify these important effects.

Sensible Weight Control Program

A sensible weight control program does the following:

- Relies on low calorie foods that are high in nutrients (fruits, vegetables, whole grains).
- Emphasizes slow weight loss—no greater than 2 pounds per week.
- Promotes exercise that increases the metabolism and builds muscle.
- Helps in beginning to understand the causes of and therefore helps to eliminate emotional eating.
- Addresses the five most common reasons for emotional eating, including boredom, stress, loneliness, filling a void, emotional turmoil, or emotional issues (including depression and early childhood trauma).
- Curbs liquid calories—Americans now drink twice as many soft drinks as they did in 1997.
- Sets realistic goals—people can typically reduce their weight by 10–15% with the best behavior modification programs. It is important to convey realistic expectations.
- Promotes finding new hobbies and interests if food has been the center of pleasurable activities. Provides sources of nurture other than food.
- Provides social support. Individuals need to determine who they want support from and how it is to be provided. Some people can undermine the patient's desires to lose weight.
- Avoids measuring success only by the scale. The body stores 3 g of water for every gram of glycogen (which is broken down during exercise).
- Incorporates self-monitoring. Food and exercise records can provide a 76% success rate for weight control.
- Looks for a weight loss strategy that works for the client. Until more studies are done, it is too early to determine which diet makes it easiest to lose weight. Some people may find it easier to cut back on bread, pasta,

Table 18.9. Dietary reference intakes for carbohydrates, fats, and protein and physical activity.

Recommended dietary ranges

Carbohydrates	45–65% of total calories
Fat	20–35% of total calories
Protein	10–35% of total calories
Exercise	One hour of accumulated physical activity per day

Translating the ranges in grams of nutrients per day for different calorie levels

	1800 calories	**2000 calories**	**2200 calories**
Carbohydrates	202–248 g/day	225–275 g/day	248–302 g/day
Fat	40–70 g/day	44–78 g/day	49–85 g/day
Protein	45–157 g/day	50–175 g/day	55–192 g/day

rice, and sweets, while others find it easier to cut back on fried foods, oils, and mayonnaise. Decreasing calories, choosing complex carbohydrates, and choosing monounsaturated fats are recommended.

• Instead of strict dieting, focuses on normalizing eating behaviors, eating healthier, becoming more physically active, and building positive self-esteem (Tables 18.9–18.12).

Table 18.10. Current daily reference values (DRV).

Sodium	2400 mg
Potassium	3500 mg
Vitamin A	5000 IU
Vitamin C	60 mg
Calcium	1000 mg
Iron	18 mg
Vitamin E	18 mg
Folate	0.4 mg
Zinc	15 mg

Table 18.11. Adequate fiber intake amounts for women.

Adults under 50 years	25 g
Adults over 50 years	21 g

Herbs and Surgery

The American Society of Anesthesiologists suggests that anyone taking herbs should discontinue them at least 2 weeks before having surgery.

At What Age to Supplement and with Which Nutrients

Age: 20s, 30s, and 40s—All women capable of becoming pregnant should take a daily multivitamin containing 400μg of folic acid to reduce the chances of having an infant affected with a neural tube defect; 1000 mg calcium and 400 IU vitamin D are needed per day.

Age: 50s—400 IU vitamin D and 1200 mg calcium are needed per day. Milk has 100 IU vitamin D per cup. To be on the safe side, take a multivitamin that contains 400 units of vitamin D or 200 units if at least two cups of milk are drunk per day.

Table 18.12. Fiber sources in various foods.

Fiber sources	Grams
½ cup kidney beans	7.3
1 large baked potato with skin	4.8
1 cup cooked oatmeal	4.0
½ cup brussels sprouts	3.4
1 medium orange	3.1
2 slices whole wheat bread	3.0
½ cup cooked spinach	2.8
1 medium banana	2.7
½ cup cooked broccoli	2.3
1 large carrot	2.2

Age: 60s—Take a multivitamin with 2.4 µg of B_{12}. An estimated one out of five people over 60 and two out of five over 80 do not get enough vitamin B_{12} because their stomachs do not have enough gastric acid to render it bioavailable; 1200 mg calcium and 400 IU vitamin D are needed per day.
Age: 70s—600 IU of vitamin D and 1200 mg calcium are needed per day.

Natural vitamin E (*d*-α-tocopherol) appears to be better retained and used by the body than synthetic vitamin E (*dl*-α-tocopherol) (Table 18.13).

Osteoporosis

Osteoporosis is a disease characterized by thin and fragile bones. Ten million people in the United States have osteoporosis and another 18 million are at risk because of low bone mass. If untreated, a postmenopausal woman can lose 10–40% of bone mass between the ages of 50 and 60 years. Hormone replacement therapy attenuates bone mass. However, contraindications exist for hormone replacement therapy in some women.

- Weight-bearing exercises such as jogging, walking, skating, tennis, and dancing strengthen bones. Some examples of nonweight-bearing exercises are swimming and bicycling.
- Avoid smoking, which lowers the estrogen content of the blood and thus weakens the bones.
- Low-fat dairy products are the most desirable way to meet calcium goals.
- For people who cannot consume enough calcium-rich foods, calcium supplements are needed.
- Women 19–50 years old need 1000 mg calcium and those over 50 years old need 1200 mg calcium per day.
- Women 19–50 years old need 200 IU vitamin D, 51–70 years old need 400 IU vitamin D, and over 70 years old need 600 IU vitamin D per day.
- Calcium carbonate and calcium citrate are good forms of calcium supplements.
- Calcium supplements are better absorbed with meals. More is absorbed from divided doses than from one high dose (more than 500 mg).
- To obtain vitamin D from the sun, expose your non-sun-screened hands, face, and arms for 10–15 minutes two to three times a week.
- Elemental calcium is the actual amount of calcium in the supplement. For example, calcium carbonate contains the largest amount of elemental calcium at 40%. Therefore, a 500-mg tablet of calcium carbonate would provide approximately 200 mg of actual calcium. Calcium citrate provides approximately 21% of elemental calcium. Aside from calcium content, the bioavailability of calcium supplements should be considered.
- Take calcium separately from iron tablets because concurrent use may decrease iron absorption.
- When consumed in excess, the following may contribute to bone loss: protein, alcohol, caffeine, phosphorus, fiber, and sodium (Table 18.14).

Table 18.13. Vitamins and minerals for women.

Nutrient	Rda	Daily value	Good sources	Upper level	Selected adverse effects
Vitamin A (retinol)	700 μg	5000 IU	Liver, fatty fish, fortified foods (milk, cereals)	10,000 IU	Liver toxicity, birth defects
Carotenoids	None	None	Fruits and vegetables	None	Smokers who took high doses had higher risk of lung cancer
Thiamine	1.1 mg	1.5 mg	Breads, cereals, pasta, pork	None	None reported
Riboflavin	1.1 mg	1.7 mg	Milk, yogurt, enriched whole grain flour	None	None reported
Niacin	14 mg	20 mg	Meat, poultry, seafood, fortified foods, liver	35 mg	Flushing (burning, tingling, redness); liver damage
Vitamin B$_6$ (pyridoxine)	Ages 19–50: 1.3 mg; 50+: 1.5 mg	2 mg	Meat, poultry, seafood, fortified cereals	100 mg	Reversible nerve damage (burning, numbness)
Vitamin B$_{12}$ (cobalamin)	2.4 μg	6 μg	Meat, poultry, seafood, dairy	None	None reported

Folate	400 µg	400 µg	Orange juice, beans, fortified cereals	1000 µg	Can mask or precipitate a B_{12} deficiency
Vitamin C (ascorbic acid)	75 mg (smokers add 35 mg)	60 mg	Citrus and other fruits, vegetables,	2000 mg	Diarrhea
Vitamin D	Ages 19–50: 200 IU Ages 51–70: 400 IU Ages 70: 600 IU	400 IU	Sunlight, fatty fish, fortified foods (milk, cereals)	2000 IU	High blood calcium, which may cause kidney and heart damage
Vitamin E (α-tocopherol)	15 mg (33 IU synthetic) (22 IU natural)	30 IU (synthetic)	Oils, whole grains, nuts	1100 IU— synthetic 1500 IU— natural	Hemorrhage
Vitamin K (phylloquinone)	90 µg	80 µg	Green leafy vegetables, oils	None	Interferes with coumadin and other anticlotting drugs
Calcium	Ages 19–50: 1000 mg Over 50: 1200 mg	1000 mg	Dairy foods, fortified, leafy green vegetables	2500 mg	May cause kidney damage; kidney stones

Continued.

Table 18.13.   *Continued.*

Nutrient	Rda	Daily value	Good sources	Upper level	Selected adverse effects
Chromium	20–25 µg	120 µg	Whole grains, bran cereals, meat, seafood	None	Inconclusive: kidney or muscle damage
Copper	900 µg	2000 µg	Liver, seafood, nuts, seeds, whole grains	10,000 µg	Liver damage
Iron	Ages 19–50: 18 mg 50+: 8 mg	18 mg	Red meat, seafood, poultry	45 mg	Gastrointestinal effects (nausea, diarrhea, constipation)
Magnesium	310–320 mg	400 mg	Green leafy vegetables, cereals	350 mg	Diarrhea
Phosphorus	700 mg	1000 mg	Dairy foods, meats, colas	Ages 19–70: 4000 mg Over 70: 3000 mg	May damage kidneys and bones
Selenium	55 µg	70 µg	Seafood, meat, grains	400 µg	Nail or hair loss or brittleness
Zinc	8 mg	15 mg	Red meat, seafood, whole grains, fortified foods	40 mg	

Table 18.14.   Calcium sources.

Food	Calcium (mg)
1 cup low fat yogurt	345–415
1 cup hard frozen yogurt	300
1 cup skim milk	302
1 cup 2% milk	297
1 cup whole milk	291
1 oz. cheddar cheese	204
1 oz. swiss cheese	272
½ cup ice cream	88
3 oz. salmon with bones	205
3 oz. sardines	372
4 oz. tofu	260
6 oz. calcium-enriched orange juice	225
½ mustard greens	97
½ cup spinach	84
½ cup macaroni and cheese	181
¼ cup almonds	83
1 tbsp. molasses	137

Eating Disorders

Clinical eating disorders, such as anorexia nervosa and bulimia nervosa, mainly occur in women and are associated with several medical problems. The chronic starvation of anorexia nervosa may lead to endocrine abnormalities, osteoporosis, delayed gastric emptying, sinus bradycardia, orthostatic hypotension, hypothermia, anemia, and a decrease in growth during adolescence.

Dehydration, renal calculi, dental caries, esophageal perforation, and metabolic alkalosis can occur in persons with bulimia nervosa who engage in chronic self-induced vomiting. Women with eating disorders who become pregnant are at increased risk for fetal complications. Psychological concerns of persons with eating disorders can include depression, diminished libido, altered sleeping patterns, and irritability.

Female athletes are at greater risk of developing eating disorders than nonathletes. The pressure to optimize performance by decreasing body fat, high self-expectations, perfectionism, and persistence place female athletes at risk for medical complications that include osteoporosis, amenorrhea, and eating disorders that compromise nutritional status.

Eating disorders are caused by genetic, neurochemical, as well as cultural and societal factors, such as fitness and thinness in women. Approximately 3% of young women have an eating disorder.

Anorexia Nervosa

1. The refusal to maintain a minimally healthy body weight (85% of that expected).
2. An intense fear of gaining weight, even though the person is underweight.
3. A disturbance about personal body weight, size, or shape. The person claims to "feel fat" even when emaciated.
4. The absence of at least three consecutive menstrual cycles in conjunction with being underweight.

Bulimia Nervosa

1. Recurrent episodes of binge eating. Large consumption of food within 2 hours, ending with vomiting, laxatives, diuretics, fasting, enemas, diet pills, or excessive exercise.
2. A minimum average of two binge-eating episodes a week for at least 3 months.
3. A feeling of lack of control over eating behavior during eating binges.
4. Persistent concern with body shape and weight.

Table 18.15 illustrates a multidisciplinary approach to meeting the nutritional needs of women.

Table 18.15. Multidisciplinary approach to meeting the nutritional needs of women.

Physician	Psychotherapist	Psychiatrist	Registered dietitian
Medical risks	Behavioral risks	Diagnosis	Provides nutrition
Critical weight	Body image	Medication	education (in
Amenorrhea	Personality	Depression	collaboration with
Blood pressure	development	Substance	client and
Hydration status	Behavior	abuse	treatment team)
Exercise program	Symptomatic		that enables client
Substance abuse	Family therapy		to normalize weight
			growth, physical
			development, and
			eating patterns

Weight Loss Case Study

Debbie is a 52-year-old retail store manager. She works long hours on her job. The dietitian knew the key to her weight loss success would be to reduce the amount of stress in her life as well as find more effective outlets for stress. First, the dietitian organized all of her eating into a three meal, two snack format. For the first time in her life she began eating breakfast. She also added healthful snacks and eliminated most of the unconscious eating that occurred at her desk. She no longer ate past 8 PM. Debbie went into the office a half hour later than usual and meditated or walked at home during this time. She also vowed not to bring work home with her, which significantly cut down on her nervous eating. Over the course of the next year, Debbie lost 35 pounds. Her weight loss was directly related to her changes in eating habits, which made her eating more of a conscious activity, as well as her lifestyle changes that removed stress from her life.

Suggested Reading

Anderson JW, Konz E, Jenkins D. Health advantages and disadvantages of weight reducing diets: a computer analysis and critical review. *J Am College Nutr* 2000;19:578–90.

Barr SI, Murphy SP, Poos MI. Interpreting and using dietary references intakes in dietary assessment of individuals and groups. *J Am Diet Assoc* 2002;102:780–88.

Deulin MJ, Yanouski SZ, Wilson GT. Obesity: what mental health professionals need to know. *Am J Psychiatry* 2000;157:854–66.

Flegal KM, Carroll MD, Kuczmarski RJ, Johnson CL. Overweight and obesity in the United States: prevalence of overweight among children, adolescents, and adults—United States: prevalence and trends, 1960–1994. *Int J Obesity* 1998;22:39–47.

Hsia JA. Cardiovascular diseases in women. *Med Clin N Am* 1998;82: 1–19.

Kelley G. Aerobic exercise and lumbar spine bone mineral density in postmenopausal women: a meta-analysis. *J Am Geriatric Soc* 1998;46: 143–52.

Monsen ER. Dietary reference intakes for the antioxidant nutrients: vitamin C, vitamin E, selenium, and carotenoids. *J Am Diet Assoc* 2000; 100:637–40.

Morris VM, Rorie AJ. Nutritional concerns in women's primary care. *J Nurse Midwifery* 1997;42(6):509–20.

Staff. Women's health and nutrition—position of ADA and Dietitians of Canada. *Can J Diet Pract Res* 1999;60(2):85–100.

Staff. Position of the American Dietetic Association: weight management. *J Am Diet Assoc* August 2002;1145–55.

Staff. What really makes you fat? *Times* September 2002;47–55.

Staff. ADA: Guidelines on the sale of dietary supplements. *J Am Diet Assoc* August 2002;1158–64.

Taylor RW, Keil D, Gold EJ, Williams SM, Goulding A. Body mass index, waist girth and waist-to-hip ratio as indexes of total and regional adiposity in women: evaluation using receiver operating characteristic curves. *Am J Clin Nutr* 1998;67:44–49.

Wiseman CV, Harris WA, Halmi KA. Eating disorders. *Med Clin N Am* 1998;82:145–59.

19

Respiratory Disorders

Roger P. Smith

Background Information

Like it or not, patients with respiratory complaints are a part of our practice. The common cold is often referred to as the most frequent illness occurring in humans: over 40% of Americans suffer from a "cold" each year, accounting for more lost productivity than any other illness. Pharyngitis affects almost 30 million patients annually, with over 10% of all school-aged children seeking medical care each year. Seventeen million patients a year are diagnosed with asthma, with more females than males among adult-onset patients. Whether it is the reason for our patient's visit or an incidental complaint, we are involved with the diagnosis and management of these problems.

Sinusitis

Sinusitis affects roughly 35 million people in the United States annually. The accumulation of purulent material in inflamed paranasal sinuses results in a feeling of fullness and pressure in and over the involved sinuses. These symptoms are worse with posture changes, bending, or with air travel—anything that alters pressure inside the sinuses. Nasal congestion and a purulent, blood-tinged discharge, general malaise, low-grade fever, and sore throat are common. These patients will have tenderness over the involved sinuses and edematous or thickened mucosa may be noted on physical examination. These findings help to differentiate sinusitis from the more common cold.

The most common cause of sinusitis is bacterial infection with *Haemophilus influenzae*, pneumococci, or streptococci. Viral and fungal infections may occur, but are less common. Upper respiratory infections, allergy, or air travel often precede the development of sinusitis, and secondary infection from a tooth abscess or from swimming in contaminated water may also create a sinus infection.

Common Cold

Affecting roughly 41% of people per year, the symptoms of the common cold are familiar. The sneezing, runny nose, and malaise usually lasts 6–10 days, but may range from 2 to 26 days. Coryza (rhinorrhea and sneezing) is present in 50–66% of patients, and almost 50% of patients experience pharyngitis with a cold. Hoarseness and cough develop in 25–50% of patients. Between 25% and 45% of patients experience headache, muscular aches, lethargy, and malaise, though only 15–30% actually develop fever or chills. Surprisingly, up to 25% of patients infected with the usual cold viruses will not develop symptoms.

The patient's symptoms generally begin with the loss of a sense of well-being, scratchy eyes, and discomfort in the nose or back of the throat (Fig. 19.1).

This is soon followed by sneezing and nasal obstruction with a clear, watery discharge. Systemic symptoms, which reach their peak in the first 2–3 days, resolve first, followed by a change in nasal discharge to a cloudy or yellow, thick character. A sore throat, cough, or hoarseness may persist up to 10 days.

Transmission of the causative virus is usually by personal contact; infected droplets of respiratory discharge are spread by coughing and sneezing, and by transfer from the hands to the eyes, nose, or face. Experimental evidence suggests that small doses of virus (1–30 particles) are sufficient to produce infection. Healthy people with normal immune systems are highly susceptible to cold virus infection once the virus enters the nose. In volunteer studies, approximately 95% of normal adults became infected when virus was dropped into the nose.

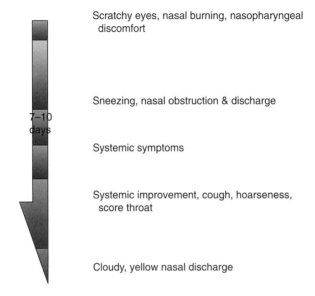

Scratchy eyes, nasal burning, nasopharyngeal discomfort

Sneezing, nasal obstruction & discharge

7–10 days

Systemic symptoms

Systemic improvement, cough, hoarseness, score throat

Cloudy, yellow nasal discharge

Fig. 19.1.   Sequence of symptoms of the common cold.

Cold viruses are carried to the back of the throat by ciliary action where they are deposited in the area of the adenoids, where the viruses attach. From the time a cold virus enters the nose, it takes 8–12 hours for the viral reproductive cycle to be completed and for new cold virus to be released in nasal secretions. Cold symptoms can begin shortly after virus is first produced in the nose (10–12 hours). The time from the beginning of the infection to the peak of symptoms is typically 36–72 hours.

There are over 100 serotypes of rhinoviruses that may cause the common cold. These account for about 15–40% of infections. Additional viral agents include coronaviruses (10–20% of cases), influenza types A, B, and C (1–5%), parainfluenza (1–5%), respiratory syncytial virus (1–5%), adenoviruses (1–5%), and others. No specific agent is known in 30–50% of cases, though it is presumed to be viral.

Any exposure to an infected person places you at risk for infection. Consequently, anything that brings larger numbers of people together, such as daycare, schools, or the work place, increases the chances of infection. The secondary attach rates in families is approximately 25%. Cold weather, fatigue, and loss of sleep do not appear to alter the risk of infection, though colds are most prevalent in the winter months. Careful hand washing may reduce the risk, especially among those chronically exposed (e.g., health care workers). Data regarding the protective effects of large doses of vitamin C are inconclusive.

Pharyngitis

Only 12–25% of all "sore throats" seen by physicians have a true pharyngitis—most are simple viral upper respiratory infections such as the common cold. Of greatest priority is the identification and treatment of those with group A streptococcal infections so as to reduce the potential for rheumatic sequelae. Despite roughly 30 million cases annually, the incidence of rheumatic fever has declined to approximately 64 cases per 100,000. Streptococcal pharyngitis has its greatest incidence between the ages of 5 and 18 years, but is still common in patients seen in a gynecology office setting. (See Fig. 19.2 for a decision tree for sore throats.)

A sore throat, tonsillar enlargement (often with exudates), soft palate petechiae, and cervical adenopathy characterize true pharyngitis. Hoarseness and lower respiratory symptoms should be absent. Streptococcal pharyngitis usually runs a 5–7 day course, with a peak fever at 2–3 days. This time course and the presence of a moderate to high fever help to differentiate true pharyngitis from the common cold. Spontaneous resolution of symptoms generally occurs, but rheumatic complications are still possible.

Viral agents, including rhinovirus, adenovirus, and parainfluenza viruses, cause most pharyngitis. *Neisseria gonorrhoeae*, *Corynebacterium diphtheriae*, and *H. influenzae* may also cause bacterial pharyngitis. The same factors that increase the risk of the common cold (close quarters, unhygienic practices) also increase the risk of pharyngitis.

Laryngitis

Viral infections with influenza A or B, parainfluenza, or adenovirus, or bacterial infections by β-hemolytic streptococcus or *Streptococcus pneumoniae* are the most common etiology for laryngitis. Excessive or improper voice use (strain) or aspiration may also result in loss of voice. An upper respiratory tract infec-

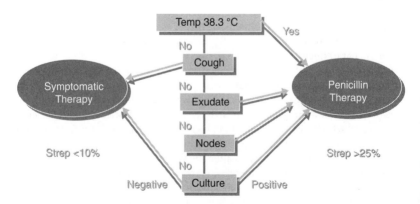

Fig. 19.2.   Decision tree for sore throat.

tion, bronchitis, or pneumonia often precedes laryngitis. Environmental causes such as smoking or being in an environment with second-hand tobacco smoke can also cause laryngitis. In the industrial or school environment, exposure to irritating chemicals can also lead to similar symptoms. The peak incidence of laryngitis parallels epidemics of the individual viruses (winter).

Laryngotracheobronchitis

This subacute viral illness is noteworthy for its barking cough, biphasic stridor, and risk of airway obstruction. While more common in children (the most common cause of stridor in children), the potential for serious complications (e.g., acute obstruction) makes it an illness that should be familiar to gynecologists. Patients with laryngotracheobronchitis often have had an upper respiratory prodromal infection in the last 1–7 days. Fatigue, malaise, low-grade to moderate fever, and a normal voice characterize the patient's symptoms. The uncomplicated disease usually wanes in 3–5 days but may persist for as many as 10 days.

Most cases of laryngotracheobronchitis are caused by viral infection (parainfluenza, influenza A, and others). Recurrent upper respiratory infections increase the risk of developing laryngotracheobronchitis. As the infection extends to the proximal trachea, diffuse inflammation with exudate and edema of the subglottic area causes narrowing of the airway. The cricoid ring of the trachea (in the immediate subglottic area) is the narrowest portion of the airway. A small amount of edema in this region can cause significant airway obstruction. (The resistance to flow through a tube is inversely proportional to the fourth power of the radius.) Air flowing through this narrowed subglottic area causes the characteristic stridor.

Asthma

With over 10 million new cases diagnosed each year, asthma affects up to one in five children in the United States—more than 4.8 million children under the age of 18. Direct health care costs for asthma (adults and children) in the United States total more than $9.8 billion annually; indirect costs (lost productivity) add another $2.8 billion for a total of $12.6 billion. Inpatient hospital services represented the largest single direct medical expenditure, over $4.2 billion. The prevalence of asthma increased 75% from 1980 to 1994, and currently affects more than 17 million Americans. Researchers have yet to pinpoint the cause for the increase in asthma. Allergic rhinitis is considered a risk factor in developing asthma, as up to 78% of people with asthma also have allergic rhinitis. While it is tempting to think of asthma as a childhood condition that is not seen in a gynecologic practice, half of all asthma cases occur in patients over the age of 10, and more women than men make up this adult onset group.

Asthma is a chronic inflammatory disorder involving constriction of the muscles lining the bronchial airways. Physical symptoms of asthma include coughing, wheezing, tightness of the chest, and shortness of breath.

Narrowing of both the large and small airways results in the wheezing, cough, and dyspnea typical of this condition. Hyperresonance and decreased breath sounds are found on clinical examination.

Allergy, exposure to smoke or other pollutants, viral infections, exercise, or even aspirin intake may induce these episodic attacks. While there is a familial association of reactive airway disease, no known genetic pattern exists. Other triggers that may play a significant role in provoking asthma attacks are shown in Table 19.1.

Asthmatic patients who become pregnant can expect their condition to remain the same or improve (75% of cases). In about 25% of cases, asthma worsens during pregnancy.

Bacterial Pneumonia

More common in adults than its viral cousin, bacterial pneumonia has an annual incidence of approximately 20 per 1000 population. Of these, approximately 60% are community acquired and 40% are acquired in a hospital or nursing home setting. Alcoholics, the debilitated, postoperative patients, patients with respiratory diseases or viral infections, and those who have weakened immune systems are at greater risk.

The cardinal signs of bacterial pneumonia are a cough, fever and chills, chest pain, and a thick dark or bloody (rusty) sputum. Malaise, myalgia, and abdominal, shoulder, or pleuritic pain may also be present. Rales and rhonchi, decreased breath sounds, and vocal fremitus may be found on examination. The tissue of part of a lobe of the lung, an entire lobe, or even most of the lung becomes completely filled with liquid (consolidation). The infection may quickly spread through the bloodstream, resulting in septicemia or bacterial seeding to other sites.

Hematogenous spread or direct inhalation of the organism (*S. pneumoniae, H. influenzae, Staphylococcus aureus, Legionella pneumophila*, and

Table 19.1.   Agents that may precipitate or provoke asthma.

Allergens such as pollens, molds, animal dander, dust mites, and
cockroaches

Irritants such as strong odors and sprays, chemicals, air pollutants, tobacco
smoke, and cold air

Viral or sinus infections including colds, pneumonia, and sinusitis

Exercise, especially in cold, dry air

Gastroesophageal reflux disease (GERD), a condition in which stomach
acid flows back up the esophagus

Medication and foods

Emotional anxiety

Table 19.2. Recommended groups for pneumonia vaccination.

Those with chronic illnesses such as lung disease, heart disease, kidney
  disorders, sickle cell anemia, or diabetes
Those recovering from severe illness
Those in nursing homes or other chronic care facilities
Age 65 or older

others) is the most common source of infection for most patients. *S. pneu-moniae* is the most frequent cause of bacterial pneumonia and is the one form of pneumonia for which a vaccine is available. Anything that diminishes the host's defenses increases the risk of becoming ill. Alcoholism and smoking, immunosuppression and AIDS, chronic disease, malnutrition, and advanced age are all associated with an increased risk. Groups for whom vaccination should be recommended are shown in Table 19.2.

Viral Pneumonia

Viral pneumonia has signs and symptoms similar to those of bacterial pneumonia, with fever, chills, and a productive cough the predominant symptoms. As with bacterial infections, a preceding upper respiratory tract infection is common. Rales, rhonchi, and altered breath sounds are typical findings on examination.

While 90% of childhood pneumonia is viral, only between 1% and 5% of adult pneumonias are caused by viral infections. Influenza A and B, as well as parainfluenza (1, 2, 3, and 4), and respiratory syncytial virus may also be common agents. Varicella, herpes simplex, and rubeola are atypical causative organisms but account for significant morbidity when they are the causative agents. Infection with the influenza virus may be severe and occasionally fatal. The virus invades the lungs and multiplies, but there are almost no physical signs of lung tissue becoming filled with fluid. Fatalities are most common among those who have preexisting heart or lung disease or are pregnant.

Mycoplasma Pneumonia

Because of its somewhat different symptoms and physical signs, and because the course of the illness differed from classic pneumococcal pneumonia, *Mycoplasma* pneumonia was once believed to be caused by one or more undiscovered viruses and was called "primary atypical pneumonia." Mycoplasmas generally cause a mild and widespread pneumonia that can affect all age groups, occurring most frequently in older children and young adults. The death rate is low, even in untreated cases.

Little separates *Mycoplasma* pneumonia from viral pneumonia except for the presence of cold agglutinins. A prodromal period of mild sore throat, low-grade fever, and malaise generally precedes the development of paroxysmal cough and blood-streaked sputum.

Confined living spaces (such as military bases, college campuses, and hospitals) increase the risk of *Mycoplasma* epidemics. Immunocompromised patients are also at higher risk for infection.

Pneumocystis carinii Pneumonia

Pneumocystis carinii pneumonia is caused by an organism believed to be a fungus and is frequently the first sign of illness in many persons with AIDS. This often insidious infection is seen almost exclusively in immunocompromised individuals. Weakness, fatigue, malaise, fever and chills, and mild dyspnea on exertion are typical. A mild nonproductive cough or a cough productive of only scant amounts of clear sputum is common.

Establishing the Diagnosis
Sinusitis

The clinical signs and symptoms present most often establish the diagnosis of sinusitis. Sinus X-rays will show cloudiness and air-fluid levels with thickened mucosa in the affected sinuses, but are not required for diagnosis in most cases. Computed tomography and magnetic resonance imaging are not indicated in these patients. Transillumination of the affected sinuses will reveal opacity. A mildly elevated white blood cell count may be found and appropriate cultures (especially in chronic sufferers) may be of help, and can help to separate cases of viral and allergic rhinitis from those of bacterial infection. The possibility of a foreign body must always be considered.

Common Cold

The diagnosis of the common cold is made on clinical grounds with testing rarely indicated and useful only when other conditions are suspected. Viral culture or isolation is not practical and should not be undertaken. Influenza, rubeola and rubella, *Mycoplasma* pneumonia, group A β-hemolytic streptococcal infections, and allergic rhinitis may all be confused with the common cold and should be considered when appropriate.

Pharyngitis

In addition to the patient's symptoms, a throat culture (on blood agar) or a rapid screening test for *Streptococcus* is indicated because history and physical examination are only 50% accurate in establishing the diagnosis. Because of a sensitivity of 80% and specificity of 95% for most rapid screening tests, a follow-up culture is indicated even if the rapid test is used for the initial screening. A fever of greater than 39.2°C (102.5°F), white blood count of greater than 12,000, or a scarlet fever rash (punctate erythematous macules with reddened flexor creases and circumoral pallor) is suggestive of a streptococcal infection and requires more aggressive evaluation and treatment. A gray pseudomembrane suggests the presence of diphtheria and vesicles should suggest herpes stomatitis as alternate diagnoses.

Laryngitis

The diagnosis of laryngitis is made primarily on the patient's symptoms. The hallmarks of laryngitis are hoarseness, abnormal sounding voice, or loss of voice. Feelings of throat tickling or rawness, coupled with a frequent urge to clear the throat, are also common. Like the cough of the common cold, laryngitis may continue after the acute infection is over. This can be recognized by noting that the fever and ill feeling have resolved, but the hoarseness continues for several days to a week or longer. Direct or indirect laryngoscopy is diagnostic but generally beyond the interest of most gynecologists.

Laryngotracheobronchitis

Laryngotracheobronchitis must be differentiated from epiglottitis, foreign body aspiration, diphtheria, and simple upper respiratory infections. X-Rays of the neck (PA and lateral) will show a characteristic narrowing in the subglottic region with a normal epiglottis (an inverted V-shaped "steeple" or "pencil" sign). Direct laryngoscopy is often required to establish the final diagnosis. Early in the course of the disease leukopenia may be present with leukocytosis occurring in later, more severe cases. Because hypoxia may be insidious and occurs in up to 80% of children with laryngotracheobronchitis, pulse oximetry should be considered. Even in adults, the condition of the patient can change rapidly, necessitating early consultation and aggressive management.

Asthma

Allergists follow the national *Guidelines for the Diagnosis and Management of Asthma* (National Asthma Education and Prevention Program, National Institutes of Health, 1997) to diagnosis and establish treatment plans for patients with asthma and other allergic diseases. The diagnosis of asthma is made mainly on the basis of the recurrent clinical pattern. Allergy testing, spirometry, and chest X-ray may support or clarify the diagnosis. Unusual conditions such as recurrent pulmonary emboli and cystic fibrosis, or more common processes such as congestive heart failure and tuberculosis, must all be considered. Special attention should be paid to the nose and sinuses for evidence of chronic infection. A spirometer may be used to objectively measure the amount of air inhaled and exhaled and to determine the level of airway obstruction, though the simple bedside test of asking the patient to blow out a match held at arm's length can provide a quick assessment of forced expiratory volume (FEV_1).

Bacterial Pneumonia

Frequently, the criteria for diagnosis have been fever, cough, and development of purulent sputum, in combination with radiologic evidence of a new or progressive pulmonary infiltrate, a suggestive Gram stain, and cultures of sputum, tracheal aspirate, pleural fluid, or blood. Unfortunately, symptoms, elevated white blood count with left shift, hemoconcentration, hyponatremia, and transaminase elevations are all nonspecific signs of bacterial pneumonia.

The onset of bacterial pneumonia can vary from gradual to sudden. In the most severe cases, the patient may experience shaking chills, chattering teeth, severe chest pain, and a cough that produces rust-colored or greenish mucus. The patient's temperature may rise as high as 105°F. The patient sweats profusely, and breathing and pulse rate increase rapidly. Lips and nail beds may demonstrate hypoxia and confusion or delirium may be present.

The chest X-ray will show air bronchograms and consolidation, with pleural effusion common. Blood cultures will be positive in 20–30% of patients with community-acquired infections. Bronchoscopic cultures with greater than 10,000 organisms are diagnostic, but beyond the capability of most gynecologists. Induced sputum for culture and Gram stain may be helpful, but are less reliable.

Viral Pneumonia

The initial symptoms of viral pneumonia are the same as influenza symptoms: fever, a dry cough, headache, muscle pain, and weakness. Within 12–36 hours, there is increasing breathlessness; the cough becomes worse and produces a small amount of mucus. There is a high fever and there may be hypoxia and cyanosis. In extreme cases, the patient has a desperate need for air and extreme breathlessness. Exclusion of the more common bacterial pneumonia and the addition of viral culture or fluorescent antigen studies establish the diagnosis of viral pneumonia.

Mycoplasma Pneumonia

The most prominent symptom of *Mycoplasma* pneumonia is a cough that tends to come in violent attacks, but produces only sparse whitish mucus. Chills and fever are early symptoms, and some patients experience nausea or vomiting. Patients may experience profound weakness that lasts for a long time. The presence of cold agglutinins in a titer of 1:64 or greater, or with a fourfold rise in titers, is found in 50% of infections. Cultures for *Mycoplasma* take 7–10 days, so are of little use in making the acute diagnosis.

Pneumocystis carinii Pneumonia

Suspicion greatly aids the diagnosis. Chest X-ray shows bilateral interstitial or perihilar infiltrates in 75% of cases, though a normal chest X-ray may be present. Serum lactate dehydrogenase (LDH) is often elevated (average 340 IU) and CD4 cell counts are generally depressed (<200) in HIV-infected patients.

Clinical Intervention
Sinusitis

Outpatient care for patients with sinusitis is appropriate except when there is involvement of the frontal or sphenoid sinuses. For simple cases involving the other sinuses, steam inhalation will provide some comfort and promote drainage. Irrigation with saline may be recommended, but is seldom required. Amoxicillin (500 mg three times a day) or trimethoprim-sulfamethoxazole twice a day for 14–21 days will generally provide good coverage for the most common causative organisms. Recent data suggest that treatment courses of as little as 3 days may be sufficient in uncomplicated cases. With proper antibiotic treatment, over 90% of cases of acute bacterial sinusitis are cured. If response is not forthcoming, a switch to an antibiotic with activity against β-lactamase-producing bacteria is prudent. Cases of acute bacterial sinusitis that do not clear after a few months of appropriate medical treatment may require sinus surgery. Analgesics, vasoconstrictors to relieve fullness, and antihistamines may all be used as needed. Patients should be advised to avoid alcohol and caffeine because both may result in swelling of the sinus membranes.

Though rare, sinusitis may lead to meningitis, extradural, subdural, or brain abscesses, osteomyelitis, or septic cavernous sinus thrombosis. Patients with chronic or recurrent sinusitis may require surgical drainage.

Common Cold

Common sense and supportive therapies are all that are required for most patients suffering from the common cold. Rest, fluids (including fruit juices), smoking cessation, and humidification may all be of some help. The best strategy for treating a cold is to start treatment as soon as there is the recognition that a cold is beginning and to continue treatment on a regular basis until it appears that the cold is over (3–7 days). Analgesics, oral decongestants (pseudoephedrine, phenylephrine, and phenylpropanolamine), antitussives (dextromethorphan, codeine) combined with mucolytics (guaifenesin), antihistamines, and topical decongestants (oxymetazoline) may all provide some relief.

Early studies of the first generation antihistamines for the treatment of colds gave negative results because of inadequate precision in symptom recording. Subsequent studies have demonstrated that first generation antihistamines are quite effective in reducing the sneezing and runny nose of colds. The use of topical decongestants should be limited to 3–4 days to avoid rebound hyperemia and congestion. Decongestants taken by mouth have less powerful and immediate activity but cause fewer problems with the cycles of recurrent nasal obstruction than topical preparations.

There is some evidence that supplemental vitamin C may reduce the duration of disability. The use of zinc gluconate lozenges has been shown to reduce the duration of symptoms but they must be used frequently and are often associated with nausea. The use of zinc (gluconate) lozenges has been shown to reduce the duration of symptoms by roughly one-half if used early in the course of the infection. In clinical trials, doses of 13–15 mg every 2 hours while symptoms persist have been used. Studies using intranasal ipratropium bromide (Atrovent) three times daily have demonstrated a reduction in rhinorrhea and sneezing. Efforts to either treat or prevent the common cold with Echinacea preparations have had variable success when subjected to randomized trials.

The use of antibiotics has only a limited role in the treatment of the common cold and should be discouraged. When a common cold has lasted for 7–10 days and is no better or worse, acute bacterial sinusitis may have developed and additional medical care may be required. For this reason, antibiotics may be indicated when symptoms continue unabated for more than 10 days. After this time, the probability of a secondary bacterial infection increases to roughly 80%. Erythromycin, amoxicillin, and sulfisoxazole-trimethoprim are reasonable empiric choices at this point.

Pharyngitis

Symptomatic treatments for pharyngitis include salt-water gargles, acetaminophen, dyclonine lozenges, and use of a cool mist humidifier. Smoking cessation and voice rest are always indicated. When a streptococcal infection is suspected (i.e., when a high fever is present), treatment with penicillin, penicillin VK (250 mg three times daily), erythromycin ethylsuccinate (300–400 mg three times daily), or cephalexin (250 mg three times daily) should be started and continued for a full 10 days. Azithromycin is also effective, with its higher cost partially offset by the shorter (5 day) course of therapy. Patients are considered noninfectious after 24 hours of antibiotic coverage.

Complications from pharyngitis are rare and are generally restricted to the bacterial forms. The greatest concern is the development of rheumatic fever and its sequellae. Poststreptococcal glomerulonephritis, peritonsillar abscess, otitis media, and systemic infections are also possible complications.

Laryngitis

Usually, laryngitis is self-limiting. However, children's croup or acute epiglottitis can present like laryngitis. The primary treatment of laryngitis is voice rest, humidity (steam or cool mist), increased fluids, antipyretics, and analgesics (Table 19.3). Smoking should be stopped. Penicillin G (250 mg every 6 hours for 10–12 days) is indicated when streptococcal or pneumococcal infections are suspected. Indications for further investigation or that a change in therapy is needed are shown in Table 19.4.

Laryngotracheobronchitis

In mild cases, outpatient treatment with humidification, fluids, rest, and analgesics may suffice. Dexamethasone has been shown to reduce symptoms in patients with moderate-to-severe croup and is frequently used in children. Because of the possibility of acute airway obstruction, more severe cases require hospitalization and intensive monitoring by those familiar with the disease.

Asthma

Although there is no cure for asthma, there are effective treatment methods. Successful management of asthma consists of four components: (1) patient education, (2) reduction of environmental triggers (allergens), (3) measurement and monitoring of pulmonary function, and (4) pharmacologic intervention.

Table 19.3. Simple interventions for laryngitis.

Suck on cough drops, a throat lozenge, or hard candy

Stop smoking

Avoid places where cigarettes are smoked

Use a humidifier (cool mist ultrasonic humidifiers are preferred—these are more expensive than the usual vaporizer, but are safer and more effective); you can also try standing in a hot shower

Use aspirin, ibuprofen, or acetaminophen for temperature, muscle discomfort, and pain; do not give aspirin to anyone less than 19 years of age—it can trigger an attack of Reyes syndrome

Gargle with warm salt solution (1/2 tsp salt in 1 cup of water)

Speak softly, but do not whisper; use a notebook and pencil to communicate

Drink warm liquids like hot Tang or honey and lemon

Medication therapies are designed to minimize the airway inflammation component of asthma as well as to treat airway narrowing. Environmental control measures are implemented to avoid or eliminate factors that induce or trigger asthma flare-ups. Immunotherapy may also be considered if allergies are known to be an asthma trigger, a condition that is most common in children.

The treatment of asthma is based on five major classes of drugs: antiinflammatory agents (cromoglycate and nedocromil), steroids (beclomethasone, prednisone), β-agonists (albuterol, terbutaline), methylxanthines (theophylline), and anticholinergics (atropine, ipratropium bromide). A sixth class has gained favor recently: antileukotrienes or leukotriene modifiers.

Table 19.4. Indications for reevaluation or a change in therapy for laryngitis.

Difficulty breathing

Fever over 101°F

Difficulty swallowing

Deep cough or, in a young child, a cough like the bark of a seal (suggestive of laryngotracheobronchitis)

Brown, green, or yellow sputum

Hoarseness that persists for 1 month or more

Inability to carry on normal activities

Symptoms of gasping or drooling

Leukotrienes are responsible for the contraction of the airway smooth muscle, increasing leakage of fluid from cells in the lung, and further promoting inflammation by attracting other inflammatory cells into the airways. Recently, new antileukotriene medications have been introduced to fight the inflammatory response typical of allergic disease. These drugs are generally limited to the treatment of chronic asthma, though recent data have demonstrated that antileukotriene therapy can be beneficial for many patients with less chronic asthma. It is likely that these newer medications will eventually have an increased role in asthma care as more studies are conducted. Comanagement with both the patient and an asthma specialist is essential when the disease is advanced.

Mild cases of asthma (brief wheezing one to two times per week) are often managed by intermittent use of β-agonists or theophylline. Bronchodilators are generally used as "rescue medications" to relieve coughing, wheezing, shortness of breath, and difficulty in breathing. Those patients with weekly symptoms that interfere with sleep, exercise, or work require a regular maintenance schedule with cromolyn qid or nedocromil bid, with inhaled steroids as an adjunct. Theophylline is added when symptoms worsen. Salmeterol is a long-acting bronchodilator that, along with an antiinflammatory medication, is used for maintenance in the long-term control of asthma symptoms.

Both patients and physicians must be aware of several potential pitfalls in management: Not recommended are mist therapy, fluid loading, breathing exercises, or intermittent positive-pressure breathing (IPPB) therapy. Erythromycin and ciprofloxacin can slow theophylline clearance resulting in increased levels of as much as 15–20% and possible toxicity.

Bacterial Pneumonia

In addition to common sense support measures, antimicrobial therapy for the most likely organisms is required. For community acquired infections, empiric treatment with erythromycin (500 IV every 6 hours) provides good coverage, including coverage for *Mycoplasma* and *Legionella*. For patients with nosocomial infections, third-generation cephalosporins (cefotaxime, ceftizoxime) plus vancomycin are recommended.

In otherwise healthy adults, improvement should occur in 1–3 days. Despite clinical improvement, it may take quite some time for the chest X-ray to clear, necessitating repeated studies for up to 6 weeks. Mortality rates for bacterial pneumonia still runs about 5%. This rate rises when the pneumonia is associated with debilitating processes such as alcoholism and AIDS. For these high-risk patients, consideration should be given to prophylaxis with polyvalent pneumococcal and influenza vaccinations (Table 19.2).

Viral Pneumonia

General supportive measures such as analgesics, antitussives, and antipyretics are appropriate. Amantadine (100 mg q 12 h) is effective for treating infections with influenza A, but not against influenza B infections. Symptoms should resolve in several days to a week. It should be noted that amantadine should be used with caution in patients with liver disease or epilepsy, and in those with a history of psychotic illness.

Mycoplasma Pneumonia

Rest, fluids, and analgesics are appropriate initial therapy. Antibiotic treatment with either tetracycline or erythromycin (500 mg every 6 hours for 7 days) provides good coverage. Azithromycin, given as 500 mg the first day, then 250 mg for days 2 through 5, may also be effective. Antibiotics such as penicillin are not effective against *Mycoplasma pneumoniae*. Symptoms often take more than 2 weeks to resolve.

A false-positive VDRL may be found in patients with *Mycoplasma pneumonia.*

Pneumocystis carinii Pneumonia

Trimethoprim/sulfamethoxazole (10–20 mg/kg/day of trimethoprim component divided every 6 hours for 21 days) with adjunctive corticosteroid therapy (prednisone) is standard, though a high percentage of AIDS patients will develop intolerance to trimethoprim/sulfamethoxazole. Trimethoprim/sulfamethoxazole has been used in pregnancy for both treatment and prophylaxis.

Pneumocystis carinii pneumonia can be successfully treated in many cases. It may recur a few months later, but treatment can help to prevent or delay its recurrence. Mortality for first episode infections is now about 10–15%, down from as high as 30–40% previously. Approximately 10% of patients develop respiratory failure and more than 85% of these succumb.

Case Study

A 23-year-old G2P2002 patient calls your office complaining of a "sinus infection" and requesting that a prescription for antibiotics be called to a local pharmacy. She reports congestion, a nasal discharge that has become thick and purulent and she has had a low-grade fever. Her symptoms began about 5 days ago. How should you proceed at this point?

This is a typical presentation for the common cold—the symptoms, their progression and the request for antibiotic therapy are all typical. Unless there is a history of previous sinus infections, or a reason to suspect that this patient is at high risk for an atypical infection or complication (e.g., immunocompromise), an office visit, additional testing, or anything other than symptomatic interventions are not warranted.

Suggested Reading

Arroll B, Kenealy T. Antibiotics for the common cold. *Cochrane Database Syst Rev* 2000;(2):CD000247.

ATS Update. Future directions for research on diseases of the lung. *Am J Respir Critical Care Med* 1998;158:320–34.

Barrett B, Vohmann M, Calabrese C. Echinacea for upper respiratory infection. *J Fam Pract* 1999;48:628–35.

Bertino JS. Cost burden of viral respiratory infections: issues for formulary decision makers. *Am J Med* 2002;112(Suppl 6A):42S–49S.

Boulet LP, Thivierge RL, Amesse A, Nunes F, Francoeur S, Collet JP. Towards excellence in asthma management (TEAM): a population disease-management model. *J Asthma* 2002;39:341–50.

Centers for Disease Control. Forecasted state-specific estimates of self-reported asthma prevalence—1998. *Morbid Mortal* 1998;47:1022–25.

Conrad DA, Jenson HB. Management of acute bacterial rhinosinusitis. *Curr Opin Pediatr* 2002;14(1):86–90.

Douglas RM, Chalker EB, Treacy B. Vitamin C for preventing and treating the common cold. *Cochrane Database Syst Rev* 2000;(2):CD000980.

Ducharme FM. Anti-leukotrienes as add-on therapy to inhaled glucocorticoids in patients with asthma: systematic review of current evidence. *BMJ* 2002;324(7353):1545.

Gern JE. Rhinovirus respiratory infections and asthma. *Am J Med* 2002;112(Suppl 6A):19S–27S.

Giles JT, Palat CT 3rd, Chien SH, Chang ZG, Kennedy DT. Evaluation of echinacea for treatment of the common cold. *Pharmacotherapy* 2000;20:690–7.

Greenberg SB. Respiratory viral infections in adults. *Curr Opin Pulmon Med* 2002;8:201–8.

Grimm W, Muller HH. A randomized controlled trial of the effect of fluid extract of Echinacea purpurea on the incidence and severity of colds and respiratory infections. *Am J Med* 1999;106:138–43.

Gwaltney JM. Clinical significance and pathogenesis of viral respiratory infections. *Am J Med* 2002;112(Suppl 6A):13S–18S.

Gwaltney JM. Viral respiratory infection therapy: historical perspectives and current trials. *Am J Med* 2002;112(Suppl 6A):33S–41S.

Henneicke-von Zepelin H, Hentschel C, Schnitker J, Kohnen R, Kohler G, Wustenberg P. Efficacy and safety of a fixed combination phytomedicine in the treatment of the common cold (acute viral respiratory tract infection): results of a randomised, double blind, placebo controlled, multicentre study. *Curr Med Res Opin* 1999;15:214–27.

Irwin RS, Madison JM. The diagnosis and treatment of cough. *N Engl J Med* 2000;343:1715–21

Jefferson TO, Tyrrell D. Antivirals for the common cold. *Cochrane Database Syst Rev* 2001;(3):CD002743.

Katz PO. Gastroesophageal reflux disease—state of the art. *Rev Gastroenterol Disord* 2001;1:128–38.

Leiner S, Mays M. Pharmacologic management of common lower respiratory tract disorders in women. *J Midwifery Womens Health* 2002;47:167–81.

Lindenmuth GF, Lindenmuth EB. The efficacy of Echinacea compound herbal tea preparation on the severity and duration of upper respiratory and flu symptoms: a randomized, double-blind placebo-controlled study. *J Altern Complement Med* 2000;6(4):327–34.

Lordan JL, Holgate ST. H1-antihistamines in asthma. *Clin Allergy Immunol* 2002;17:221–48.

Marshall I. Zinc for the common cold. *Cochrane Database Syst Rev* 2000;(2): CD001364.

Meadows M. Beat the winter bugs. How to hold your own against colds and flu. *FDA Consum* 2001;35(6):11–17.

Melchart D, Walther E, Linde K, Brandmaier R, Lersch C. Echinacea root extracts for the prevention of upper respiratory tract infections: a double-blind, placebo-controlled randomized trial. *Arch Fam Med* 1998;7: 541–5.

Mitchell JL. Use of cough and cold preparations during breastfeeding. *J Hum Lact* 1999;15:347–9.

Monto AS. Epidemiology of viral respiratory infections. *Am J Med* 2002; 112(Suppl 6A):4S–12S.

Mossad SB, Macknin ML, Medendorp SV, Mason P. Zinc gluconate lozenges for treating the common cold. A randomized, double-blind, placebo-controlled study. *Ann Intern Med* 1996;125(2):81-88.

Neuzil KM, Reed GW, Mitchell EF Jr, Griffin MR. Influenza-associated morbidity and mortality in young and middle-aged women. *JAMA* 1999; 281:901.

Peebles RS, Hartert TV. Highlights from the annual scientific assembly: patient-centered approaches to asthma management: strategies for treatment and management of asthma. *South Med J* 2002;95(7):775–9.

Potter YJ, Hart LL. Zinc lozenges for treatment of common colds. *Ann Pharmacother* 1993;27(5):589-592.

Powrie RO. Drugs in pregnancy. Respiratory disease. *Best Pract Res Clin Obstet Gynaecol* 2001;15(6):913–36.

Recommendations of prophylaxis against PCP for adults and adolescents with human immunodeficiency virus. *MMWR*, Recommendations and Reports, 41 RR-4 (April 10, 1992).

Rodrigo GJ, Rodrigo C. Continuous vs intermittent beta-agonists in the treatment of acute adult asthma: a systematic review with meta-analysis. *Chest* 2002;122:160–5.

Singh M. Heated, humidified air for the common cold. *Cochrane Database Syst Rev* 2000;(2):CD001728.

Smucny J, Fahey T, Becker L, Glazier R, McIsaac W. Antibiotics for acute bronchitis. *Cochrane Database Syst Rev* 2000;(4):CD000245.

Taverner D, Bickford L, Draper M. Nasal decongestants for the common cold. *Cochrane Database Syst Rev* 2000;(2):CD001953.

Tuffaha A, Gern JE, Lemanske RF Jr. The role of respiratory viruses in acute and chronic asthma. *Clin Chest Med* 2000;21:289–300.

Van Cauwenberge PB, van Kempen MJ, Bachert C. The common cold at the turn of the millennium. *Am J Rhinol* 2000;14:339–43.

West JV. Acute upper airway infections. *Br Med Bull* 2002;61:215–30.

20

Sexual Dysfunction

Jean D. Koehler

Background Information

Female sexual dysfunction or dissatisfaction is a common complaint among obstetric-gynecology patients. These complaints may result from medical treatments and procedures, or may secondarily complicate the management and patient compliance of treatment for other medical issues. Therefore, it is important that clinicians treating females obtain basic information regarding human sexual function and dysfunction. This chapter presents an integration of the clinical research as well as the author's experience regarding sexual function and the management of sexual problems often presented in an obstetric-gynecology practice.

Sexual Functioning

The Sexual Response Cycle

Sexual functioning is often described through the sexual response cycle, which includes sexual drive (libido), arousal, orgasm, and resolution. Each phase interacts with and influences the presence or absence of the other, and does not necessarily proceed in a linear fashion. Each is affected by psychological, sociological, and relational processes. However, natural sexual function throughout the whole sexual response cycle is physiologically dependent on adequate hormone levels—particularly estrogen and testosterone, enzymes that convert precursor hormones to the above-mentioned hormones, nonhormonal neurotransmitters like dopamine, adequate blood supply, and adequate central and peripheral nerve conduction. The clinician who assesses all of the physiologic and nonphysiologic areas, when presented with a patient with sexual dysfunction, will obtain a better diagnosis and treatment plan.

Sexual drive is the urge to obtain sexual stimulation. It can take the form of an urge to masturbate, watch or hear erotica, experience sexual dreams, or engage in stimulation with another person.

Sexual arousal occurs in two basic forms: mental and physiologic. Mental arousal occurs when a person reports feeling "turned on" or pleasure to erotic stimuli. Physiologic arousal usually includes genital vasocongestion, vaginal lubrication, increased genital erotic sensitivity, and the presence of prostatic-type secretions in the bladder and urethra as well as increases in respiration, pulse, and blood pressure. Mental arousal and physiologic arousal do not always occur together, as is sometimes the case with rape or unwanted stimulation, where vaginal lubrication may occur without any sense of subjective arousal. Physical reactions of sexual arousal in the female are presented in Table 20.1. Not all of these are observed in every woman.

The orgasmic phase of the sexual response cycle mainly consists of the 0.8-second involuntary contractions of the vaginal canal and uterus, accompanied by a subjective sense of sudden heightened pleasure. Some

Table 20.1.   Physical reactions during female sexual arousal.

1. Swelling of the labia, clitoris, and introitus
2. Lubrication of the vaginal canal—a "sweating phenomenon" through the mucous membranes lining the vaginal walls
3. Minor secretions of the Bartholin glands
4. Erythema of the genitalia
5. Lengthening, ballooning, and involuntary spasms of the vagina
6. Lifting of the uterus into the false pelvis
7. Descending of the uterus with G-spot stimulation
8. Swelling of the breasts
9. Nipple erections
10. Reddening of the neck and chest of some women
11. Increase in heart rate, blood pressure, and respiration
12. Milky, prostatic-like fluid from the paraurethral gland either emitted out of urethra or present in the bladder or urethra poststimulation

Table 20.2. Physical reactions during orgasm.

1. 0.8 second contractions of the vaginal canal
2. Possible contractions of the uterus, rectum, urethra, perineum, and lower abdomen
3. Milky, prostatic-like fluid from the paraurethral gland either ejaculated out of urethra or present in the bladder or urethra poststimulation
4. Heart rate increases to 110–180 beats per minute
5. Systolic blood pressure increases 30–80 mm Hg
6. Diastolic blood pressure increases 20–40 mm Hg
7. Respiratory rate increases up to 40 breaths per minute
8. Muscular tension (different from anxious tension) throughout the whole body

women with strong vaginal and uterine muscle strength will ejaculate the milky prostatic-type fluid that is already present in the arousal phase, from the urethra during orgasm. When not ejaculated externally, this fluid can be found in the bladder poststimulation. The clitoris is probably the most reliable source of stimulation for female orgasm, although some women report a preference and facility for orgasms mediated primarily by vaginal or cervical stimulation. Even women with complete spinal cord injuries have reported laboratory-documented orgasms. The G-spot (an area felt through the anterior wall of the vagina, halfway between the back of the pubic symphysis and cervix, along the urethra) is a common site of intravaginal orgasmic stimulation. If a patient is unsure as to whether she has ever experienced orgasm, preorgasmic sensations may be described as a wave of pleasure that extends over her pelvic area much like the sensation of going over a roller coaster hill followed by the sensation of vaginal contractions and then a feeling of satisfaction. Intense orgasm can be compared to the sudden pleasure and intensity of a sneeze, usually accompanied by a throbbing sensation in the vagina. The vaginal sensations of less intense orgasms feel more like a ripple than an intense series of contractions.

Table 20.2 lists the typical physiologic reactions during the orgasm phase. Orgasm contractions usually last from 3–5 seconds and will be followed either by a sense of physiologic satisfaction (especially in the case of an intense orgasm) or by an urge to continue the stimulation (possibly resulting in more orgasms). When orgasm occurs in a very positive context, the woman often has subjective feelings of satisfaction and/or emotional bonding toward her partner. However, these positive feelings can also result without experiencing the orgasm phase of sexual response, a phenomenon that is difficult for many men to relate to.

After orgasm, all of the physiologic changes return to the unstimulated state in most women. This is called the resolution phase. A few women will retain the vasocongestion, sometimes resulting in an uncomfortable condition called pelvic congestion syndrome or persistent sexual arousal syndrome.

Establishing the Diagnosis: Sexual Dysfunctions and Problems

This section lists the definitions, etiologies, and treatment of sexual dysfunctions and problems. The information on pharmacologic and medical causes of dysfunctions cannot be considered all-inclusive, because all conditions and medications listed have not been supported by controlled research, especially in women. Many of the conditions and drugs listed have been supported by research, while others are included because of clinical experience that is consistent with mechanisms of action known to influence sexual response. However, medication effects vary across individuals, with higher dosage levels and greater length of use increasing the incidence of sexual side effects. The clinician is encouraged to refer to the two sexual pharmacology compendia in the reference section to obtain information on the sexual effects of specific drugs as well as preferred alternatives within classes of drugs.

Definitions and Physical Etiologies

The sexual dysfunctions of female patients are (1) hypoactive sexual desire disorder; (2) arousal disorders; (3) orgasmic disorders; (4) dyspareunia and noncoital sexual pain disorders; (5) vaginismus; and (6) sexual aversion. Other sexual problems that might be encountered include (1) sexual drive discrepancy between the patient and her partner, (2) concern over types of sexual activities, and (3) sexually compulsive behavior in the patient or her partner. In addition, heterosexual patients may seek advice about sexual dysfunction in their male partners, including (1) hypoactive sexual desire disorder, (2) erectile dysfunction, (3) premature ejaculation, and (4) delayed or absent ejaculation.

Hypoactive Sexual Desire Disorder

This disorder is characterized by a persistent absence or near absence of sexual drive and receptivity that cause personal and/or interpersonal distress. In the general population, about one-third of women reported low sexual drive in the immediate past year of their lives. The range of normality is affected by the patient's age, length and quality of sexual and emotional relationship with her current partner, and her health status. In population-based studies, most women aged 18–29 years engage in partnered sex between two times a week and a few times a month. In contrast, almost a third of women aged 50–59 years claim to be sexually inactive with partners, while 57% engage in partnered sex a few times a month to a few times a year. Of those who are sexually active with partners, the average frequency of sex ranges from seven times a month for young women to four times a month for women in their fifties.

Potential physical causes of low sex drive are listed in Table 20.3. Androgen insufficiency has become increasingly recognized as an important cause of this disorder, and is present in women following oophorectomy or ovarian shutdown from medications or radiation, the binding of free testosterone from oral estrogen medications, hypothyroidism, hypopituitarism, and adrenal insufficiency. Table 20.4 lists psychotropic drugs, Table 20.5 outlines antihypertensives, and Table 20.6 provides information on miscellaneous drugs that have been shown to lower sex drive in some patients.

Sexual Arousal Disorders

One type of sexual arousal disorder is the persistent or recurrent inability to attain or maintain sufficient sexual excitement as noted by a lack of genital vasocongestion, erotic genital sensitivity, and vaginal lubrication. Another type involves a failure to mentally perceive sexual stimulation as arousing or pleasurable despite adequate physiologic indications. In a study of the general population, around 20% of women complained either of unpleasurable sex or difficulty with lubrication. Vaginal lubrication and elasticity are highly dependent on estrogen. Likewise, lubrication is dependent indirectly on cholinergic transmitter activity. External genital vasocongestion is also dependent on nonadrenergic/noncholinergic neurotransmitters like nitric oxide synthetase and polypeptides, such as vasoactive intestinal peptide. Therefore estrogen levels and a review of medications that might interfere with transmitter action are warranted. Also, the conditions or medications that affect sexual desire or orgasmic capacity can affect arousal through a negative feedback loop. In other words, if a woman does not desire to be sexually active because of a testosterone deficiency, she may comply with her partner's initiations but fail to lubricate because of disinterest. There are drugs and conditions believed to inhibit arousal directly and they are listed in Tables 20.7 and 20.8, respectively.

A third type of arousal disorder is persistent sexual arousal syndrome or "PSAS." Prevalence statistics are not available for this disorder. In PSAS, the physiologic responses characteristic of sexual arousal mentioned above may persist for hours or days, and are not necessarily triggered by sexual stimulation or resolved by orgasm. Most, but not all women complaining of this disorder find the symptoms intrusive, worrisome, and sometimes depressing. The research into this syndrome is so new that much is not known about the cause or treatment. All treatments reported to date have failed, but occasionally a patient's symptoms will remit spontaneously.

Orgasmic Disorders

Orgasm dysfunction occurs when a woman fails to reach that peak level of pleasurable release accompanied by vaginal contractions after sufficient genital stimulation. She is considered dysfunctional only if the condition is persistent and causes her distress. Over 20% of women in the general population claimed

Table 20.3.   Physical causes of low sex drive.

1. Causes of hormonal imbalances or deficiencies or excesses (involving estrogen, androgens, prolactin)
   a. Surgeries—oophorectomy, hypophysectomy, adrenalectomy
   b. Chemotherapy that destroys ovarian function
   c. Chronic depression or stress
   d. Renal dialysis
   e. Pituitary tumors—especially craniopharyngiomas and prolactinomas
   f. Hypopituitarism
   g. Oral contraceptives
   h. Alcohol and drug abuse
   i. Opiate abuse
   j. Oral estrogen replacement therapy
   k. Deficiencies of adrenal androgens—dehydroepiandrosterone (DHEA), DHEA-S, androstenedione
   l. Rheumatoid arthritis
   m. Systemic lupus erythematosis
   n. Hypothyroidism
   o. Androgen insensitivity syndrome
   p. Antiandrogen medications (e.g., for endometriosis)
2. Any disease process or injury that affects the sex centers of the brain
   a. Epilepsy—all forms but especially right-sided temporal lobe epilepsy in women
3. Illnesses that affect a woman's general feeling of well-being or her ability to respond sexually
   a. Cancer
   b. Anemia
   c. Diabetes
   d. Addison's disease
   e. Chronic active hepatitis
   f. Chronic renal failure
   g. Cirrhosis
   h. Cardiomyopathy and other cardiovascular conditions
   i. Cushing's syndrome
   j. Hemochromatosis
   k. Kallman's syndrome
   l. Myotonic dystrophy
   m. Parkinson's disease
   n. Tuberculosis

Continued.

Table 20.3.   *Continued*.

o. Chronic obstructive pulmonary disease
p. Chronic pain syndrome
q. Hypertension—treated and untreated
4. Conditions that are often associated with lowered drive
   a. Pregnancy and postpartum
   b. Perimenopause and menopause
   c. Infertility
   d. Alcoholism
5. Surgery
   a. Any disruption to the nervous or vascular supply to the genitalia can indirectly lead to low sex drive because of the loss of pleasurable feedback to the brain (i.e., colon and rectal surgery for cancer)
   b. Any surgery that disrupts the sex centers of the brain
6. Injury—any injury that disrupts the nervous and vascular supply to the pelvis or sex centers of the brain

difficulty with orgasm in the prior year, whereas only 4% claimed to have never orgasmed. A woman is considered dysfunctional if she fails to achieve orgasm under any circumstance, if her orgasms come so infrequently that sex is disappointing to her, or if orgasm requires such prolonged stimulation that sex becomes a chore. Although many women can learn to reach orgasm with sexual intercourse, failure to reach orgasm regularly with penetration is common and

Table 20.4.   Psychotropic drugs that can lower sex drive.

1. Sedatives/hypnotics
2. Antianxiety agents
3. Antidepressants
   a. Tricyclic antidepressants
   b. Monoamine oxidase inhibitors
   c. Selective serotonin reuptake inhibitors
   d. Lithium
4. Antipsychotics/neuroleptics
5. Stimulants/anorectics

Source: Adapted with permission from Crenshaw T, Goldberg J. *Sexual Pharmacology: Drugs That Affect Sexual Function.* New York: Norton; 1966.

Table 20.5.   Antihypertensives that may lower sex drive.

1. Diuretics
2. Reserpine
3. Methyldopa
4. Guanethidine (Ismelin)
5. β-Blockers
6. α_2-Agonists
7. Calcium channel blockers—unlikely unless secondary to depression

Source: Adapted with permission from Crenshaw T, Goldberg J. *Sexual Pharmacology: Drugs That Affect Sexual Function.* New York: Norton; 1966.

Table 20.6.   Miscellaneous medications and treatments that can lower sex drive.

1. Anticonvulsants
2. Anticancer drugs
3. Cardiac drugs
4. Hemodialysis
5. Ophthalmic solutions

Source: Adapted with permission from Crenshaw T, Goldberg J. *Sexual Pharmacology: Drugs That Affect Sexual Function.* New York: Norton; 1966.

Table 20.7.   Drugs known to inhibit vaginal lubrication.

1. Tricyclic antidepressants
2. Anticholinergics, such as those used for asthma
3. Tamoxifen
4. Chemotherapy
5. Monophasic oral contraceptives
6. Any drug that lowers available estrogen
7. Antihistamines

Table 20.8. Conditions known to inhibit vaginal lubrication.

1. Perimenopause
2. Menopause
3. Vaginitis
4. Expansively growing pituitary adenoma
5. Postpartum-nursing
6. Multiple sclerosis

appears to be normal. However, coital orgasmic capacity is correlated with very strong pubococcygeal muscles. Medical conditions that might cause orgasm dysfunction are listed in Table 20.9 and drugs that can block the orgasmic reflex are listed in Table 20.10.

Table 20.9. Medical conditions that can cause orgasmic dysfunction.

1. Neuropathy
   a. Multiple sclerosis
   b. Amyotrophic lateral sclerosis
   c. Diabetic neuropathy
   d. Spinal cord tumors
   e. Spinal cord trauma
2. Endocrine disorders
   a. Addison's disease
   b. Cushing's syndrome
   c. Hypothyroidism
   d. Hyperthyroidism
   e. Hypopituitarism
   f. Expansively growing pituitary adenoma
   g. Diabetes mellitus
   h. Androgen insufficiency
3. Epilepsy
4. Gynecologic factors
   a. Surgery that disrupts the pelvic nerve supply
   b. Any vaginal condition that causes pain upon stimulation
   c. Any chronic illness can indirectly lower orgasmic capacity through malaise, chronic fatigue, or chronic pain

Table 20.10.   Drugs that can inhibit orgasm.

1. Antidepressants—tricyclics, monoamine oxidase inhibitors, selective serotonin reuptake inhibitors
2. Antipsychotics/neuroleptics
3. Stimulants–anorectics
4. Tamoxifen
5. Sedatives/hypnotics

Source: Adapted with permission from Crenshaw T, Goldberg J. *Sexual Pharmacology: Drugs That Affect Sexual Function.* New York: Norton; 1966.

Dyspareunia and Noncoital Sexual Pain

Dyspareunia (coital pain), which occurs in about 15% of women in the general population, and noncoital sexual pain can be the result of a variety of physical sources. Types of pain range from itching, burning, or friction of the mucosa, pinpoint sharp pain upon light touch, tightness, and pain upon deep penetration. Even psychological sources can eventually lead to a physiologic cause. For example, failure to arouse mentally can prevent vaginal lubrication causing friction, and fear of pain may cause the vaginal muscles to tighten, making the canal too small to accommodate the penis comfortably. Table 20.11 lists conditions that may cause dyspareunia.

Vaginismus

Vaginismus is an involuntary contraction of the perivaginal musculature making vaginal penetration impossible, or nearly impossible without significant discomfort or pain. Its prevalence is unclear due to the lack of sampling in population-based studies. However, clinical experience suggests that this problem is being presented at increasing rates to health care providers due to the impact of vulvodynia. Vaginismus is often caused by a prior history of dyspareunia for reasons listed in Table 20.11, by fear of painful intercourse learned from folklore, or by a history of sexual abuse. This condition can be worsened by the gynecologist who is too eager to complete a pelvic examination, despite the patient's warnings of prior painful penetrations or painful protestations during the pelvic examination. Women with vaginismus sometimes retain normal sex drive and the ability to achieve orgasm by noncoital methods.

Sexual Aversion/Phobia

Sexual aversion is the negative or phobic reaction to sexual activity or to the anticipation of sexual activity. Sometimes aversion to a particular sexual activity, like fellatio, or to a sexual part, like the penis, makes the woman avoid all sexual activity. When aversion is of phobic proportions, physical reactions are those of panic disorder: overwhelming anxiety, sweating, nausea, vomiting, diarrhea, or palpitations. Once sexual activity begins, some women proceed through the sexual response cycle. A previous history of dyspareunia and low testosterone could be physical precursors to this condition, though most causes are believed to be psychological.

Table 20.11.   Physical conditions that can cause dyspareunia.

1. Rigid hymen
2. Painful hymeneal tags
3. Endometriosis
4. Pelvic inflammatory disease
5. Atrophic vaginitis
6. Relaxation or laceration of broad ligaments supporting the uterus
7. Pelvic tumors
8. Poor episiotomy repair
9. Vulvodynia
10. Interstitial cystitis
11. Ectopic ureter
12. Vaginal stenosis
13. Urethral caruncle
14. Hemorrhoids
15. Vaginal disease—herpes, candidiasis, human papilloma virus, etc.
16. Allergic reaction to rubber products used in condoms and diaphragms
17. Allergic reaction to contraceptive chemicals
18. Allergic reaction to semen
19. Repeated douching upsetting the vaginal pH value
20. Pelvic surgery
21. Estrogen deficiency during the postpartum nursing phase
22. Forced intercourse causing tearing of the vaginal mucosa
23. Levator ani myalgia from overuse of Kegel exercises
24. Urethritis
25. Radiation therapy
26. Pelvic adhesions
27. Adnexal pathology (i.e., ovarian cyst)
28. Symptomatic uterine retroversion
29. Pelvic floor disorders

Other Sexual Problems

Sexual drive differences between partners constitute one of the most common sexual concerns presented to sex therapists. It is not necessarily accompanied by sexual dysfunction in either partner. When drive differences cause significant problems, it is often because one partner believes that his or her drive is the norm and the other partner's drive is abnormal. Physicians can educate their patients about the wide range of normal sexual frequencies and discuss options for compromise.

Another sexual problem commonly encountered is the discrepancy between a woman and her partner over the type of sexual activity they enjoy. The inclusion of oral sex is a common source of disagreement between partners. These discrepancies, if left unresolved, can lead to sexual dysfunction. The physician can assess whether the patient needs accurate information about the normality of a given activity, how to engage in sexual practices effectively, or how to prevent injury or disease. Oral sex participants should know that many sexually transmitted diseases can be transmitted orally and condoms or dental dams should be used when there is a risk of disease. Additionally, there is a statistically significant, positive association between oral sex and repeated vulvovaginal candidiasis.

Likewise, anal sex recipients should be encouraged to lubricate and gradually dilate their anal openings before penetration with a penis or dildo to prevent tears of the mucosa. Frequent anal eroticism is associated with anorectal pain, ulcers or fissures, rectal prolapse or leakage, and hemorrhoids. Condoms should be used to prevent transmission of sexually transmitted diseases (STDs). There should be no penetration of the vagina with anything that has just been in the rectum because normal bacterial flora in the rectum will cause infection.

Sexual Addiction/Compulsion

The physician may encounter sexually compulsive behavior in the patient or her partner. This problem is defined as a pathologic need for sexual activity that gradually replaces the desire to have healthy relationships and activities. And while compulsive sexual activity can be secondary to other compulsive, addictive, mood, or posttraumatic stress disorders, it may also be a primary comorbid condition. Clues to sexual compulsivity that may present in the gynecologist's office include genital injury from compulsive masturbation, repeated STDs or unplanned pregnancies, a history of multiple sexual partners in a short period of time, or a demanding attitude about frequency or activity. This patient may also be seductive with her physician.

More often, the patient is the victim of her partner's sexual compulsions. In this situation she may present with genital injury, STDs, a loss of sex drive due to the excessive demands of her partner, or a complaint of infrequent sex due to the partner acting compulsively outside of the relationship. Use of Internet pornography has become an increasing complaint of sex therapy patients, with research showing some participants spending over 20 hours a week in such activities—neglecting family, job, or the need for adequate sleep. Patients with simply high sex drives, or practices that are not part of the cultural norm, can be misdiagnosed as compulsive by conservative partners or clinicians. Such diagnoses should be left to sexual specialists. Furthermore, true sexual compulsion is a very complex problem to treat and almost always warrants a referral to a sex therapist.

Male Sexual Dysfunction

Sexual dysfunction in the heterosexual patient's partner may lead to her own sexual dysfunctions. A patient may also seek guidance for the partner's dysfunction. It is important for the gynecologist to know how to diagnose and refer these patients. (Lesbian partner's dysfunctions can have similar effects on your patient and likewise need to be addressed.) Male sexual dysfunctions are listed in Table 20.12.

Hypoactive Sexual Desire Disorder

Hypoactive sexual desire disorder in a male is essentially the same phenomenon as in women in definition and causes (see related tables). One main difference is in the role of estrogen, which, when excessive in the male, lowers his drive. Some diseases, such as alcoholism, result in a relative increase of estrogen in a man's body because of the pathologic state of the liver. In other cases, medications may raise his estrogen levels to sexually dysfunctional proportions. A man with a global decline in sex drive should be evaluated by his primary care physician. However, the man whose sex drive has remained intact in general but is turned off only by his current partner can be referred for couples therapy or to a sex therapist.

Erectile Dysfunction

Erectile dysfunction is a failure to attain an erection during genital stimulation, or failure to maintain an erection until ejaculation or the man's desire to stop. This label also applies to erections lacking adequate rigidity for penetration. The ability to maintain an erection to ejaculation with manual stimulation, or with an alternate partner's stimulation, is a good indicator that there is no

---

Table 20.12.   Common male sexual dysfunctions.

1.   Hypoactive sexual desire disorder
2.   Erectile failure
3.   Premature ejaculation
4.   Delayed or absent ejaculation

physical cause. Decreasing frequency of morning erections or inability to keep morning erections with body movement may be signs of organic etiology. Referral to a urologist who specializes in sexual dysfunction is the safest way to ensure diagnostic accuracy. As psychogenic erectile dysfunction is more adequately treated if it is addressed sooner, prompt referral to an appropriate specialist is important.

Premature Ejaculation

Premature ejaculation occurs when a man lacks the ability to exert some control over his ejaculatory latency. Usually this diagnosis is more appropriate when the man ejaculates sooner than several minutes after penetration. The human male would naturally ejaculate within 2 minutes of vaginal thrusting if he were not purposefully delaying this reflex. A patient might complain of the partner's premature ejaculation because she has not reached orgasm with vaginal penetration, even after as much as 10 minutes of thrusting. This patient merely needs to be educated about the relative differences in vaginal and penile sensitivity and the importance of clitoral stimulation and increased foreplay before penetration. Premature ejaculation is rarely a result of medical conditions, and unless the man is complaining of other symptoms indicative of urinary tract infection or prostatitis, referral to a sex therapist is appropriate.

Delayed Ejaculation

Delayed ejaculation occurs when a man or his partner complains of his inability to ejaculate after sufficient stimulation to the penis. The inability to ejaculate within 5–10 minutes (when a man is not intentionally suppressing this reflex to please his partner) can be considered dysfunctional. As with female orgasmic dysfunction this definition is subjectively defined by the couple, and especially the man's subjective sense of a failure to progress to orgasm. When the man has no difficulty ejaculating with noncoital stimulation, the problem is assumed to be psychogenic and referral to a sex therapist is appropriate. However, diseases such as diabetes and medications such as selective serotonin reuptake inhibitors (antidepressants) are often associated with this symptom and referral to an internist or urologist is recommended.

Psychological Causes of Sexual Dysfunction

Table 20.13 lists the five main categories of psychological causes of sexual dysfunction: immediate, relational, psychiatric, historical, and societal.

Immediate Causes

Immediate causes of sexual dysfunction are those that occur during the love-making process and include the following.

Spectatoring

This phenomenon occurs when a person mentally stands outside herself and watches during sexual activity. As she watches, she will often internally criticize

Table 20.13.   Psychological causes of sexual dysfunction.

1. Immediate—spectatoring, performance anxiety, need to please, negative focus, ineffective stimulation, lack of attraction, distracting fantasies/thoughts
2. Relational—anger, power struggle, infidelity, mistrust, lack of emotional intimacy, fear of pregnancy, divergent preferences, sexual addiction/compulsion
3. Psychiatric—depression, anxiety, posttraumatic stress disorder, some personality disorders
4. Historical—religious repression, sexual trauma, negative parental input
5. Societal—myths, media, double standard

herself whether or not that evaluation has any basis in reality. These mental processes lower her mental pleasure and send inhibitory messages to the pelvic nerves, thus damping her sexual reflexes.

Performance Anxiety
This occurs when a woman has certain expectations of the "right" way to respond sexually and does not live up to her own expectations.

Excessive Need to Please
A woman may have trouble responding if she is focused so much on her partner's pleasure that she does not attend to the type of stimulations or conditions she needs to be aroused.

Focusing on Negative Aspects
Sometimes a woman focuses on certain negative characteristics of her lover during or just before the sexual experience—body type, manner of dress, etc. Although perhaps justifiable, this may also stem from being a perfectionist and thus unable to focus on the total love-making experience.

Lack of Proper Stimulation
Although commonalities exist, each woman is unique in her preferences. Furthermore, the same stimulation may produce opposite reactions in the same woman at different times. Thus, it is very important that the woman be free to communicate her sexual preferences to her partner. The clinician should urge the patient to be a good communicator.

Lack of Physical/Chemical Attraction to Partner
Research demonstrates that women are less likely to require sexual attraction when selecting their committed partners versus their dates. After the newness of a relationship wears off, a woman may find sex with her partner of decreasing appeal. An often overlooked factor in women's arousal is the bodily scent of

her partner. Therefore, a woman turned off by her partner's scent will be negatively affected by a common precursor to women's sexual receptivity—the physically affectionate touching that precedes sexual interaction. Such partners should pay strict attention to their hygiene to minimize this impact.

Unwanted Fantasies/Thoughts
Sometimes disruptive fantasies and thoughts occur during sex. They may include images of prior sexual abuse causing anxiety and disgust, images of other desirable sexual partners or taboo, but arousing sexual activities inducing guilt, or simply images or thoughts of which chores need to get done.

Relational Causes
Relational causes of sexual dysfunction, which occur with one's sexual partner, are characterized by the following.

Displaced Anger. Unresolved anger often affects the ability and desire to respond to one's partner sexually.

Power Struggle. Some individuals withhold sex to punish or engage in sex to manipulate their partner, in response to a lack of power or agreement in other aspects of the relationship.

Infidelity. If the patient has had an affair, her drive toward her committed partner may decrease out of guilt, a sense of loyalty to her other lover, or fear of infecting her committed partner with an STD. Likewise, if her partner has been unfaithful, her drive may decrease as a result of a feeling of betrayal, depression, anger, or fear of contracting a disease.

Mistrust. In addition to the mistrust that results from an affair, women's drives may be decreased by their inability to trust their partners with the intimate physical and verbal reactions that come from uninhibited sex. Similarly, they may refuse sex because they are not certain that the relationship will last.

Lack of Emotional Intimacy. Women tend to respond best when they feel emotionally close to their partners. Poor communication patterns and lack of personal differentiation can prevent emotional intimacy from developing in a couple.

Fear of Pregnancy. For a woman to respond best during sex, she must be uninhibited and free of fears. The woman who is not ready to risk a pregnancy may keep herself "in check" so that she will not have intercourse or forget to use contraception.

Divergent Preferences
Some women avoid sex because of the fear of being pressured into unappealing sexual activity (such as anal sex). Others may not respond well because their partners do not want to touch them the way they most prefer. Remind the

patient that a healthy partner appreciates not having to guess, is aroused by his or her partner's forthrightness, and is willing to find sexual activities that appeal to both.

Sexual Compulsivity
Compulsive tendencies may cause a decrease in responsiveness as a result of oversatiation. Likewise, sexual activity may not be particularly pleasurable because the goal may be to numb negative emotions rather than to express sexual urges. The woman with a sexually compulsive partner may become less responsive because of the pressure to be sexual regardless of her feelings or needs. Conversely, some compulsive partners engage in sex elsewhere, leaving the woman to complain of infrequent sex.

Psychiatric Disorders
Psychiatric disorders can produce sexual problems. The most frequent associations are with depression, anxiety disorders, posttraumatic stress syndrome, and alcoholism or drug addiction. Other common psychiatric disorders, such as personality disorders, can be related to sexual dysfunction, but not necessarily.

Historical Inputs

Historical inputs to sexual dysfunction, including events in the individual's upbringing that have negatively affected current sexual attitudes, may occur through the following ways.

Religion
The Judeo-Christian ethic has traditionally been sexually repressive, assigning negative attitudes to sexual pleasure. While this message has changed in some religions, the current trend of sexual conservatism has resulted in mixed messages, leaving young newlyweds with sexual anxiety and guilt, aging couples with the belief that sex solely for pleasure is inappropriate, and homosexual individuals struggling to function within heterosexual marriages.

Sexual Trauma
An estimated one-third of women have experienced sexual abuse in their past. This is most often associated with subsequent sexual dysfunction, but compulsive and irresponsible sexual activity can also result. Adolescent girls who have been abused are more likely to attempt to or to become pregnant and to initiate sex at a younger age than their nonabused peers.

Parental Influences
Parents convey sexual attitudes to their children whether they refer to sex directly or not. By not educating children positively about the sexual aspects of their bodies and feelings, or by conveying only the consequences of sex, parents inadvertently convey a negative or shameful attitude about sex and sexual body parts.

Societal Causes

Societal causes, which are those generalized beliefs and behaviors within a culture that affect women's sexual self-image and self-esteem, are conveyed through the following.

Myths. Our society has a history of withholding sexual information, and myths develop out of this ignorance. A very common myth is that women should find sexual intercourse as physically stimulating as men. Another is that what stimulates one person will automatically stimulate that person's partner.

Media. Use of beautiful, slender models in media advertising has resulted in a negative body image in some women. These women tend to focus on their perceived bodily imperfections during sex rather than on their pleasure.

Double Standard. The double standard still exists, causing women confusion about claiming their sexuality. Sexually assertive men may be revered, whereas the same behavior in women may be seen as "loose." This double standard extends to some medical sexual studies when it ignores the research on the complexity of female sexual function and satisfaction, and how often the sexual responses of females are attained differently from those of males.

Management of Sexual Problems

Sexual History

Taking a thorough sexual history of a patient is the key to accurate diagnosis and treatment. Three types of histories, listed in Table 20.14, are appropriate in an obstetric-gynecology practice: one occurs within a routine review of systems during an annual examination or request for a physical; the second occurs when the physician is consulted about physical symptoms that may be related to sexual activity; and the third occurs when a patient specifically discloses a sexual dysfunction and asks for help. A sex history can be covered in several minutes.

Although a high percentage of patients (85–91%) believe it is appropriate for physicians to take sexual histories, studies show that physicians are generally reluctant to initiate questions concerning sex with their patients for fear of seeming inappropriate, because they feel unskilled, or because they believe they do not have time to cover this area. Other physicians are reluctant

Table 20.14. Types of sexual histories.

1. Routine review of systems
2. Secondary to pelvic symptomatology
3. Sexual dysfunction

to bring up sex because of their own embarrassment or lack of skill in discussing sex or because they do not want to make their patients uncomfortable. Because research shows that more than half of women admit to sexual problems when specifically asked, and because STDs can have far-reaching health consequences for women, it is imperative that clinicians initiate these discussions.

Effective sexual history taking requires more sensitivity than other reviews. A patient is more likely to be honest if she believes that her physician is interested, nonjudgmental, and comfortable with the topic. Physicians who are uncomfortable are encouraged to seek guidance from an experienced sex therapist and/or attend a "Sexual Attitude Reassessment" seminar (for a list of SARs call The American Association of Sex Educators, Counselors, and Therapists—804-752-0026). Questions should be worded in a way that makes no assumptions about sexual orientation or monogamy.

Sexual History Taking During a Routine Examination

The form of sexual history taking shown in Table 20.15 is used as a screening device for sexual activities that may affect a woman's health or sexual satisfaction. In addition, it can provide a baseline of functioning that can be used for comparison in later years to more effectively assess the impact of gynecologic surgeries, medication, menopause, or pregnancy on the patient's sexuality.

This sexual data gathering seems to flow best at the end of a menstrual history. Using the same matter of fact tone of voice and pacing, proceed with the questions in Table 20.15. If you are fearful of being misunderstood, begin with something like this: "Ms. Jones, I'd like to ask you some questions about your sexual functioning if you don't mind. Sexual activity can affect your health and your health can affect your sexual activity. I want to make sure I don't miss anything important. I am not here to judge you, so please feel free to be candid with me."

Some of the questions in Table 20.15 are best asked the first time a patient is seen. For ongoing patients, use judgment to modify questions based on what is already known about the patient. For example, a long-term patient whose previous history shows she is monogamous and heterosexual might be insulted by questions that suggest she is not. It is best to review the sexual functioning questions in terms of whether the patient has developed any new symptoms or concerns since the last visit. Try to assess the patient's level of sophistication with vocabulary and modify questions using the terms with which she seems comfortable. It may be necessary to define some terms, especially if the patient seems confused. Likewise, begin questions with "how often do you" or "when you." Phrases such as "have you ever" suggest that such a practice is unusual and is likely to elicit a false-negative reply.

If the patient seems unusually uncomfortable with sexual history taking, stop and note her discomfort and ask her if she would like to talk about it. She may reveal that she experienced sexual abuse as a child and has kept this a secret. Be sure to stop the history taking and show appropriate

Table 20.15. Questions for a detailed sexual history.

Are you currently sexually active? Have you ever been?

Are your partners men, women, or both?

How many partners have you had in the past month? Six months? Lifetime?

How satisfied with your (and/or your partner's sexual functioning are you?

Has there been any change in your (or your partner's) sexual desire or the frequency of sexual activity?

Do you have, or have your ever had, any risk factors for HIV? (List blood transfusions, needlestick injuries, IV drug use, STDs, partners who may have placed you at risk.)

Have you ever had any sexually related diseases?

Have you ever been tested for HIV? Would you like to be?

What do you do to protect yourself from contracting HIV?

What method do you use for contraception?

Are you trying to become pregnant (or father a child)?

Do you participate in oral sex? Anal sex?

Do you or your partner(s) use any particular devices or substances to enhance your sexual pleasure?

Do you ever have pain with intercourse?

Women: Do you have any difficulty achieving orgasm?

Men: Do you have any difficulty obtaining and maintaining an erection? Difficulty with ejaculation?

Do you have any questions or concerns about your sexual functioning?

Is there anything about your (or your partner's) sexual activity (as individuals or as a couple) that you would like to change?

HIV = human immunodeficiency virus; IV = intravenous; STDs = sexually transmitted diseases.

Source: From "The Proactive Sexual Health History" Nusbaum M, Hamilton C, (authors) American Family Physician Vol. 66(9): November 1, 2002.

concern. The patient may feel she is taking a major risk in revealing this information. Another patient may be uncertain of the physician's motives in asking sexually explicit questions. If the prologue mentioned above was not used, now is the time to briefly explain that sexual symptoms and dissatisfaction can affect a woman's health and how well she takes care of herself. After explaining this to the uncomfortable patient, always ask her permission to continue with the sexual history. If she will not allow it, nonjudgmentally suggest that if she ever wants to discuss her concerns in the future, you are willing to do so. Likewise, offer a referral to a therapist if she reveals a history of abuse or dysfunction. It may take multiple visits for a patient to build enough trust to reveal her sexual concerns. By opening the door each time with sexual questions, it allows her to address these issues when she is ready, without having to openly admit that she withheld information in the past.

Most physicians' concerns about sexual history taking can be alleviated by showing their patients they care about their health and are sensitive to the embarrassment that many have in discussing sex.

Sexual History Taking following Patient Presentation of Vaginal Symptoms

Parts of the same sexual history used for routine examinations noted in Table 20.15 can be used for the patient with pelvic symptomatology. Just preface these questions differently, such as, "Ms. Johnson, sometimes the symptoms you are having are related to a woman's sexual practices. I'd like to ask you some questions that could help me treat your symptoms more successfully. Please feel free to be honest. I just want to help you get over these symptoms."

Sexual Dysfunction History

Table 20.16 lists general questions to ask when a patient presents with a sexual dysfunction or when you have uncovered a problem in a routine screening. Note that a patient with no personal or interpersonal distress about her sexual responses needs no treatment unless she specifically wants to improve her functioning. Obtain information on the entire sexual response cycle of the patient and her partner, as one dysfunction may be at the root of another. For example, a patient who presents with low sex drive may have dyspareunia as the causative factor. Assess desire, lubrication/erection, orgasm/ejaculation, presence of sexual pain, and satisfaction regardless of which dysfunction is initially presented. If the patient shows distress in discussing these problems, be sure to make empathic statements such as "this has really bothered you, hasn't it?"

If the patient's complaints include decreased sexual desire, she should always be screened for depression. Table 20.17 lists the appropriate questions. A positive reply in several areas indicates a need for further evaluation by an internist and possibly a referral to a psychiatrist or experienced nonmedical therapist. Reassure the patient that she will get a thorough assessment and appropriate treatment.

Office Management of Sexual Dysfunction

It should be noted that diagnostic tools for identifying organic causes of female sexual dysfunction are greatly underresearched and lag far behind those for male sexual dysfunction. Vaginal photoplethysmography is of some benefit and other measures of clitoral and labial temperature and blood flow are being developed. Well-researched neurologic tools for genital sensitivity are needed as well as greater understanding of hormonal and other neurochemical mediators. Furthermore, current testosterone assays for normal female levels are unreliable at the lower ranges and laboratory ranges are not correlated with good sexual functioning. Therefore the recommendations given below may change greatly over the next few years.

Table 20.16. Sexual dysfunction history.

1. Describe your symptoms. (Be very explicit about this, especially with dyspareunia)
   a. Dyspareunia. Where do you feel the pain—general, localized, with deep penetration, upon entry? Describe the pain—sharp, raw, burning, too small for anything to enter?
2. When did this problem begin?
3. Describe the circumstances at the time of onset
   a. With masturbation or with which partner
   b. Patient's mental health—depression, anxiety, stress, etc.
   c. Medical problems or surgeries
   d. Intoxication with mood-altering drugs by patient or her partner (i.e., alcohol, marijuana)
   e. Nature of relationship to partner
   f. Use of prescription drugs, herbal medicines, or over-the-counter drugs
   g. Pregnancy, infertility treatments, menopause/perimenopause
   h. Concurrence with sexual pain
4. Does this problem change in severity or frequency? If so, what makes it better or worse?
5. Do you or your partner have difficulty in other sexual responses—desire, lubrication/erection, or orgasm/ejaculation?
6. What do you believe caused this problem? (for example, differences in sexual style, frequency, ineffective stimulation, coincidental with medication or illness onset, history of sexual trauma)
7. Have you sought other professional help for this? If so, what was done? Results? May I consult with that professional?
8. What treatments have you tried on your own?
9. Do you have any ideas about what should be done to help you overcome this symptom?

Table 20.17.   Depression screening.

---

1. Do you feel depressed? (A negative reply does not necessarily rule out depression)
2. Is your sleep disrupted in any way, such as difficulty getting to sleep within 10–15 minutes, waking during the night with difficulty getting back to sleep easily, awakening 1–2 hours earlier than you need or want to?
3. Has your appetite greatly increased or decreased?
4. Has your weight fluctuated more than 10 pounds without effort on your part (not due to smoking cessation)?
5. Do you experience constipation? Diarrhea?
6. Has your drive for sex been lowered under all circumstances?
7. Has your energy decreased a lot?
8. Has your concentration decreased a lot?
9. Are you feeling excessively guilty about something?
10. Do you feel inadequate or like a failure?
11. Do you have persistent thoughts of death or suicide? (A positive reply to this question warrants immediate referral to a psychiatrist.)

Low Sex Drive

If the history and physical examination suggest it, laboratory studies should be done to screen out physical causes of low sex drive, especially hypothyroidism and hypopituitarism. Androgen deficiency is emerging as a likely medical cause of this disorder, especially if the patient is well estrogenized. A woman with insufficient androgens will give a history of persistent absent or almost absent sexual drive for partnered sex, masturbation, and erotica, and few if any sexual dreams. Additionally, she may complain of a persistent unexplained fatigue, lowered mood, and decreased sexual receptivity, orgasm, and pleasure. Recommended laboratory screening for low sex drive is presented in Table 20.18. There are no large-scale studies documenting minimum androgen levels needed for adequate sexual functioning, however, when androgen insufficiency needs to be ruled out. The Princeton Conference on Androgen Insufficiency in Women (2002) provides us with our current guidelines listed in Tables 20.19 and 20.20. (Androgen insufficiency should be suspected when women complain of the symptoms listed in Table 20.19. The diagnosis of androgen insufficiency can be made using the guidelines in Table 20.20.) There are no large-scale studies to determine androgen levels adequate for sexual function; however, Table 20.21 contains a range of levels correlated with good sexual functioning in a small sample of reproductive aged women. Androgen levels

Table 20.18.   Suggested laboratory screening for low sex drive.

1. Estradiol or follicle-stimulating hormone (if symptoms of deficiency)
2. Serum testosterone
3. Free testosterone—equilibrium dialysis preferred or calculated free T
4. Dehydroepiandrosterone sulfate (DHEAS)
5. Thyroid profile
6. Prolactin (if symptoms warrant)

should be obtained in the morning, but there is lack of consensus as to whether they should be drawn in the follicular phase, when androgens are lowest, or in the midcycle, when testosterone peaks at ovulation.

Treatment for most physical causes of low sex drive listed in the tables is well documented. However, treatment recommendations for androgen insufficiency are just emerging and thus it will be discussed in detail here. It has been suggested that because testosterone assays are not sensitive at lower levels of female normal ranges, a free testosterone level in the lower quartile of the normal range accompanied by symptoms of testosterone deficiency warrants a trial of replacement therapy. Ironically, because oral contraceptives lower free testosterone, replacing them with nonhormonal methods may be all that is needed in some women. Likewise, women on oral forms of estrogen (replacement) therapy should switch to a transdermal approach, which does not bind free testosterone except at high doses. If sexual symptoms persist 6–12 weeks after these medication changes, laboratory tests should be repeated to rule out continued androgen deficiency. Options for androgen replacement therapy are presented in Table 20.22.

Research results indicate that injectable forms of testosterone produce reliably positive sexual drive effects in oophorectomized women and have not

Table 20.19.   Symptoms of androgen insufficiency.

1. Decreased sexual drive, pleasure, genital sensitivity, or orgasm
2. Persistent, unexplained fatigue
3. Low mood
4. Decreased vaginal lubrication even when adequately estrogenized
5. Changes in cognition and memory
6. Decreased muscle strength
7. Bone loss
8. Hot flashes despite adequate estrogen

Table 20.20.   Criteria for diagnosing androgen insufficiency.

1. Clinical symptoms are present
2. Adequate estrogen—regular menstrual periods or estrogen replacement therapy
3. Free testosterone is in the lowest quartile (or lower) for norms based on women aged 20–40 years

Table 20.21.   Androgen laboratory norms[a] correlated with positive female sexual function.

	Age range		
Age	20–29 (17)	30–39 (23)	40–49 (20)
Total T (ng/dl)	45–57	28–40	27–39
Free T (pg/ml)	1.4–1.6	1.0–1.2	0.9–1.1
DHEA-S (μg/dl)	177–214	139–171	125–156
SHBG (nmol/liter)	44–59	45–52	47–58

[a] Drawn in the morning on days 8–15 for premenopausal women with no sexual dysfunction. T, testosterone; DHEA, dehydroepiandrosterone; SHBG, sex hormone-binding globulin.
Source: Reproduced with permission from Guay A. Androgen values in premenopausal women without sexual dysfunction. Podium #6. *Proceedings of the International Society for the Study of Women's Sexual Health Annual Meeting.* 2002.

Table 20.22.   Androgen therapy options for women.

1. 1.25–2.50 mg/day methyltestosterone
2. 75 mg testosterone enanthate IM for 28 days postoophorectomy
3. 200 mg dihydroandrosterone IM for 28 days postoophorectomy
4. 300 mg testosterone patch for a month
5. 50–100 mg dehydroepiandrosterone (DHEA) daily am

been shown to adversely affect high-density lipoprotein (HDL) and liver toxicity like oral forms. While clinical experience attests to the efficacy of injectable routes of testosterone administration in premenopausal, testosterone-deficient women, there are no published data to support this approach while keeping testosterone levels within physiologic ranges. Once replacement begins, laboratory tests need to be repeated every few months to make sure the patient stays within normal ranges. Though not well supported by controlled research results, methyltestosterone (oral form) dosed at 1.25–2.50 mg/day is effective for some women and is available for hormone therapy (HT) either as Estratest or can be individually compounded. Surgically menopausal women have not demonstrated any hepatotoxicity at dosages of 2.5 mg of methyltestosterone daily, but have demonstrated adverse trends in lipoproteins. Furthermore, research on higher replacement dosages of methyltestosterone (often in men) reports significantly lower HDL cholesterol, liver toxicity, and polycythemia. Therefore, pretreatment laboratory measures of hepatic function, lipid profile, triglycerides, and hematocrit, as listed in Table 20.23, are indicated with repeat studies in intervals of several months to 1 year once replacement begins.

In controlled studies, dehydroepiandrosterone (DHEA) tablets have been shown to be effective in raising sex drive and responsiveness for pre- and postmenopausal women with documented adrenal insufficiency and for premenopausal women with hypopituitarism. The overall efficacy of DHEA for premenopausal women with androgen insufficiency remains to be clarified. Effective dosages ranged from 30–50 mg/day. However, finding a brand of DHEA with guaranteed potency is difficult since it is unregulated by the Food and Drug Administration (FDA). Both oral forms of androgen replacement—DHEA and methyltestosterone—appear to be safe in the short run in the dosages mentioned. Controlled research on testosterone gels in this population so far shows positive sexual effects only when free testosterone was elevated to supraphysiologic ranges.

Anecdotally, a 2% testosterone cream has also been used with mixed feedback as to its effectiveness for libido problems, possibly because some patients tend to use insufficient doses to bring testosterone into normal ranges. The lack of controlled studies on this route of administration leaves the clinician with only experiential guidelines and repeated laboratory assays

Table 20.23. Laboratory tests prior to and during androgen replacement.

1. Lipid profile—total, high-density lipoprotein, low-density lipoprotein
2. Hepatic function
3. Triglycerides
4. Hematocrit

to determine if dosages are producing improved levels of circulating androgens. The same is true for testosterone gels, modified from male dosages that are currently available. However, controlled research does support the efficacy of a testosterone patch in raising several sexual function parameters in oophorectomized women, but this approach currently lacks FDA approval until longer term safety studies can be conducted. This product has excellent short-term safety results. No matter which route of hormone administration is used, patients will likely need several months—possibly 4–6—of consistent treatment, with regulation of dosages often based on repeated laboratory assays and symptom relief, before positive effects can be seen or androgen replacement therapy can be considered ineffective.

The most common side effects of any form of testosterone replacement therapy include weight gain, increased facial hair, and acne. However, when levels are kept within normal ranges, these side effects are not common and do not require discontinuation of treatment. Lipid profiles may worsen, especially with oral routes, and therefore need to be monitored before administration and at intervals of several months during usage. Dosages can be lowered to obtain a balance between sexually enhancing effects and unwanted side effects.

If desire stays low despite several months of documented normal androgen values, the couple should be referred for sex therapy. Replacement therapy can be continued during the course of psychotherapy to see if the combination produces effective results. However, couples with long-term desire difficulties and androgen insufficiency often benefit from combining sex therapy and androgen replacement therapy at the beginning of treatment, to counteract negative attitudes and ineffective coping strategies.

Reproductive aged women who choose androgen replacement therapy should be informed of the potential masculinizing risks to a fetus and be encouraged to use highly reliable birth control methods. Until long-term studies can document the safety of androgen replacement therapy, women with an already adverse lipoprotein profile, documented atherosclerotic cardiovascular disease, or a marked family history of cardiovascular disease, diabetes, or breast cancer should be informed of the potential for exacerbation of these diseases or their side effects with androgen replacement therapy.

Patients with no discernible medical cause for low sex drive should be referred with their partners to a sex therapist. Sometimes the patient presents with a complaint of low sex drive based only on the discrepancy of drives between partners. When no sexual dysfunction is present, couples should be encouraged to use the following paradigm. If the patient is approached for sex but would resent participation, her partner can be encouraged to masturbate, if that is within the partner's value system. If the patient is neutral, she might propose a sexual encounter where no expectations about outcome would be the ground rule. That way, if she does not become aroused, her partner need not take it personally, but can nonetheless benefit from the stimulation received. Similarly, the sexually neutral patient can offer to stimulate her partner without receiving any stimulation in return. Of course, if any of these solutions become the norm, or if both people are not willing to be flexible, a referral for sex therapy is warranted.

For all the sexual dysfunctions, the obstretic-gynecologic clinician can provide immediate help in the form of accurate information, permission to be sexual, or encouragement to communicate the patient's sexual needs to her partner. However, because low drive tends to be a multifactorial problem, treatment often requires a trained sex therapist who may recommend a combination of psychotherapy, couples therapy, bibliotherapy, and at-home sexual exercises. If there is sexual abuse in the patient's history, direct referral to a psychotherapist is indicated.

Arousal Disorder

Standard applications of vaginally inserted estrogen cream or tablets in those with laboratory documented serum deficiencies of estrogen or who otherwise show signs of vaginal atrophy should be prescribed for those lacking genital vasocongestion and lubrication. If coincident with androgen insufficiency, lack of genital sensitivity can be treated with a topical testosterone cream applied to the vulva, though its effectiveness is yet to be documented with controlled research. Other androgen replacement options mentioned above could be considered as well. In selected cases, oral vasodilators such as Sildenafil have increased genital vasocongestion with sexual stimulation. Clinical trials are under way to determine the effectiveness of Sildenafil and other vasodilators such as L-arginine, yohimbine, apomorphine, and phentolamine. Topical prostaglandin E_1 and vasoactive intestinal peptide are also under investigation for arousal disorder.

If physical causes of this disorder have been ruled out, and the patient's sexual attraction for her partner is intact, her problem may be caused simply by a lack of proper stimulation. The patient should be encouraged to communicate the type of touch she wants to her partner. If not already known from prior experience, this can be learned through masturbation or by reading books designed to help women to orgasm. Often she will need emotional connection or a different type of initiation to become receptive, but she has failed to communicate to her partner how that can be established. Women who are unable to follow through with communication or whose arousal disorder is not amenable to simple education and permission giving by their physician will need psychotherapy to address the more complex causes such as relationship problems or sexual trauma.

Orgasm Disorder

Orgasmic dysfunction may be medical in etiology. Certainly physicians should assess for symptoms indicative of medical causes listed in the tables, for example, unregulated diabetes or diabetic neuropathy, androgen deficiency, and selective serotonin reuptake inhibitor (SSRI) antidepressants. Sexual dysfunction in diabetics may subside once blood sugar levels are brought under control.

Androgen insufficiency should be treated using the guidelines in the low sex drive section. Preliminary controlled trials show that the testosterone/estrogen patch can significantly improve orgasm and pleasure beyond estrogen replacement alone in surgically menopausal women; however, not all women low in testosterone have difficulties with orgasm. Likewise, Tibolone, a drug with androgenic, estrogenic, and progestogenic activity (not available in the United States) is showing significantly positive sexual effects on orgasm and responsivity in surgically menopausal women compared to estrogen replacement therapy alone. However, its adverse impact on lipid profiles is a concern.

A 2% testosterone cream can be applied to the vulva prior to sexual activity in those who complain of decreased genital sensitivity and delayed orgasm, though its effectiveness remains anecdotal. Since many patients are on antidepressants, management of SSRI-induced orgasmic delay will often be warranted. Options include waiting for tolerance to develop, reducing the dosage, switching to a different antidepressant like the dopamine-agonist bupropion, or taking drug holidays on the weekends. Augmenting SSRIs with $5\text{-}HT_2$, $5\text{-}HT_3$, α_2-adrenergic receptor antagonists, PDE5 inhibitors, and dopamine receptor agonists has been proposed. Such drugs include buspirone, Sildenafil, and yohimbine and may show potential once large-scale studies are undertaken. However, their safety in combination with SSRIs is currently in question. Because genital sexual arousal and orgasm depend on adequate nerve conduction involving the pudendal, pelvic, hypogastric, and sensory vagus nerves, gynecologic surgeons should be careful to spare those nerve pathways.

Patients with primarily nonmedical causes of orgasm disorder should be educated about the importance of clitoral and G-spot stimulation and the relative insensitivity of the back two-thirds of the vagina for the average woman. Women tend to learn how to achieve orgasm most easily through their own masturbation, followed by teaching these techniques to their partners. Furthermore, patients should be taught Kegel exercises as vaginal muscle strength is correlated with orgasmic potential. The stronger her vaginal muscles, the more likely the woman is to be orgasmic with intercourse. The patient should be informed that most women do not easily reach orgasm with intercourse and that only with effective stimulation and communication will she find out whether she will be coitally orgasmic. Books written for anorgasmic women can be recommended. Preorgasmic women need to be encouraged to engage in prolonged stimulation, perhaps 30–60 minutes, to break through the emotional barriers to responding. Vibrators work for most preorgasmic women, but learning to achieve orgasm by less intense methods is preferable. Women unable to benefit from these suggestions should be referred to therapy—with their partners if possible.

Vaginismus

When a patient presents with vaginismus, physicians should proceed with the pelvic examination very slowly, *if at all*, ideally using a pediatric speculum.

Sometimes the patient is so phobic that an internal examination to rule out physical causes is inadvisable until the patient has benefited from psychotherapy. If the patient has other symptoms indicative of a pelvic floor disorder, such as painful defecation, then referral to a pelvic floor physical therapist is also indicated. Vaginismus is sometimes accompanied by pelvic pain disorders such as vulvodynia. The physician should be thorough in ruling out and/or treating these medical precursors to vaginismus, although sometimes a combined approach has been shown to be effective.

Physicians should educate the patient with nonmedical vaginismus symptoms by explaining the spasm of paravaginal muscles and stressing that she can learn to relax them. Physician-assigned relaxation exercises and Kegel exercises followed by the insertion of lubricated dilators of graduated circumference may be all that is needed in milder cases. Dilator insertion may be done by the physician in multiple office visits or at home by the patient and her partner. However, vaginismus is often associated with such a phobic element that a psychotherapy background is needed to treat it successfully. A combination of sex therapy and pelvic floor physical therapy has been shown to be highly effective. Assuring the patient that pain is not involved will help her take that first step.

Sexual Aversion/Phobia

This condition should be treated by a psychotherapist because of the complexity involved. If the patient is amenable, rule out both physical causes of dyspareunia via a pelvic examination as well as medical causes of low sex drive. Psychotherapy, often involving treatment for sexual abuse, and couples therapy may be warranted.

Referral

Because sexual disorders may require diagnosis and management beyond the usual training and focus of the obstetric-gynecologic clinician, it is important to develop referral sources in internal medicine, endocrinology, urogynecology, psychiatry/psychotherapy, and pelvic floor physical therapy. For a listing of pelvic floor physical therapists in your area, call The American Physical Therapy Association at 800-999-2782 and ask for the "women's health division." For nonmedical causes of sexual dysfunction, the most effective referral is to a psychotherapist who has been extensively trained to do sex therapy and couples therapy. Since Florida is the only state that currently licenses sex therapists, the most reliable credential of a good sex therapist is certification by a national organization. Currently, the American Association of Sexuality Educators, Counselors, and Therapists (AASECT) is the oldest, largest, and most nationally recognized certifying organization for sex therapists. Referrals can be reached online at www.aasect.org or by calling the national office at 804-752-0026. Likewise, clinical members of the American Association for Marriage and Family Therapy (go to www.aamft.org for a list of clinical members) will have training in couples therapy, although not necessarily in sex therapy.

Therapists from all disciplines—psychiatry, social work, psychology, marriage and family therapy, and psychiatric nursing—can be credentialed in these areas with the appropriate training.

The referral will be more effective if the clinician (1) can assure the patient that this therapist has been effective with other patients; (2) reassures the patient that no sexual touching is done or demonstrated by the therapist; (3) knows that this therapist is comfortable with the subject and will not judge the patient; (4) stresses that the patient's partner (if she has a steady, committed one) often needs to be involved in the therapy for therapy to be most effective; and (5) assures the patient that the therapist will make every effort to work within the patient's value system.

Case Study

Tara, a 31-year-old working mother of two toddlers, was married for 5 years. She was referred to sex therapy for a total loss of sex drive with onset after her first delivery 3 years earlier. In addition to her loss of sex drive, she was usually anorgasmic, though she was able to achieve orgasm with coital stimulation within 5 minutes of penetration and within 1 minute of vibrator stimulation about two times a month. In addition, she reported that she resented her husband's initiations. She was taking low-dose desogesterel containing oral contraceptives for ovarian cysts, Zyrtec, and methyltestosterone for her low drive. She complained of excessive fatigue, which she attributed to raising small children. The only benefit she obtained from methyltestosterone was the eradication of her dyspareunia and restoration of vaginal lubrication. Her initial laboratory results revealed a very low total and free testosterone. (No other laboratory results were reported but there were no additional symptoms of other endocrine malfunctions.)

Tara's husband was involved in the initial evaluation but was unable to attend therapy due to work conflicts. However, the couple seemed to have a warm, cooperative marriage and she appeared to have no substantial psychopathology. Tara's history included some features that clinicians often correlate with sexual repression in adulthood. As a child she had been forced to watch her babysitter sexually stimulate her little brother and felt guilty for not protecting him. She also reported that her father was unusually negative about anything to do with sex throughout her rearing.

Despite having been informed of the probable effect of her oral contraceptives on her free testosterone, Tara chose to remain on them because of significant consequences from prior ovarian cysts. Her methyltestosterone was discontinued and she was started on a regimen of testosterone injections every 3 weeks coinciding with weekly psychotherapy. After stabilizing her dosage in the physician's office, she continued with at-home injections. Tara began to notice a positive change after the second injection, and by the fourth month her drive had substantially risen. She began to initiate sex and was receptive to her husband's initiations most of the month. She began to achieve orgasm in 100% of her sexual encounters, and felt comfortable with proposing a variety of sexual acts. In psychotherapy Tara worked through her traumatic feelings from the sexual abuse incident and confronted her father on the negative impact of his sexual attitudes. She learned a variety of sexual techniques and was reassured of their normalcy.

However, by the fourth month, her total testosterone (T) was rising above physiologic range though her free T remained in midrange. She lowered her dosage at her endocrinologist's request, reducing her total testosterone to normal range and her free T to just below normal range. After 2 months on the lower dosage, she had maintained her level of sexual desire and responsivity, felt emotionally satisfied with her sexual relations, and satisfactorily terminated psychotherapy. At no time did she complain of any unwanted side effects.

Tara's case illustrates how the combination of androgen insufficiency and sexual trauma and repression can cause sexual dysfunction at all stages—drive, arousal, orgasm, and satisfaction. The combination of testosterone replacement and psychotherapy restored her to consistently satisfactory sexual functioning.

Summary

Sexual dysfunctions can be caused by organic, psychogenic, or mixed etiologies. Obstetric-gynecologic clinicians are often the frontline in diagnosing and treating organic causes of female sexual disorders and are crucial in referring patients whose disorders involve psychogenic and mixed etiologies. Too often, clinicians use their own experiences and value systems to guide the treatment of sexual issues, an approach that may delay effective treatment. Scientifically based knowledge is essential in effective management and collaboration with related specialists is often warranted. Women's sexual medicine suffers from a lack of adequate diagnostic techniques, laboratory tests, and treatment norms. Some treatment regimens, especially androgen replacement therapy, are still considered experimental and lack well-done studies with long-term safety data to back up clinical experience. However, research in this area is rapidly increasing and clinicians are encouraged to obtain further training by attending meetings hosted by the American Association of Sexuality Educators, Counselors, and Therapists—AASECT (www.aasect.org), The International Society for the Study of Women's Sexual Health—ISSWSH (www.isswsh.org), The Society for Sex Therapy and Research—SSTAR (www.sstarnet.org), and The Society for the Scientific Study of Sexuality—SSSS (www.sexualscience.org). Furthermore, by joining these organizations, the clinician will also have access to publications and Web-based case discussion groups. Those with a special interest in treating female sexual dysfunction are encouraged to obtain certification from The American Association of Sexuality Educators, Counselors, and Therapists. When done with up-to-date, scientifically based information, obstetric-gynecologic clinicians can play an educational and therapeutic role in the lives of their patients with sexual problems. Those who do will find it a rewarding area of medicine.

Reading for the Female Patient

Barbach L. *For Yourself.* 1976 (for orgasm disorders).

Ellison CR. *Women's Sexualities.* 2000 (for general understanding).

Foley S, Kope S, Sugrue D. *Sex Matters For Women—A Complete Guide for Taking Care of Your Sexual Self.* 2002.

Goldstein A, Brandon M. *Reclaiming Desire: 4 Keys to Finding Your Lost Libido.* 2004.

Heiman J, LoPiccolo J. *Becoming Orgasmic.* 1988 (book and video).

Katz D, Tabisel RL. *Private Pain.* 2002 (for vaginismus).

Ladas A, Whipple B, Perry JD. *The G Spot: And Other Discoveries About Human Sexuality.* 2005.

Maltz W. *The Sexual Healing Journey.* 1991 (for sexual abuse survivors).

McCarthy B, McCarthy E. *Rekindling Desire: A Step by Step Program to Help Low-Sex and No-Sex Marriages.* 2003.

Zilbergeld B. *The New Male Sexuality—Revised Edition.* 1999 (for the male partner).

Additional Suggested Web Sites

www.aasect.org—listing of certified sex therapists

www.SexualHealth.com—for sexuality information

www.vaginismus@yahoogroups.com—for vaginismus patients only

www.lvaginismus@yahoogroups.com—for vaginismic patients, their partners, and treating professionals

www.sexualitytutor.com—links to vaginismus information, especially non-English-speaking patients

See list within Maurice W. *Sexual Medicine in Primary Care* (referenced below)

Acknowledgments. The author would like thank Beverly Whipple, Ph.D., R.N. and Michael Plaut, Ph.D. for their editorial input. Note: Dr. Koehler was a paid consultant of Procter & Gamble on their third stage clinical trials of the testosterone patch in women and a paid consultant on female sexual dysfunction for Ortho-McNeill.

Suggested Reading

Allolio B, Arlt W. DHEA treatment: myth or reality? *Trends Endocrin Metab* 2002;13(7):288–94.

Androgen Insensitivity in Women. The Princeton Conference. *Fertil Steril* 2002;77(4).

Arlt W, et al. Dehydroepiandrosterone replacement in women with adrenal insufficiency. *N Engl J Med* 1999;341(14):1013–20.

Barrett-Conner E. Efficacy and safety of estrogen/androgen therapy—menopausal symptoms, bone, and cardiovascular parameters. *J Reprod Med* 1998(suppl);43(8):746–52.

Barrett-Connor E, et al. A two-year, double-blind comparison of estrogen-androgen and conjugated estrogens in surgically menopausal women—effects on bone mineral density, symptoms, and lipid profiles. *J Reprod Med* 1999;44(12):1012–20.

Basson R. The complexities of female sexual arousal disorder. *World J Urol* 2002;20(2):119–26.

Basson R, et al. Report of the International Consensus Development Conference on Female Sexual Dysfunction: Definitions and Classifications. *J Urol* 2000;163(3):888–99.

Basson R, et al. Summary of the Recommendations on Sexual Dysfunctions in Women. *J Sex Med* 2004;1(1):24–34.

Berman J, Bassuk J. Physiology and pathophysiology of female sexual function and dysfunction. *World J Urol* 2002;20:111–18.

Castelo-Branco C, et al. Comparative effects of estrogens plus androgens and tibolone on bone, lipid pattern and sexuality in postmenopausal women. *Maturitas* 2000;34(2):161–8.

Crenshaw T, Goldberg J. *Sexual Pharmacology: Drugs That Affect Sexual Function.* New York: Norton; 1966.

Davis S, et al. Endocrine aspects of female sexual dysfunction. *J Sex Med* 2004; 1(1):82–6.

Geiger AM, Foxman B. Risk factors for vulvovaginal candidiasis: a case-control study among university students. *Epidemiology* 1996;7(2): 182–7.

Guay A. Androgen values in premenopausal women without sexual dysfunction. Podium #6. *Proceedings of the International Society for the Study of Women's Sexual Health Annual Meeting.* 2002.

Hatzichristou D, et al. Clinical evaluation and management strategy for sexual dysfunction in men and women. *J Sex Med* 2004;1(1):49–57.

Hellberg D, Zdolsek B, Nilsson S, Mardh PA. Sexual behavior of women with repeated episodes of vulvovaginal candidiasis. *Eur J Epidemiol* 1995;11(5):575–9.

Johannsson G, et al. Low dose dehydroepiandrosterone affects behavior in hypopituitary androgen-deficient women: a placebo-controlled trial. *J Clin Endocrinol Metab* 2002;87(5):2046–52.

Leiblum SR, Nathan SG. Persistent sexual arousal syndrome: a newly discovered pattern of female sexuality. *J Sex Marital Ther* 2001;27(4): 365–80.

Leiblum S, Wiegal M. Psychotherapeutic interventions for treating female sexual dysfunction. *World J Urol* 2002;20(2):127–36.

Lewis CE. *The 60 second interview* (video). Los Angeles: UCLA Center for Health Promotion and Disease Prevention; 1993.

Maurice W. *Sexual Medicine in Primary Care.* St. Louis: Mosby; 1999.

Michael RT, et al. *Sex in America.* Boston: Little, Brown & Co.; 1994.

Munarriz R, et al. Androgen replacement therapy with dehydroepiandrosterone for androgen insufficiency and female sexual dysfunction: androgen and questionnaire results. *J Sex Marital Ther* 2002;28(s):165–73.

Segraves RT, Balon R. *Sexual Pharmacology: Fast Facts.* New York: W.W. Norton; 2003.

Simon JA. Safety of estrogen/androgen regimens. *J Reprod Med* 2001; 46(3):281–90.

Sipski M, Alexander C. *Sexual Function in People with Disability and Chronic Illness.* Gaithersburg, MD: Aspen Publications; 1997.

Whipple B. Beyond the G spot: new research on human female sexual anatomy and physiology. *Scand J Sexol* 2000;3(2):35–42.

Whipple B, Gerdes CA, Komisaruk BR. Sexual response to self-stimulation in women with complete spinal cord injury. *J Sex Res* 1996; 33(3):231–40.

Zaviacic M. *The Human Female Prostate.* Brastislava: Slovak Academic Press; 1999.

21

Sports Medicine and Injuries in the Athletic Woman

Tanya J. Hagen and Freddie H. Fu

Background Information

There is a general trend toward increased participation of females in sports and physical activity across the lifespan. While women were banned from the first modern Olympic games in 1896, they comprised 35.1% of the participants in 1996. There were a few early pioneers, including Olympic champions Charlotte Cooper and Mildred "Babe" Didrikson, but World War II probably had a greater influence on society's acceptance of the female athlete. With men away at war, the women were called upon to accomplish all types of physical tasks on the home front. In World War II the depiction of "Rosie the Riveter" as well as the success of the All American Girl's Baseball League redefined "appropriate" roles for women. The trend of increased female participation in athletics escalated in the last half of the twentieth century when in 1972, Title IX of the Educational Amendment Act allowed equal access to all federally funded activities including school-sponsored sports. In the 1980s there was a 700% increase in participation of women and girls in sports and another 50% increase was seen in the 1990s. One in 27 high school girls participated in sports in 1972. This number increased to 1 in 3 by 1998 and continues to grow. More and more research is revealing the tremendous benefits of exercise in women. Physicians will continue to play a key role in encouraging and even prescribing physical activity. Given the explosion of female athletic participation, it is imperative that physicians understand not only the benefits, but also the orthopedic and medical challenges that specifically apply to women in sports.

Benefits of Exercise in Females

There are an estimated 200,000 deaths annually in the United States related to a sedentary lifestyle. Several studies have revealed that physical fitness is associated with dramatic reductions in all-cause mortality. While patients and physicians alike are most familiar with the positive cardiovascular affects of exercise, the benefits extend beyond the heart. Increased physical activity is associated with additional benefits such as decreased risk of diabetes, breast cancer, and even depression. High school girls who are active in sports have higher graduation rates, fewer unwanted pregnancies, and greater self-esteem than those who are not active. Physical activity positively influences almost every aspect of a woman's health from her physiology to her social interactions and mental health (see Table 21.1).

Table 21.1. Probable benefits of exercise in females.

Decreased all-cause mortality
Decreased risk of coronary disease, cardiac events, and death
Improved lipid profile and control of obesity
Slower progression of early carotid atherosclerosis and a reduction in stroke
  risk
Improved blood pressure control
Improved glycemic control and prevention of type 2 diabetes
Decreased rate of cholelithiasis
Modest protection against breast cancer
Improved bone mineral density
Less dysmenorrhea and premenstrual tension syndrome
Decreased disability and improved cognitive function and autonomy in
  older women
In young females, decreased risky behavior including involvement with
  drugs, smoking, and teen pregnancy
Improved self-image, self-esteem, and mental health
Improved immunity
Decreased health-related costs

Orthopedic Issues in Active Women

Evaluation of an Active Female with Musculoskeletal Complaints

History

Though athletes with orthopedic problems occasionally present with a sense of joint instability, early muscle fatigue, or decreased power, the usual complaint is "pain." With this in mind, the majority of the musculoskeletal history is not that different from the history taken for chest or abdominal pain. It is necessary to ask about onset, quantity, quality, and duration of the pain, contributing and alleviating factors, and associated symptoms. A few unique, yet important historical questions to ask include the mechanism of injury, predisposing factors, and goals of treatment. The mechanism of injury refers to the inciting event that caused the current complaint. With traumatic events, this is typically straightforward. The patient athlete with an acute wrist fracture, for example, may describe a fall onto an outstretched hand. Someone with a meniscus tear may describe a twisting injury of the knee. The mechanism of injury can be a key component in developing a differential diagnosis and will help guide the physical examination. For overuse injuries, the mechanism of injury may not be as important per se as predisposing factors. Factors that may influence these conditions include previous injury, anatomical and biomechanical issues, and a change in routine, equipment, or training intensity. In addition to questions regarding the patient's current and previous status, it is extremely important to ask patients about their goals of treatment. Because many of these problems are not life-threatening, different treatment options may be acceptable depending on the injury. A "jammed" finger for a soccer player may be a mild annoyance whereas the same injury for a softball pitcher can be devastating. Does a patient with knee pain hope to run a marathon or simply desire pain-free sleep? The patient's goals will help decide the appropriate level of aggressiveness. A review of systems, focusing on neurologic, rheumatologic, and systemic complaints, should be included. Additionally, sources of referred pain should be considered, such as cholelithiasis causing shoulder pain.

Physical Examination

Key components of the musculoskeletal physical examination are listed in Table 21.2. In addition to these essential items, a general examination for signs of rheumatologic or other systemic illness should be considered. Also, a brief evaluation of the joints above and below the injured area/joint should be performed.

Common Injuries in Female Athletes

As with men, the overuse to traumatic injury ratio for women is approximately 50:50. The type of injury is most closely linked to the type of sport. Knee and

Table 21.2. Components of the musculoskeletal physical examination.

Inspection	Look for deformity, ecchymosis, muscle atrophy
Palpation	Feel for swelling/effusion, tenderness, warmth
Range of motion (ROM)	Test for pain/disability with both active and passive motion
Manual muscle testing (MMT)	Evaluate for weakness (and pain) by resistance muscle action
Special tests	Check the integrity of a specific structure (ligament, cartilage, tendon, bone) by challenging its function or by "aggravating" the structure and reproducing pain
Neurovascular tests	In acute injury, rule out nerve and vessel damage; in overuse injuries, evaluate for associated or contributing neuropathy

ankle problems are common in running sports, whereas shoulder complaints are more common in swimming, crew, and throwing sports.

Despite similar injury rates in comparable sports, there are data to suggest that females may be at increased risk for specific injury types and patterns. Aside from obvious anatomic differences, factors that may influence injury patterns include differences in metabolism, circulation, and cardiorespiratory capacity, body shape, size, and composition, and others. It has been proposed, for example, that an increased quadriceps angle (Q-angle), a less developed vastus medialis, and a greater degree of genu valgum in the female knee contribute to the higher rate of patellofemoral disorders. Hormonal influences and differing neuromuscular reflex patterns among other factors have been implicated in the 2- to 8-fold increased risk for noncontact anterior cruciate ligament (ACL) injuries.

While a full tutorial on the evaluation and treatment of specific injuries is beyond the scope of this chapter, Table 21.3 shows the typical presentation, signs, and symptoms of some of the more common injuries seen in female athletes. There are a number of excellent resources/texts to further complement knowledge in these areas. With overuse or traumatic injury, early recognition, treatment, and, if necessary, sports medicine or orthopedic consultation are paramount to prevent further injury and minimize time lost from sport participation. It is important to note that for overuse injuries, rest alone is typically not sufficient. Addressing inflammation, muscle weakness, inflexibility, and/or biomechanical factors allows return to activity with decreased risk of reinjury. Many traumatic injuries, even some fractures and ligament tears, are best treated nonsurgically, but good outcomes require early

Table 21.3. Some common injuries in female athletes.

Diagnosis	Presentation	Examination findings	Radiographs	Initial treatment
Overuse injuries				
Patellofemoral Pain/lateral patella tracking	Peripatellar/anterior knee pain exacerbated by running, stairs, prolonged sitting Occasional swelling after activity	I: +/− Genu valgus overpronation P: Peripatellar tenderness MMT: Weak quads; +/− hip weakness, tight IT band Spec tests: Apprehension and pain with lateral patellar glide	X-rays: Weight-bearing AP and lateral and merchant views—evaluating for joint space narrowing and patella position	PRICE (protect, rest, ice, compress, elevate) PT (quad strengthening) Patellar stabilization brace Address biomechanical factors
Shoulder instability	Shoulder pain or fatigue after overhead activity +/− Hx of episodic subluxation or frank dislocation	I: +/− Scapulothoracic dysrhythmia P: Minimal tenderness ROM: May be increased MMT: RTC weakness Spec tests: Apprehension with Jobe dislocation/relocation test, increased anterior/posterior translation, + O'Brien's test for labral tear if associated NV: Rule out cervical spine pathology	X-rays: (may include true AP, axillary lateral, west point view, strycher notch view) to evaluate for bony pathology MRA if labral injury is suspected	PRICE PT (RTC strengthening, scapular stabilization) Consider surgery for unidirectional, involuntary instability, or failed conservative treatment

Continued.

Table 21.3. *Continued.*

Diagnosis	Presentation	Examination findings	Radiographs	Initial treatment
Tibial stress fracture	"Stabbing" shin pain that initially was with impact activity only, now with any activity. No obvious acute injury +/− night pain	**I:** +/− Swelling, ecchymosis. **P:** Point tenderness. **MMT:** Anterior tibial weakness. **Spec tests:** Bony pain at tender site with tapping either proximally or distally	X-rays: AP and lateral to evaluate for obvious fracture. Bone scan or MRI for early diagnosis	Rest from impact activity. Pneumatic compression (e.g., "aircast"). PT. Address predisposing factors. Anterior tibial stress fx: nonweight bearing, immobilize, refer to specialist
Spondylolysis (pars fracture)	Low back pain worse with hyperextension. No radicular symptoms	**P:** +/− Tenderness over lumbar spine. **Spec tests:** Increased pain with single leg hyperextension maneuver, straight leg raise; FABER if associated sacroiliac joint pain	X-rays: AP, lateral and oblique lumbosacral films to evaluate for fx, spondylolisthesis. Bone scan for early diagnosis and evaluation of healing	Avoid hyperextension. Brace when bone scan is positive and to allow healing. PT when pain free (or immediately with negative bone scan)

Traumatic injuries

ACL tear	Sudden onset of swelling and pain (deep, medial or lateral depending on associated injuries) after a twisting injury to the knee Often there is a sense of instability	**I**: Effusion **P**: Tenderness depends on associated bony, meniscal, and collateral ligament injury **ROM**: Limited (by effusion or mechanical block) **Spec tests**: Lachman and anterior drawer (increased anterior tibial translation on femur), pivot shift (rotational instability) **MMT**: Decreased quad strength	X-rays: AP, lateral and merchant views to r/o fracture, assess growth plates in adolescents MRI may be used to confirm diagnosis and evaluate for other pathology	PRICE Brace if there is significant instability PT (increase ROM, decrease swelling, quad atrophy) Orthopedic referral

Continued.

Table 21.3. *Continued.*

Diagnosis	Presentation	Examination findings	Radiographs	Initial treatment
Ankle sprain	90% are lateral/inversion injuries +/− Inability to bear weight depending on severity Complaints of instability, swelling, ecchymosis is variable	**I:** Swelling, ecchymosis **P:** Tender over affected ligaments; suspect fx with bony tenderness **ROM:** Limited **Spec tests:** +/− Anterior drawer and talar tilt tests for lateral ligament injury; note, with anterior/medial pain, special tests for syndesmotic injury ("high ankle sprain") should be performed **MMT:** Decreased strength **NV:** R/o peroneal nerve injury with inversion sprains	X-rays: AP, lateral and mortise views to r/o fracture if bony tenderness is present Weight-bearing mortise view to evaluate syndesmotic injury	PRICE Crutches prn comfort Walking boot vs. pneumatic compression (e.g., aircast) for stability PT (ROM, strength, balance) Consider functional brace for accelerated return to activity
Patella dislocation	Acute, severe anterior knee pain and swelling	**I:** Swelling, erythema **P:** Effusion, severe peripatellar tenderness	X-rays: to r/o Fx and evaluate patellar position	PRICE Immobilize in extension Consider early specialist

	after the patella "shifts out of place" Traumatic vs. noncontact Continued sense of instability	**ROM**: Limited by pain, effusion **Spec tests**: Apprehension (and pain) with lateral patellar glide test **MMT**: Quad weakness, r/o tendon rupture	Consider MRI if chondral injury is suspected	(sports medicine or orthopedic) referral for conservative vs. surgical management
Concussion	Reported (or observed) symptoms after minor head injury may include headache, nausea, fatigue, dizziness, light or noise sensitivity, memory or concentration problems, and others	LOC may or may not be observed Cognitive testing may reveal retrograde or anterograde amnesia, problems with concentration, decreased reaction time, etc. Findings can be subtle Neurologic exam is usually nonfocal	CT (or MRI) should be considered in cases of LOC, amnesia, severe, accelerating or prolonged symptoms, or in cases with focal neurological findings on exam	Remove from exertion/ sport until symptom free Consider formal neuro-psychological testing with refractory symptoms

[a] MMT, manual muscle testing; Spec tests, special tests; NV, next visit; ROM, range of motion; Hx, history; fx, fracture; r/o, rule out; IT, iliotibial; AP, anteroposterior; PT, physical therapy; MRA, magnetic resonance angiography; RTC, rotator cuff; FABER, flexion in abduction and external rotation; MRI, magnetic resonance imaging; CT, computed tomography; ACL, anterior cruciate ligament; LOC, loss of consciousness.

Table 21.4.   Injury management.

1. PRICE = Protect, Rest, Ice, Compress, Elevate. PRICE is initiated to minimize initial injury

   Decrease pain and swelling

   Prevent further tissue damage
2. Maintain flexibility, strength, and proprioception, and overall fitness during healing
3. Functionally rehabilitate injured patient to enable return to activity
4. Assess and correct any predisposing factors to decrease the likelihood of recurrence

appropriate management. If there is any question as to whether a patient athlete would benefit from surgical management, referral to a specialist should not be delayed.

General Guidelines for Injury Management

Whether injury is secondary to acute trauma or overuse, the general management principles hold true. These are listed in Table 21.4.

Medical Issues in Active Women
The Female Athlete Triad

The term female athlete triad refers to the combination of disordered eating, amenorrhea, and osteoporosis. These conditions are often interrelated and associated with athletic training. The exact prevalence of the female athlete triad is unknown, but studies have reported disordered eating behavior in 15–75% of adolescent athletes. Many athletes do not meet the strict *DSM-IV* criteria for anorexia or bulimia but will manifest a wide range of harmful behaviors, from food restriction to binging, purging, and diet pill or laxative abuse to lose weight or maintain a thin physique. Disordered eating can be seen in athletes participating in all sports, but women and girls involved in sports that emphasize low body weights are especially vulnerable. Particularly "high-risk" sports include gymnastics, crew, swimming, dance, running, and equestrian sports. Disordered eating can impair athletic performance and increase the risk of injury. Medical complications can include menstrual dysfunction and irreversible bone loss (as in the female athlete triad) as well as some potentially fatal changes in the cardiovascular, endocrine, and thermoregulatory systems.

Amenorrhea occurs in 3.4–66% of adult female athletes (depending on the population studied and inclusion criteria used), compared with only 2–5% of women in the general population. These issues often go unreported and unrecognized because of the secretive nature of disordered eating behavior and because of the commonly held belief that amenorrhea is a normal consequence of exercise. Athletic amenorrhea (primary or secondary) is typically classified as hypothalamic-induced menstrual dysfunction, identified with abnormal luteinizing hormone (LH) and gonadotropin-releasing hormone (GnRH) levels. Contributing factors likely include psychological stress, genetic predisposition, low body fat, and overtraining. One of the main theories as to the etiology of athletic amenorrhea, however, is that nutritional needs are not met, causing an "energy drain" and resultant hypothalamic dysfunction. Delayed menarche, prolonged secondary amenorrhea, and even oligomenorrhea may represent a prolonged hypoestrogenemia that can contribute to decreased bone density, osteopenia, and eventually osteoporosis.

The majority (50–63%) of the peak bone mass is achieved during childhood and the rest (37–50%) during adolescence. Thus, young women who lose bone mineral density due to the hypoestrogenism associated with amenorrhea may never recoup that loss. Low bone mineral density puts the athlete at risk for stress fractures as well as more devastating fractures of the hip or vertebral column.

Treatment of the female athlete triad requires a multidisciplinary and multifactorial approach. Estrogen replacement [in the form of oral contraceptive pills (OCPs)] remains controversial. Some research suggests that hormonal replacement (with >50 ng estrogen per day) will preserve some bone loss. The criteria for initiating estrogen replacement therapy and the optimal dosing schedule have not been determined, but the American Academy of Pediatrics recommends supplementation for amenorrheal adolescents if they are 3 years postmenarche and older than 16 years of age. A younger age is permitted for initiation if she has had a stress fracture. Other treatment considerations should include a change in activity to decrease overall energy expenditure, nutrition consultation, calcium and vitamin D supplementation, and psychological counseling. In addition to health care professionals, the role of family members, teachers, trainers, and coaches in the athlete's recovery should not be underestimated.

Pregnancy

The literature notes that exercise in general is not harmful to the pregnant female or her fetus. There is also evidence to suggest that regular exercise throughout an uncomplicated pregnancy can be beneficial to both mother and baby. Maternal benefits may include improved mental state, limited weight gain, and decreased risk of gestational diabetes, easier delivery, and improved overall fitness. Fetal benefits may include improved stress tolerance, decreased body fat, and advanced neurobehavioral maturation. Concerns have been raised that fetal hypoxia could occur as a result of blood being shunted from the placenta to exercising muscles or that exercise will raise the core temperature and harm the fetus. Current data do not support these concepts. The morphologic and physiologic changes of pregnancy may, however, interfere with sports performance and safety. The American College of Obstetricians and Gynecologists' guidelines for exercise during pregnancy state that "in absence of either medical or obstetric complications, 30 minutes or more of moderate exercise a day on most, if not all, days of the week is recommended for pregnant women." Absolute contraindications to exercise in pregnancy are listed in Table 21.5. Activities with a high risk of trauma should be avoided as well as scuba diving and exertion at extreme altitude. The supine position and prolonged motionless standing should be discouraged after the first trimester because of decreased venous return and subsequent decreased cardiac output. Women participating in jumping activities should be advised that they may be predisposed to pelvic ligamentous injury. This is thought to be due to the effects of the hormone relaxin. Return to full activity after delivery may decrease the risk of postpartum depression and is known to be safe for both mother and the breastfeeding baby. Return to athletics should be gradual because of deconditioning and the known 4- to 6-week period it takes to get back to the prepregnancy physiologic and morphologic state.

Anemia in the Athlete

There are several causes of decreased hematocrit (HCT) in athletes, including pseudoanemia (decreased HCT secondary to plasma expansion), iron deficiency anemia, "foot-strike" or exertional hemolysis, anemia of malnutrition (in eating disordered athletes), and exercise-related gastrointestinal (GI) bleeding. Of these, the most common cause of true anemia in athletic females, as in the general population, is iron deficiency. Many female athletes, especially "low weight" athletes (e.g., ballet dancers, distance runners, gymnasts), consume fewer calories and insufficient iron to make up for their menstrual loss. The small amounts of iron lost in urine and sweat during exercise is likely

Table 21.5. Absolute contraindications to exercise in pregnancy.

Hemodynamically significant heart disease
Restrictive lung disease
Incompetent cervix/cerclage
Multiple gestation at risk for premature labor
Persistent second or third trimester bleeding
Placenta previa after 26 weeks gestation
Premature labor during current pregnancy
Ruptured membranes
Preeclampsia/pregnancy-induced hypertension

ACOG Committee Opinion January 2002.
Source: From American College of Obstetricians and Gynecologists: ACOG Committee Opinion number 267, January 2002: Exercise during pregnancy and the post partum period. Obstet Gynecol 2002; 99(1): 171–173.

Table 21.6. Recommendations for prevention of iron deficiency anemia.

Increase intake of lean red meat, dark chicken, and iron fortified cereals, etc.

Combine poultry or seafood with dried beans or peas

Enhance iron absorption by avoiding caffeine and increasing vitamin C intake

Cook acidic foods in cast iron cookware

Consider menstrual manipulation with oral contraceptive pills in cases of menorrhagia

Consider supplementation with ferrous sulfate (325 mg three times per week) in the athlete with recurrent anemia

---

insignificant. Minor GI bleeding can occur in some distance runners, cyclists, and triathletes from superficial stomach "stress ulcers" or from "ischemic colitis" when blood is shunted from the gut to working muscles. The diagnosis of iron deficiency anemia is made with serum findings of low hematocrit, ferritin, and mean cell volume (MCV), and blood smear findings of hypochromic, microcytic erythrocytosis. Low ferritin without anemia has not been found to affect sports performance, but true iron deficiency anemia, even mild, can affect athletic performance and treatment should be considered. To differentiate between iron deficiency anemia and pseudoanemia with low ferritin, a 2-month trial of iron therapy is appropriate, looking for a minimum 1 g/dl increase in hemoglobin. See Table 21.6 for recommendations for prevention of iron deficiency anemia.

Pelvic Floor Dysfunction and Stress Urinary Incontinence

In some studies, stress urinary incontinence has been identified in up to 28% of young female athletes. Incontinence in general is thought to be grossly underreported. Exercise-related stress incontinence is most often a benign condition, but should be addressed as it can be quite troublesome to the athlete. It can occur during various physical activities, but especially in exercise involving chronic repetitive motion, high impact landings, jumping, and running. Other risk factors for stress incontinence during sports include obesity, hypoestrogenic amenorrhea, and increased age and parity. Evaluation for pelvic floor dysfunction is warranted. In the absence of anatomic defects, management includes education, avoidance of excessive fluids before exercise, and sanitary napkins. Kegel exercises with or without biofeedback therapy may be helpful. Pharmacologic therapy includes tricyclics and α-mimetics. Anticholinergic agents should be avoided (particularly in hot, humid conditions) because of the potential for exercise-induced heat disorders.

The Breast and Sports

Exercise can lead to breast injury and discomfort through increased motion, friction, and, less commonly, blunt trauma.

Pain from excessive breast motion is very common in active women, particularly those with larger breasts. In one study, 31% of female athletes surveyed reported general exercise-induced breast discomfort, whereas 52% of the same group noted specific injury and pain secondary to sport involvement. Several sports such as running, basketball, volleyball, and equestrian activities can lead to significant breast displacement and painful stress on the fascial attachments to the pectoralis muscle. Such breast injury can be reduced and often prevented by wearing a properly fitted sports bra. The bra should lift and separate the breasts, limiting motion as much as possible. It should be made of nonabrasive, "breathable" material. Bra and shoulder strap padding may be necessary depending on breast size and type of sports activity.

The nipple is a common site of abrasion injury in active females. This is especially true for women involved in running or other sports where the activity leads to strong repetitive rubbing. The resultant irritation and excoriation have been termed "jogger's nipple" because of the propensity in runners. Cold wind exposure further promotes bleeding, raw, severely painful nipples. This can be an issue in events such as cycling, crew, and multisport competitions. Prevention of exercise-induced nipple injury also includes a properly fitted sports bra. Additional interventions include coating the nipples with petroleum jelly or applying plastic bandages (e.g., Band-aid) before activity, and avoiding cold and wind exposure with appropriate clothing.

Injuries from breast trauma include lacerations, contusions, and hematomas that may result in abscess formation, thrombophlebitis, and fat necrosis. Although it is beyond the scope of this chapter, physicians should be familiar with the management of these issues. It is of course also important to note that many exercise-related injuries can mimic more serious illness. Although a patient is active in sports, other diagnoses such as intraductal papilloma and carcinoma must be considered.

Prevention and Return to Play

The Preparticipation Examination Targeted for the Female Athlete

The purpose of the preparticipation physical examination is to detect medical conditions and musculoskeletal problems that may lead to illness or injury. Theoretically, the examination is not intended to be a substitute for regular health maintenance visits, but in a great majority of cases, this is the athlete's only exposure to the health care system. The medical history is truly the most important part of the examination. In the female athlete the history should go beyond the usual past medical history, cardiovascular risk, and previous injury questions. Because of the high risk of disordered eating and female athlete triad, a survey of the athlete's body image, nutritional habits, and menstrual history can be extremely important. In addition to the general physical examination, a comprehensive musculoskeletal assessment should be performed. Muscle weakness, inflexibility, and other factors that may predispose an athlete to injury should be evaluated. Education about illness and injury risk factors is the most powerful tool the physician has in terms of preventing problems in the female athlete. The preparticipation examination additionally provides an appropriate setting for counseling on issues such as smoking and sexually transmitted diseases.

Return to Activity After Injury or Illness

Timing and aggressiveness of return to full activity are based on multiple factors including type of injury/illness, degree of disability, interventions (e.g., surgery, injections, medications, etc.), compliance with rehabilitation, and cardiovascular condition. For certain injuries and illnesses, there are specific time guidelines for return to play that are considered standard of care. A full review of these issues is beyond the scope of this chapter, but an example is returning to sports 3 weeks after mononucleosis infection (provided there is no splenic enlargement). The athlete should progress through the steps of rehabilitation as outlined above in "injury management." In general, she is able to return to activity gradually once the risk of worsening the injury is low and she is able to perform sports-specific functional activities without pain or problems.

Suggested Reading

ACOG Committee Opinion No. 267. Exercise during pregnancy and the postpartum period. *Obstet Gynecol* 2002;99:171.

Blair SN, Kohl HW, Paffenbarger RS, et al. Physical fitness and all-cause mortality: a prospective study of healthy men and women. *JAMA* 1989; 262:2395.

Clapp JF. Exercise during pregnancy: a clinical update. *Clin Sports Med* 2000; 19:273.

Committee on Sports Medicine, American Academy of Pediatrics. Amenorrhea in adolescent athletes. *Pediatrics* 1989;84:394.

Frankovich RJ, Lebrun CM. Menstrual cycle, contraception, and performance. *Clin Sports Med* 2000;19:251,

Hobart JA, Smucker DR. Cardiovascular medicine update: the female athlete triad. *Am Family Physician* 2000;61(11).

Kibler WB, Chandler TJ, Uhl T, et al. A musculoskeletal approach to the preparticipation physical examination. *Am J Sports Med* 1989;17:525.

Loud KJ, Micheli LJ. Common athletic injuries in adolescent girls. *Curr Opin Pediatr* 2001;13(4):317.

22

Thyroid Disease

Mary Korytkowski and Haruko Akatsu Kuffner

Introduction

Thyroid hormone plays a role in the regulation of body temperature, reproduction, growth, and metabolism. The importance of the thyroid gland to the obstetrician/gynecologist is based on several factors. One is the role this hormone plays in regulating menstruation, ovulation, and fertility. Another is the contribution of normal thyroid hormone levels to fetal development and pregnancy outcome. And finally, as the obstetrician/gynecologist is often the only physician to see many women, this group of physicians has a key role in the detection and ongoing treatment of these disorders, which affect women with a much greater frequency than men.

This chapter will briefly review basic thyroid physiology, the epidemiology of thyroid disorders, and diagnosis and treatment of commonly encountered abnormalities of thyroid function. These abnormalities include hypothyroidism, hyperthyroidism, and thyroid nodules. A section on thyroid function testing and disorders during pregnancy is also included.

Regulation of Thyroid Hormone Synthesis and Secretion

There are two major circulating thyroid hormones, thyroxine (T_4) and triiodothyronine (T_3). Both T_4 and T_3 are produced, stored, and secreted by follicular cells within the thyroid gland. The release of T_4 and T_3 is regulated by the pituitary hormone, thyroid-stimulating hormone (TSH), and the hypothalamic hormone, thyrotropin-releasing hormone (TRH). The release of T_4 and T_3 is regulated by a regulatory feedback system (Fig. 22.1). A decrease in T_4 leads to an increase in TSH, while an increase in T_4 will result in a reduction in TSH.

All circulating T_4 and 15% of T_3 are secreted by the thyroid gland in response to stimulation by TSH. The remaining 85% of circulating T_3 is derived from peripheral conversion of T_4 to T_3.

Both T_4 and T_3 circulate in the bound and free forms. Only 0.03% of T_4 and 0.3% of T_3 circulate in the free or active form, while the remainder of each hormone is bound to the thyroid-binding proteins: thyroid-binding globulin (TBG), albumin, and prealbumin (transthyretin). Any factor that increases or decreases the amount of thyroid binding proteins can affect the

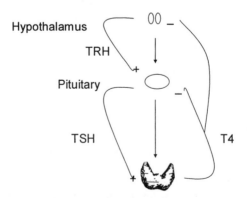

Fig. 22.1. This illustrates the normal feedback regulation of thyroid hormone secretion by thyroid-stimulating hormone (TSH) in the pituitary gland and thyrotropin-releasing hormone (TRH) in the hypothalamus.

Table 22.1.   Causes of euthyroid hyperthyroxinemia due to an increase in thyroid-binding proteins and hypothyroxinemia due to a decrease in thyroid-binding proteins.

Increased thyroid-binding proteins	Decreased thyroid-binding proteins
Pregnancy	Androgens
Hormone therapy	Glucocorticoids
Oral contraceptive pills	Nephrotic syndrome
Acute viral hepatitis	Cirrhosis
Primary biliary cirrhosis	Critical illness
Hepatocellular carcinoma	Starvation
Collagen vascular disease	Protein-losing enteropathy
Myeloma	
Acute phase of HIV	

total T_4 and T_3 while leaving the free hormone levels unchanged (Table 22.1).

Thyroid Function Tests

The tests available for monitoring thyroid function are outlined in Table 22.2. Laboratory testing is available for measurement of total T_4 (TT_4), total T_3 (TT_3), and TSH. The free thyroxine index (FTI) is calculated as the product

Table 22.2.   Thyroid function studies.

Thyroid-stimulating hormone
Total T_4 (TT_4)
Total T_3 (TT_3)
Free T_4 (FT_4) by analog assays
Free T_4 (FT_4) by equilibrium dialysis
Free T_3 (FT_3)
Thyroid hormone binding ratio
Free thyroxine index (FTI)
Thyroid-stimulating immunoglobulins
Thyrotropin inhibitory immunoglobulins
Thyroid peroxidase antibodies
Thryoglobulin antibodies

of TT_4 and thyroid hormone binding ratio (THBR) ($TT_4 \times$ THBR = FTI). Clinical assays are also available for measurement of a free T_4 level alone. The gold standard for measurement of a free T_4 is by equilibrium dialysis, which is more expensive and not necessary for the majority of women who are being screened or tested for an underlying thyroid disorder. Analog assays for free T_4 are also available; however, these assays have not had the same reliability as the thyroid panel described above (TT_4, THBR, and FTI).

Possibly the most difficult of the thyroid tests to understand is that of the THBR, also referred to as the T_3 resin uptake (T_3RU) by many clinical laboratories. Both the THBR and the T_3 uptake are indirect measures of circulating thyroid-binding proteins. An elevated THBR occurs in the setting of low thyroid-binding proteins. Conversely, a low THBR occurs in the setting of high thyroid-binding proteins. Situations associated with abnormalities in thyroid-binding proteins are listed in Table 22.1.

Interpretation of Thyroid Function Studies

Table 22.2 lists available thyroid function tests (TFTs). A guide to interpretation of TFTs appears in Table 22.3. Women with true hypothyroidism will have a low TT_4, a low THBR, and a low FTI. Women with a low TT_4 due to

Table 22.3.   Interpretation of thyroid function testing.[a]

	TSH	Total T_4	THBR	Free T_4 (index)
Primary hypothyroidism	High	Low	Low	Low
Secondary hypothyroidism	Low normal or nondetectable	Low	Low	Low
Primary hyperthyroidism	Low or nondetectable	High	High	High
High binding proteins	Normal	High	Low	Normal or slightly increased
Low binding proteins	Normal	Low	High	Normal or slightly decreased

[a]TSH, thyroid-stimulating hormone; THBR, thyroid hormone binding ratio.

low thyroid-binding proteins will have a low TT_4, a high THBR, and a normal FTI and TSH This is referred to as euthyroid hypothyroxinemia.

Patients with true hyperthyroidism will have a high TT_4, a high THBR, and a high FTI. Women with a high TT_4 due to high thyroid-binding proteins will have a high TT_4, a low THBR, and a normal FTI and TSH. This is referred to as euthyroid hyperthyroxinemia.

Epidemiology and Screening for Thyroid Disorders

The prevalence of thyroid disorders is greater in women than in men. In the United States, overt hypothyroidism is five times more likely to occur in women, affecting an estimated 2–7%. Subclinical hypothyroidism (discussed below) affects up to 17% of all women. Hyperthyroidism affects approximately 1–2% of the overall adult population with a 10-fold greater incidence in women than in men.

These high prevalence rates for thyroid disorders prompted the publication of guidelines for screening by the American Thyroid Association (ATA). It is recommended that all adults older than 35 years of age have a screening TSH performed at 5-year intervals. The ATA suggests that this recommendation is particularly compelling for women. Individuals with any of the symptoms listed in Tables 22.4 and 22.5 should be screened at presentation for an underlying thyroid disorder.

The cost of measuring a TSH is cost-effective. Individuals with a TSH outside the normal range should undergo additional testing.

Table 22.4.   Clinical manifestations of hypothyroidism.

Symptoms	Signs
Cold intolerance	Bradycardia
Weight increase	Hypothermia
Fatigue	Delayed deep-tendon reflex relation phase
Dry skin	Dry skin
Hair loss	Brittle hair and nails
Constipation	Thick tongue and skin
Apathy	Edema
Memory impairment	Pericardial effusion
Depression	Elevated cholesterol
Menstrual irregularities (menorrhagia)	Anemia
Dyspnea	Hyponatremia

Table 22.5. Clinical manifestations of hyperthyroidism.

Symptoms	Signs
Palpitations	Tachycardia
Weight loss	Atrial fibrillation
Heat intolerance	Wide pulse pressure
Hyperphagia	Proximal muscle weakness
Hyperdefecation	Thyroid enlargement
Anxiety/nervousness	Smooth warm diaphoretic skin
Insomnia	Tremor
Tremor	Palmar erythema
Menstrual irregularities (oligoamenorrhea)	Stare with lid retraction
Infertility	Hyperreflexia

Hypothyroidism

Signs and Symptoms

The clinical manifestations of thyroid hormone excess are listed in Table 22.4.

Etiology

Hypothyroidism can be primary or secondary. Primary hypothyroidism is caused by a disorder that results in the failure of thyroid hormone production by the gland. Secondary hypothyroidism results from a defect in the production of TSH from the pituitary gland.

Primary Hypothyroidism

The most common cause of primary hypothyroidism is Hashimoto's autoimmune thyroiditis. More than 90% of patients with Hashimoto's disease have circulating antibodies against thyroid peroxidase (previously known as the microsomal antigen). Antithyroglobulin antibodies occur with a lower frequency (Table 22.2). Primary hypothyroidism can also occur following ablative therapy with radioactive iodine therapy for treatment of hyperthyroidism and after thyroidectomy for goiter or thyroid cancer.

Thyroiditis can present as primary hypothyroidism. There are three types of thyroiditis: subacute thyroiditis, silent thyroiditis, and postpartum thyroiditis. Subacute thyroiditis results from inflammation of the thyroid follicles attributed to viral infection. Patients typically present with thyroid tenderness. There is frequently a hyperthyroid period due to thyroid hormone release from the damaged follicles, a transition through euthyroidism, followed by a hypothyroid phase. Silent thyroiditis and postpartum thyroiditis are more common in women with underlying autoimmune conditions such as Hashimoto's thyroiditis. Unlike subacute thyroiditis, women with silent thyroiditis or postpartum thyroiditis do not have thyroid tenderness. Hypothyroidism can be transient or permanent.

Several medications, such as lithium, iodide, amiodarone, and cytokines, can cause hypothyroidism in susceptible individuals. Lithium results in hypothyroidism in approximately 5% of individuals by inhibiting the release of thyroid hormones. Iodine, which is present in many drugs (vitamins, amiodarone, radiology contrast agents), can acutely inhibit iodide organification. In normal persons, this effect is transient and hypothyroidism will not occur. Amiodarone contains 37% iodine by weight and also has a structural similarity to thyroxine. It is associated with both hypothyroidism and hyperthyroidism. Interferon-α used to treat hepatitis B, C, or malignant disease may also cause hypo- or hyperthyroidism. The mechanism may be via induction of thyroid autoantibodies; however, some patients develop thyroid abnormalities without autoantibody formation.

Secondary Hypothyroidism

Secondary hypothyroidism results from a defect in the production of TSH from the pituitary gland, usually due to the presence of a pituitary tumor that interferes with normal hormone production and secretion. Most commonly, patients present with other pituitary hormone deficiencies in addition to a deficiency in TSH secretion. It is rare to have an isolated TSH defect where other pituitary hormones, including follicle-stimulating hormone (FSH) and luteinizing hormone (LH), are normal.

Establishing the Diagnosis

Clinical evaluation together with thyroid function testing will establish the diagnosis in the majority of cases. In primary hypothyroidism, TSH will be increased and TT_4, THBR, and FT_4 will be decreased. In secondary hypothyroidism, TSH will be low normal or decreased and TT_4, THBR, and FT_4 will be decreased. In euthyroid hypothyroxinemia, thyroid hormone-binding proteins are low causing low TT_4, increased THBR, and normal FT_4 and TSH. The pattern of thyroid hormone abnormalities associated with primary and secondary hypothyroidism is presented in Table 22.3.

Clinical Intervention

Hypothyroidism is treated with thyroid hormones. Thyroid hormone is commercially available as either levothyroxine (T_4), liothyronine (T_3), or a combination of T_4 and T_3. Standard practice is to give T_4. Since 85% of circulating T_3 comes from peripheral tissue conversion of T_4 to T_3, both T_4 and T_3 become available even if only T_4 is given. The dose has to be individually tailored. The rough estimate for T_4 dosing is $1–2\,\mu g/kg/day$ or 75% of weight in pounds. In elderly or cardiac patients, the initial dose should be decreased with slow and careful titration as tolerated. Since the half-life of T_4 is 7 days, it takes 6–8 weeks before reaching steady state. Therefore, it is appropriate to check the thyroid function tests approximately 6–8 weeks after initiation or change of thyroid hormone treatment to assess the adequacy of the dose.

There is no clear evidence supporting the superiority of T_4 and T_3 combination therapy over T_4 alone. Of note, commercially available T_4 and T_3 combination preparations have a nonphysiologic ratio of T_4:T_3 of approximately 4:1. The normal molecular ratio of T_4 and T_3 is 14:1. Since T_3 has a short half-life, its administration can cause supraphysiologic T_3 levels several hours after ingestion, causing transient hyperthyroid symptoms such as tachycardia, tremor, or nervousness.

Hyperthyroidism

Signs and Symptoms

The clinical manifestations of thyroid hormone excess are listed in Table 22.5.

Etiology

Hyperthyroidism is defined as a clinical syndrome due to an increase in circulating levels of thyroid hormone. Thyrotoxicosis is another term used to describe the clinical manifestations of hyperthyroidism. The major causes of hyperthyroidism are outlined in Table 22.6.

Subclinical hyperthyroidism refers to a condition characterized by a suppressed level of TSH by the pituitary gland in association with normal levels of T_4 and T_3. These patients may have one or more of the symptoms associated with overt thyrotoxicosis listed in Table 22.5 but are frequently asymptomatic. In subclinical hyperthyroidism, these symptoms, if present, are manifested to a milder degree.

Establishing the Diagnosis

Thyroid disease is a common cause of disturbances in weight, mood, and menstruation in women. When the diagnosis of hyperthyroidism is suspected based on the presence of one or more of the symptoms listed in Table 22.5, or if a woman has a suppressed TSH on a screening test, further diagnostic testing (TT$_4$, THBR, FTI, T$_3$) is recommended. T$_3$ toxicosis is a form of Graves' disease characterized by a normal TT$_4$, a suppressed TSH, and an elevated TT$_3$. Measurement of TT$_3$ can help establish this diagnosis.

If the suspicion for an underlying thyroid disorder is low, a screening TSH may be adequate. If the TSH is in the normal range, the patient does not have hyperthyroidism.

There are rare situations in which TSH can be inappropriately normal or mildly elevated. These include hyperthyroid patients with a TSH-secreting pituitary adenoma or patients with pituitary resistance to thyroid hormone. Anyone with a detectable TSH in the setting of an elevated FTI

Table 22.6. Causes of hyperthyroidism.

Suppressed or nondetectable thyroid-stimulating hormone (TSH)
  Inadvertent overreplacement with exogenous thyroid hormone
  Graves' disease (autoimmune mediated toxic diffuse goiter)
  Toxic multinodular goiter
  Toxic adenoma
  Iodine induced
  Thyroiditis
    Postpartum
    Subacute (De Quervains)
  Iatrogenic
    "Hamburger" induced
  Factitious
  Trophoblastic tumors
  Struma ovarii
  Widely metastatic follicular carcinoma of the thyroid
Inappropriately normal or elevated TSH
  TSH secreting pituitary adenoma
  Pituitary resistance to thyroid hormone

---

and symptoms of hyperthyroidism should be referred to an endocrinologist for additional testing.

Radioactive Iodine Uptake and Scan

A 24-hour radioactive iodine uptake (RAIU) and scan can help in distinguishing among the more common forms of hyperthyroidism. Thyroiditis (see the section on the etiology of hypothyroidism) and factitious and iodine-induced hyperthyroidism are usually associated with a low or nondetectable uptake of tracer, whereas Graves' disease, toxic multinodular goiter (TMNG), and toxic nodules are associated with an increased or normal uptake (Fig. 22.2). In Graves' disease, this uptake is diffuse and homogeneous; in TMNG, the uptake is diffuse and nonhomogeneous; and in toxic nodules, the uptake is isolated to the area of hyperfunction with suppression of the remainder of the gland.

Clinical Intervention

When the etiology of the hyperthyroidism is not readily apparent, definitive therapy should be withheld pending a full diagnostic evaluation. β-Blockers may be used to ameliorate the adrenergic symptoms associated with hyperthyroidism (i.e., tachycardia, tremor, anxiety) unless these agents are contraindicated because of a history of asthma or obstructive airway disease. The

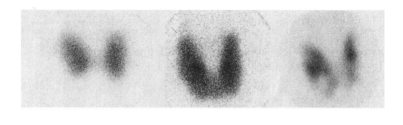

A   B   C

Fig. 22.2. (A) Normal thyroid scan. (B) Graves' disease with increased uptake. (C) A cold nonfunctioning nodule in the lower pole of the right lobe of the thyroid.

therapeutic strategies for the treatment of hyperthyroidism are outlined below.

Antithyroid Drugs

The antithyroid drugs (ATD), propylthiouracil (PTU) and methimazole, interfere with the intrathyroidal synthesis of thyroid hormone. In high doses (300 mg qid), PTU will also interfere with the conversion of T_4 to T_3, making it useful in the treatment of life threatening thyrotoxicosis or thyroid storm. The ATDs are useful in treating hyperthyroidism that is due to an overproduction of thyroid hormone, such as Graves' disease, TMNG, or a toxic adenoma. These agents can also be useful in treating iodine-induced thyrotoxicosis. Some patients with Graves' disease will enter a period of remission following treatment for 6–12 months with an ATD. Individuals with a small goiter and a mild elevation in TFTs are most likely to experience a remission; however, it is difficult to predict the course for any one individual. The majority of patients will require definitive therapy with radioactive iodine or surgery.

Radioactive Iodine

Remissions do not occur when hyperthyroidism occurs in the setting of a toxic adenoma or a TMNG. In these cases, levels of circulating thyroid hormone will increase once the ATD is discontinued. Therefore, definitive therapy with radioactive iodine (RAI) or surgery (thyroidectomy) is recommended. RAI ablation can also be used as definitive therapy for patients with Graves' disease or for those individuals who experience an exacerbation of their thyrotoxicosis following a period of remission. This treatment is successful in more than 80% of patients. For those who have persistent hyperthyroidism, a second dose may be required 6 months to 1 year later. The dose is calculated to deliver sufficient radiation to result in destruction of a hyperfunctioning thyroid gland, and is usually based upon the size of the gland and RAIU. In some institutions, a dose of 5–10 mCi ^{131}I is given to any patient with a suppressed TSH and a positive uptake and scan.

RAI is absolutely contraindicated for use in women who are pregnant. The iodine can cross the placenta and ablate the fetal thyroid (which is present at 10–12 weeks gestation), with subsequent cretinism. A pregnancy test is recommended for all women for whom either an RAI scan or uptake or RAI therapy is planned.

Surgery

Where RAI is the favored therapeutic strategy for treatment of hyperthyroidism due to Graves' disease, TMNG, and toxic adenoma in the United States, surgery is the favored therapeutic strategy of many endocrinologists in Europe. Some patients prefer to have surgery as the definitive and curative procedure over RAI or ATD. Patients must be euthyroid prior to surgery to avoid or minimize the risk of thyroid storm. β-Blockers are used perioperatively to reduce the risk of thyroid storm in those individuals who may not be able to tolerate use of ATD.

Treatment following Definitive Therapy

Hypothyroidism frequently occurs following RAI therapy or surgery, necessitating lifelong therapy with ḷ-thyroxine to maintain euthyroidism (see the section on the treatment of hypothyroidism).

Treatment of Hyperthyroidism Due to Thyroiditis

For thyrotoxicosis due to thyroiditis, treatment is usually supportive. In the case of subacute thyroiditis, therapy with antiinflammatory medications such as aspirin or nonsteroidal antiinflammatory drugs (NSAIDs) can relieve some of the painful symptoms. β-Adrenergic blockade can help to control symptoms of tachycardia and tremor. In more severe and prolonged cases, a trial of glucocorticoid therapy can help reduce thyroid hormone levels and reduce inflammation.

Thyroid Nodules

Epidemiology

The prevalence of thyroid nodules increases steadily with advancing age. More than 50% of women in their 60s and more than 80% of those in their 90s have a thyroid nodule at autopsy. Thyroid nodules detected by physical examination are present in 2–7% of the U.S. population, again affecting women more frequently than men.

Although thyroid nodules are extremely common, malignant lesions are relatively uncommon. Thyroid carcinomas constitute less than 1% of all human malignant tumors. Women have a 3-fold greater incidence of thyroid malignancies compared to men. The peak incidence is in the third and fourth decades of life.

Signs and Symptoms

Typically, nonfunctioning thyroid nodules are found incidentally on a routine physical examination in asymptomatic patients. If a nodule is toxic (producing excessive thyroid hormone), hyperthyroid signs and symptoms are likely to be present. Thyroid nodules do not cause hypothyroidism.

Etiology

Different classifications can be used to differentiate thyroid nodules: nodules can be solitary or multiple, benign or malignant, and hormonally active or nonfunctioning (silent). The presence of a solitary nodule or a dominant nodule in a multinodular gland raises the suspicion for a malignancy and requires evaluation with fine needle aspiration biopsy (FNAB).

Approximately 5–8% of nonfunctioning or "cold" nodules are malignant. The majority of malignant nodules are well-differentiated thyroid cancers [i.e., papillary (75–85%) or follicular (10–20%)] and can be associated with a good prognosis if detected and treated in a timely manner. Other thyroid malignancies include medullary (5%) and anaplastic thyroid carcinomas (rare). Painless rapid enlargement of the thyroid can be the primary manifestation of lymphoma, and is more common in women with underlying Hashimoto's thyroiditis (rare).

Establishing the Diagnosis

In evaluating patients with thyroid nodules, it is important to determine whether the nodule is associated with hyperthyroid symptoms, whether it is causing any tracheal and/or esophageal obstruction, and whether it is malignant. (See hyperthyroidism for establishing the diagnosis.)

To differentiate benign from malignant nodules, FNAB is necessary. It is a relatively easy procedure, done either at an office setting or under ultrasound guidance. The sensitivity of FNAB varies from 68 to 98% (mean, 83%) and specificity from 72 to 100% (mean, 92%), usually depending on the skill of the physician performing the aspirate.

Ultrasound is useful in obtaining the size of the overall thyroid gland and the nodules of interest. It is also useful in guiding FNA biopsy and following the nodule over time. However, the value of ultrasound for diagnosing malignancy is limited.

RAIU and scanning can be used to distinguish "hot" nodules (more than a normal amount of iodine localized) from "cold" nodules (less than a normal amount of iodine localized) (Fig. 22.2C). For practical purposes, it is extremely rare for an autonomously functioning "hot" nodule to harbor a malignancy.

Clinical Interventions
Benign Nodules

In patients with a toxic or "hot" nodule, RAI is the treatment of choice. Thyroid lobectomy is appropriate for some patients. Clinical judgment is important in the management of patients with toxic nodules and subclinical hyperthyroidism (i.e., a normal T_4 with a suppressed TSH). Referral to an endocrinologist is recommended in these situations.

Asymptomatic, euthyroid patients with a benign thyroid nodule by cytology can be monitored at periodic intervals. The evaluation should include a careful interval history and physical examination with palpation of the thyroid gland to determine whether there has been an increase in the size of the nodule. Enlargement of a nodule raises the concern for a malignancy with need for repeat FNAB or surgical referral.

There is a controversy as to the role of l-thyroxine suppression treatment for patients with benign thyroid nodules. Proponents argue that this treatment reduces the size of some nodules, but opponents refute its efficacy.

Malignant Nodules

Patients with malignant thyroid nodules by FNAB should be referred to a thyroid surgeon and an endocrinologist for management.

The Thyroid During Pregnancy
Changes in Thyroid Function Tests with Normal Pregnancy

Changes in thyroid function occur in the majority of women during pregnancy. In women without underlying thyroid disease, these are physiologic changes that require no intervention. Normal pregnancy is associated with an increase in levels of circulating thyroid-binding proteins, resulting in an increase in total T_4, low THBR, and normal FTI.

β-Human chorionic gonadotropin (HCG) has 85% sequence homology with TSH and can thus bind to and stimulate the TSH receptor. Sufficient stimulation of thyroid hormone secretion that transiently suppresses the TSH to a level of $0.1–0.5\,\mu U/ml$ occurs during the first trimester in up to 15% of normal women.

Treatment of Hypothyroidism During Pregnancy

Although thyroid hormone crosses the placenta poorly, clinical and biochemical euthyroidism contributes to the ability of a woman to carry the pregnancy to term. In women treated with exogenous thyroid hormone for hypothyroidism, an increase in the dose of levothyroxine is usually required to compensate for the increase in thyroid hormone binding. Monitoring of TFTS with TSH is recommended during each trimester of pregnancy with appropriate dose adjustments of L-thyroxine therapy to maintain the TSH at a low normal range (i.e., 1–2 µIU/ml).

Hyperemesis Gravidarum

Hyperemesis gravidarum (HG) is defined as the persistence of severe nausea and vomiting in association with weight loss (>5% prepregnancy weight) and ketonuria (likely secondary to starvation) that can be associated with an increase in TT$_4$ and a decrease in TSH. It may occur as a result of the higher serum concentrations of HCG, which has intrinsic thyroid-stimulating activity. HG can be distinguished from true thyrotoxicosis by the presence of severe nausea and vomiting, the absence of a goiter or ophthalmopathy, and the absence of other symptoms and signs of hyperthyroidism (Table 22.5).

Treatment of Thyrotoxicosis During Pregnancy

The obstetrician/gynecologist may be faced with the need to treat a woman with thyrotoxicosis during pregnancy. Some women decline therapy with RAI or surgery prior to pregnancy. Other women may have their thyrotoxicosis first diagnosed during pregnancy. For these women, treatment with the ATD, PTU, has the greatest track record. PTU is more highly protein bound than methimazole, and thus is less likely to cross the placenta. Doses of PTU or methimazole should be titrated to keep the TT$_4$ just above the upper limit of the normal range. Remission of the preexisting hyperthyroidism during pregnancy is not uncommon. This can allow discontinuation of antithyroid medication in some women.

Thyroid-stimulating immunoglobulins and TBII present in many women with Graves' disease cross the placenta, especially in the late second and third trimester. Measurement of these immunoglobulins is recommended during the third trimester as elevated levels can predict risk for neonatal thyrotoxicosis.

Postpartum Hyperthyroidism/Thyroiditis

Abnormalities in thyroid function occur during the postpartum period in approximately 5–10% of women in the United States. One-third of all cases of postpartum hyperthyroidism are due to an exacerbation of Graves' disease, one-third are due to new onset Graves' disease, and another third are due to the thyrotoxic phase of postpartum thyroiditis (see the section on the etiology of hypothyroidism). It is reasonable to measure a TSH at the 6-week postpartum visit in women with and even those without a prior or family history of thyroid disease.

Case Studies

Case 1. A 24-year-old G1P1 woman presents with a 10 lb weight loss despite an increase in appetite and a 6-month history of oligoamenorrhea and 3 months of amenorrhea. She delivered her first and only baby 1 year ago. She reports feeling energetic with a decrease in the number of hours of required sleep. On physical examination, her blood pressure (BP) is 138/60 and heart rate (HR) is 104. Her body mass index (BMI) is $19 \, kg/m^2$. She has a stare, a smooth enlarged thyroid gland at approximately 50 g (normal 10–20), palmar erythema, a tremor, and smooth moist skin.

What testing should be ordered? If this patient were presenting only with oligoamenorrhea, a TSH as a screen for an underlying thyroid disorder would be the recommended test. In this case, she has both signs and symptoms of thyrotoxicosis, which raises the suspicion for one of the disorders listed in Table 22.4. Therefore, a TT_4, THBR, FTI, TSH, and a TT_3 should be obtained.

The following results are obtained:

TT_4	$16 \, \mu g/dl$	(normal 5–11)
THBR	1.6	(normal 0.85–1.1)
FTI	25.6	(normal 4.2–12.1)
TT_3	$456 \, ng/dl$	(normal 80–180)
TSH	$<0.018 \, \mu U/ml$	(normal 0.3–5.0)

Once you confirm that she is not pregnant by a serum pregnancy test (this test was likely done as part of the evaluation for amenorrhea), an RAIU and scan can be obtained to establish whether this is due to Graves' disease (which is suggested by the physical examination), a TMNG, a toxic adenoma, or painless thyroiditis (this can occur up to 1 year following delivery).

In addition, measuring TSI or TBII can help establish Graves' disease as the likely etiology of her symptoms. Results are as follows:

RAIU	80%	(normal 10–30%)
TBII	45%	(normal <10%)

You confirm that she has Graves' disease and decide to treat her. She is reluctant to take RAI as she is breastfeeding her baby and would have to discontinue this for at least 1 week, as well as avoid any intimate contact with the baby. She declines surgery because this would also interrupt her breastfeeding. This is a difficult but not uncommon situation. The patient states that she will do whatever you recommend short of surgery. The only remaining choice at this time is the use of an ATD. There is limited but reassuring evidence that the use of methimazole in doses of ≤20 mg/day or PTU < 450 mg/day does not affect thyroid function in the baby. If PTU is used, it is recommended that doses of PTU, which has a shorter half-life, be given immediately after a breastfeeding session.

Case 2. A 28-year-old woman presents with a 1-month history of cold intolerance, fatigue, and weight gain. Her past medical history is significant for Hashimoto's disease diagnosed 8 years ago. She has been stable and well on levothyroxine 100 μg po qd for the past 5 years. Her last thyroid function tests were normal 4 months ago. On physical examination, her BP

= 105/60, pulse = 68, height = 5 feet 3 inches, and weight = 150 lb. Generally, the patient was not in acute distress. Her physical examination was normal including a normal thyroid examination.

Laboratory evaluation revealed the following:

TSH	8.5 µU/ml	(normal 0.3–5.0)
TT$_4$	5.7 µg/dl	(normal 5.0–12.0)
THBR	1.0	(normal 0.8–1.2)
FTI	5.7	(normal 5.0–12.0)

Why is she hypothyroid now? This case illustrates a patient who was stable on the same dose of levothyroxine replacement for many years and who suddenly became hypothyroid. Differential diagnosis includes the following:

1. Decreased thyroid hormone intake
   Noncompliance with medication.
2. Decreased thyroid hormone absorption due to
   Malabsorption
   Medications that can decrease thyroid hormone absorption: iron, calcium, sucraflate, cholestyramine.
3. Increased thyroid hormone metabolism
   Medications that can increase thyroid hormone metabolism: phenytoin, carbamazepine, rifampin, phenobarbital.
4. Increased thyroid hormone requirement
   Weight gain
   Pregnancy (especially during the first and second trimesters).

In this patient's case, she started taking multivitamin pills that contained iron and calcium 4 months prior to presentation. She was taking them together with levothyroxine, which decreased its absorption. She was instructed to take levothyroxine either 1 hour before or 4 hours after her multivitamin pills. Without any change in her levothyroxine dose, thyroid function tests rechecked 2 months later returned to normal.

Acknowledgments. We thank Dr. Frank Torok for contributing the thyroid scans to illustrate aspects of thyroid function and dysfunction in this chapter and Dr. Maja Stefanovic for her careful review and suggestions.

Suggested Reading

AACE/AAES. Medical/surgical guidelines for clinical practice: management of thyroid carcinoma. *Endocrine Pract* 2001;7(3):203–20.

AACE. Clinical practice guidelines for the diagnosis and management of thyroid nodules. *Endocrine Pract* 1996;2(1):80–4.

Adlersberg MA, Burrow GN. Thyroid function and dysfunction in women. *Obstet Gynecol Surv* 2002;57(3, Suppl):S1–S7.

American College of Physicians. Screening for thyroid disease. *Ann Intern Med* 1998;129(2):141–3, 144–58.

Becker K. *Principles and Practice of Endocrinology.* Philadelphia: Lippincott Williams & Wilkins; 2001.

Besser GM, Thorner MO. *Comprehensive Clinical Endocrinology.* London: Mosby; 2002.

Braverman LE, Utiger RD. *The Thyroid.* Philadelphia: Lippincott-Raven; 1996.

Burch HB. Evaluation and management of the solid thyroid nodule. *Endocrinol Metab Clin N Am* 1995;24(4):663–710.

DeGroot LJ, Jameson LJ. *Endocrinology.* Philadelphia: W.B. Saunders; 2001.

Ezzat S, Sarti DA, Cain DR, Braunstein GD. Thyroid incidentalomas. *Arch Intern Med* 1994;154:1838–40.

Ladenson PW, Singer PA, Ain KB, et al. American Thyroid Association Guidelines for detection of thyroid dysfunction. *Arch Intern Med* 2000;160:1573–75.

Mandel SJ, Cooper DS. The use of antithyroid drugs during pregnancy and lactation. *J Clin Endocrinol Metab* 2001;86(6):2354–59.

Mazzaferri EL. Management of a solitary thyroid nodule. *N Engl J Med* 1993;328(8):553–59.

Smallridge RC, Ladenson PW. Hypothyroidism in pregnancy: consequences to neonatal health. *J Clin Endocrinol Metab* 2001;86(6):2349–53.

Weetman AP. Grave's disease. *N Engl J Med* 2000;343(17):1236–48.

Appendix: Ready Reference Tables for Preventive Health Care and Health Maintenance

Joseph S. Sanfilippo

Cardiovascular Disease

Table A.1.   Risk factors for coronary heart disease.

Positive Predictors
- Male: Age >45 years
- Female: Age >55 years
  No estrogen replacement therapy (ERT)
  Pemature menopause without ERT
- Cigarette smoking
- Hypertension (blood pressure of >140/90 or on treatment)
- Diabetes
- HDL-cholesterol <35 mg/dL
- Family history of myocardial infarction or sudden death prior to 55 years in first-degree male relative, or 65 in first-degree female relative

Negative Risk Factor
- HDL-cholesterol >60 mg/dL (also allows subtraction of one risk factor)

Source: Adapted from National Institutes of Health Publication 93-3095. Second report of the expert panel on detection, evaluation, and treatment of high blood cholesterol in adults. Page I–11.

Table A.2. ATP III classification of LDL, total, and HDL cholesterol (mg/dL)*.

LDL cholesterol	
<100	Optimal
100–129	Near or above optimal
130–159	Borderline high
160–189	High
≥190	Very high
Total cholesterol	
<200	Desirable
200–239	Borderline high
≥240	High
HDL cholesterol	
<40	Low
≥60	High

*ATP indicates Adult Treatment Panel: LDL, low-density lipoprotein; and HDL, high-density lipoprotein.

Source: Executive Summary of the Third Report of the National Cholesterol Education Program (NCEP) Expert Panel on Detection, Evaluation and Treatment of High Blood Cholesterol in Adults (Adult Treatment Panel III). JAMA, May 16, 2001, Vol. 285; pg. 2487. Used with permission.

Table A.3.   **Blood pressure classification.**

Category	Systolic (mm Hg)	Diastolic (mm Hg)
Normal	<130	<85
High normal	130–139	85–89
Hypertension		
Stage 1 (mild)	140–159	90–99
Stage 2 (moderate)	160–179	100–109
Stage 3 (severe)	180–209	110–119
Stage 4 (very severe)	≥210	≥120

Source: Joint National Committee on the Detection, Evaluation, and Treatment of High Blood Pressure. The fifth report of the Joint National Committee on the Detection, Evaluation, and Treatment of High Blood Pressure (JNCV). *Arch Intern Med* 1993;153:161.

Nutrition

Table A.4A. Dietary reference intakes (DRIs): recommended intakes for individuals, vitamins (Food and Nutrition Board, Institute of Medicine, National Academies)

Life Stage Group	Vit A (μg/d)[a]	Vit C (mg/d)	Vit D (μg/d)[b,c]	Vit E (mg/d)[d]	Vit K (μg/d)	Thiamin (mg/d)
Infants						
0–6 mo	400*	40*	5*	4*	2.0*	0.2*
7–12 mo	500*	50*	5*	5*	2.5*	0.3*
Children						
1–3 y	300	15	5*	6	30*	0.5
4–8 y	400	25	5*	7	55*	0.6
Males						
9–13 y	600	45	5*	11	60*	0.9
14–18 y	900	75	5*	15	75*	1.2
19–30 y	900	90	5*	15	120*	1.2
31–50 y	900	90	5*	15	120*	1.2
51–70 y	900	90	10*	15	120*	1.2
>70 y	900	90	15*	15	120*	1.2
Females						
9–13 y	600	45	5*	11	60*	0.9
14–18 y	700	65	5*	15	75*	1.0
19–30 y	700	75	5*	15	90*	1.1
31–50 y	700	75	5*	15	90*	1.1
51–70 y	700	75	10*	15	90*	1.1
>70 y	700	75	15*	15	90*	1.1
Pregnancy						
14–18 y	750	80	5*	15	75*	1.4
19–30 y	770	85	5*	15	90*	1.4
31–50 y	770	85	5*	15	90*	1.4
Lactation						
14–18 y	1200	115	5*	19	75*	1.4
19–30 y	1300	120	5*	19	90*	1.4
31–50 y	1300	120	5*	19	90*	1.4

Note: This table (taken from the DRI reports, see www.nap.edu) presents Recommended Dietary Allowances (RDAs) in **bold** type and adequate Intakes (AIs) in ordinary type followed by an asterisk (*). RDAs and AIs may both be used as goals for individual intake. RDAs are set to meet the needs of almost all (97 to 98 percent) individuals in a group. For healthy breastfed infants, the AI is the mean intake. The AI for other life stage and gender groups is believed to cover needs of all individuals in the group, but lack of data or uncertainty in the data prevent being able to specify with confidence the percentage of individuals covered by this intake.

[a] As retinol activity equivalents (REAs) 1 RAE = 1 μg retinol, 12 μg β-carotene, 24 μg α-carotene, or 24 μg β-cryptoxanthin. The RAE for dietary provitamin A carotenoids is twofold greater than retinol equivalents (RE), whereas the RAE for preformed vitamin A is the same as RE.

[b] As cholecalciferol. 1 μg cholecalciferol = 40 IU vitamin D.

[c] In the absence of adequate exposure to sunlight.

[d] As α-tocopherol. α-Tocopherol includes RRR-α-tocopherol, the only forms of α-tocopherol that occurs naturally in foods, and the $2R$-stereoisomeric form of α-tocopherol (RRR-, RSR-, RRS-, and RSS-α-tocopherot) that occur in fortified foods and supplements. It does not include the $2S$-stereoisomeric forms of α-tocopherol (SRR-, SSR-, SRS- and SSS-α-tocopherol), also found in fortified foods and supplements.

Table A.4A. *Continued.*

Riboflavin (mg/d)	Niacin (mg/d)[c]	Vit B$_6$ (mg/d)	Folate (μg/d)[f]	Vit B$_{12}$ (μg/d)	Pantothenic Acid (mg/d)	Biotin (μg/d)	Choline[g] (mg/d)
0.3*	2*	0.1*	65*	0.4*	1.7*	5*	125*
0.4*	4*	0.3*	80*	0.5*	1.8*	6*	150*
0.5	6	0.5	150	0.9	2*	8*	200*
0.6	8	0.6	200	1.2	3*	12*	250*
0.9	12	1.0	300	1.8	4*	20*	375*
1.3	16	1.3	400	2.4	5*	25*	550*
1.3	16	1.3	400	2.4	5*	30*	550*
1.3	16	1.3	400	2.4	5*	30*	550*
1.3	16	1.7	400	2.4[i]	5*	30*	550*
1.3	16	1.7	400	2.4[i]	5*	30*	550*
0.9	12	1.0	300	1.8	4*	20*	375*
1.0	14	1.2	400[i]	2.4	5*	25*	400*
1.1	14	1.3	400[i]	2.4	5*	30*	425*
1.1	14	1.3	400[i]	2.4	5*	30*	425*
1.1	14	1.5	400	2.4[h]	5*	30*	425*
1.1	14	1.5	400	2.4[h]	5*	30*	425*
1.4	18	1.9	600[j]	2.6	6*	30*	450*
1.4	18	1.9	600[j]	2.6	6*	30*	450*
1.4	18	1.9	600[j]	2.6	6*	30*	450*
1.6	17	2.0	500	2.8	7*	35*	550*
1.6	17	2.0	500	2.8	7*	35*	550*
1.6	17	2.0	500	2.8	7*	35*	550*

[c] As niacin equivalents (NE). 1 mg of niacin = 60 mg of tryptophan; 0–6 months = preformed niacin (not NB).

[f] As dietary folate equivalents (DFE). 1 DFE = 1 μg food folate = 0.6 μg of folic acid from fortified food or as a supplement consumed with food = 0.5 μg of a supplement taken on an empty stomach.

[g] Although AIs have been set for choline, there are few data to assess whether a dietary supply of choline is needed at all stages of the life cycle, and it may be that the choline requirement can be met by endogenous synthesis at some of these stages.

[h] Because 10 to 30 percent of older people may malabsorb food-bound B$_{12}$, it is advisable for those older than 50 years to meet their RDA mainly by consuming foods fortified with B$_{12}$ or a supplement containing B$_{12}$.

[i] In view of evidence linking folate intake with neural tube defects in the fetus, it is recommended that all women capable of becoming pregnant consume 400 μg from supplements or fortified foods in addition to intake of food folate from a varied diet.

[j] It is assumed that women will continue consuming 400 μg from supplements or fortified food until their pregnancy is confirmed and they enter prenatal care, which ordinarily occurs after the end of the periconceptional period—the critical time for formation of the neural tube.

Table A.4B. Dietary reference intakes (DRIs): recommended intakes for individuals, elements (Food and Nutrition Board, Institute of Medicine, National Academies)

Life Stage Group	Calcium (mg/d)	Chromium (μg/d)	Copper (μg/d)	Fluoride (mg/d)	Iodine (μg/d)	Iron (mg/d)	Magne-sium (mg/d)
Infants							
0–6 mo	210*	0.2*	200*	0.01*	110*	0.27*	30*
7–12 mo	270*	5.5*	220*	0.5*	130*	11	75*
Children							
1–3 y	500*	11*	**340**	0.7*	**90**	**7**	**80**
4–8 y	800*	15*	**440**	1*	**90**	**10**	**130**
Males							
9–13 y	1300*	25*	**700**	2*	**120**	**8**	**240**
14–18 y	1300*	35*	**890**	3*	**150**	**11**	**410**
19–30 y	1000*	35*	**900**	4*	**150**	**8**	**400**
31–50 y	1000*	35*	**900**	4*	**150**	**8**	**420**
51–70 y	1200*	30*	**900**	4*	**150**	**8**	**420**
>70 y	1200*	30*	**900**	4*	**150**	**8**	**420**
Females							
9–13 y	1300*	21*	**700**	2*	**120**	**8**	**240**
14–18 y	1300*	24*	**890**	3*	**150**	**15**	**360**
19–30 y	1000*	25*	**900**	3*	**150**	**18**	**310**
31–50 y	1000*	25*	**900**	3*	**150**	**18**	**320**
51–70 y	1200*	20*	**900**	3*	**150**	**8**	**320**
>70 y	1200*	20*	**900**	3*	**150**	**8**	**320**
Pregnancy							
14–18 y	1300*	29*	**1000**	3*	**220**	**27**	**400**
19–30 y	1000*	30*	**1000**	3*	**220**	**27**	**350**
31–50 y	1000*	30*	**1000**	3*	**220**	**27**	**360**
Lactation							
14–18 y	1300*	44*	**1300**	3*	**290**	**10**	**360**
19–30 y	1000*	45*	**1300**	3*	**290**	**9**	**310**
31–50 y	1000*	45*	**1300**	3*	**290**	**9**	**320**

Note: This table presents Recommended Dietary Allowances (RDAs) in **bold** type and Adequate Intakes (AIs) in ordinary type followed by an asterisk (*). RDAs and AIs may both be used as goals for individual intake. RDAs are set to meet the needs of almost all (97 to 98 percent) individuals in a group. For healthy breastfed infants, the AI is the mean intake. The AI for other life stage and gender groups is believed to cover needs of all individuals in the group, but lack of data or uncertainty in the data prevent being able to specify with confidence the percentage of individuals covered by this intake.

Table A.4B. *Continued.*

Manganese (mg/d)	Molyb- denum (μg/d)	Phos- phorus (mg/d)	Selen- ium (μg/d)	Zinc (mg/d)	Potas- sium (g/d)	Sodium (g/d)	Chloride (g/d)
0.003*	2*	100*	15*	2*	0.4*	0.12*	0.18*
0.6*	3*	275*	20*	3	0.7*	0.37*	0.57*
1.2*	17	460	20	3	3.0*	1.0*	1.5*
1.5*	22	500	30	5	3.8*	1.2*	1.9*
1.9*	34	1250	40	8	4.5*	1.5*	2.3*
2.2*	43	1250	55	11	4.7*	1.5*	2.3*
2.3*	45	700	55	11	4.7*	1.5*	2.3*
2.3*	45	700	55	11	4.7*	1.5*	2.3*
2.3*	45	700	55	11	4.7*	1.3*	2.0*
2.3*	45	700	55	11	4.7*	1.2*	1.8*
1.6*	34	1250	40	8	4.5*	1.5*	2.3*
1.6*	43	1250	55	9	4.7*	1.5*	2.3*
1.8*	45	700	55	8	4.7*	1.5*	2.3*
1.8*	45	700	55	8	4.7*	1.5*	2.3*
1.8*	45	700	55	8	4.7*	1.3*	2.0*
1.8*	45	700	55	8	4.7*	1.2*	1.8*
2.0*	50	1250	60	12	4.7*	1.5*	2.3*
2.0*	50	700	60	11	4.7*	1.5*	2.3*
2.0*	50	700	60	11	4.7*	1.5*	2.3*
2.6*	50	1250	70	13	5.1*	1.5*	2.3*
2.6*	50	700	70	12	5.1*	1.5*	2.3*
2.6*	50	700	70	12	5.1*	1.5*	2.3*

Source: Dietary Reference Intakes for Calcium, Phosphorous, Magnesium, Vitamin D, and Fluoride (1997); *Dietary Reference Intakes for Thiamin, Riboflavin, Niacin, Vitamin B$_6$, Folate, Vitamin B$_{12}$, Pantothenic Acid, Biotin, and Choline* (1998); *Dietary Reference Intakes for Vitamin C, Vitamin E, Selenium, and Carotenoids* (2000); *Dietary Reference Intakes for Vitamin A, Vitamin K, Arsenic, Boron, Chromium, Copper, Iodine, Iron, Manganese, Molybdernum, Nickel, Silicon, Vanadium, and Zinc* (2001); and *Dietary Reference Intakes for Water, Potassium, Sodium, Chloride, and Sulfate* (2004). These reports may be accessed via http://www.nap.edu.
Source: Reprinted with permission (Dietary Reference Intakes) © (2004) by the National Academy of Sciences, Courtesy of the National Academics Press, Washington, D.C.

Immunization

Table A.5A Recommended childhood and adolescent immunization schedule.

DEPARTMENT OF HEALTH AND HUMAN SERVICES • CENTERS FOR DISEASE CONTROL AND PREVENTION

Recommended Childhood and Adolescent Immunization Schedule · UNITED STATES · 2006

Vaccine ▼ / Age ▶	Birth	1 month	2 months	4 months	6 months	12 months	15 months	18 months	24 months	4–6 years	11–12 years	13–14 years	15 years	16–18 years
Hepatitis B[1]	HepB	HepB		HepB[1]		HepB					HepB Series			
Diphtheria, Tetanus, Pertussis[2]			DTaP	DTaP	DTaP		DTaP	DTaP		DTaP	Tdap	Tdap	Tdap	Tdap
Haemophilus influenzae type b[3]			Hib	Hib	Hib[3]	Hib	Hib							
Inactivated Poliovirus			IPV	IPV	IPV	IPV		IPV		IPV				
Measles, Mumps, Rubella[4]						MMR	MMR			MMR	MMR			
Varicella[5]						Varicella	Varicella	Varicella			Varicella	Varicella		
Meningococcal[6]									MPSV4	MPSV4	MCV4	MCV4	MCV4	MCV4
Pneumococcal[7]			PCV	PCV	PCV	PCV	PCV		PCV	PCV	PPV	PPV		
Influenza[8]					Influenza (Yearly)	Influenza (Yearly)					Influenza (Yearly)	Influenza (Yearly)		
Hepatitis A[9]									HepA Series	HepA Series				

Vaccines within broken line are for selected populations

This schedule indicates the recommended ages for routine administration of currently licensed childhood vaccines, as of December 1, 2005, for children through age 18 years. Any dose not administered at the recommended age should be administered at any subsequent visit when indicated and feasible. ▨ Indicates age groups that warrant special effort to administer those vaccines not previously administered. Additional vaccines may be licensed and recommended during the year. Licensed combination vaccines may be used whenever any components of the combination are indicated and other components of the vaccine are not contraindicated and if approved by the Food and Drug Administration for that dose of the series. Providers should consult the respective ACIP statement for detailed recommendations. Clinically significant adverse events that follow immunization should be reported to the Vaccine Adverse Event Reporting System (VAERS). Guidance about how to obtain and complete a VAERS form is available at www.vaers.hhs.gov or by telephone, 800-822-7967.

1. **Hepatitis B vaccine (HepB).** *AT BIRTH:* All newborns should receive monovalent HepB soon after birth and before hospital discharge. Infants born to mothers who are HBsAg-positive should receive HepB and 0.5 mL of hepatitis B immune globulin (HBIG) within 12 hours of birth. Infants born to mothers whose HBsAg status is unknown should receive HepB within 12 hours of birth. The mother should have blood drawn as soon as possible to determine her HBsAg status; if HBsAg-positive, the infant should receive HBIG as soon as possible (no later than age 1 week). For infants born to HBsAg-negative mothers, the birth dose can be delayed in rare circumstances but only if a physician's order to withhold the vaccine and a copy of the mother's original HBsAg-negative laboratory report are documented in the infant's medical record. *FOLLOWING THE BIRTHDOSE:* The HepB series should be completed with either monovalent HepB or a combination vaccine containing HepB. The second dose should be administered at age 1–2 months. The final dose should be administered at age ≥24 weeks. It is permissible to administer 4 doses of HepB (e.g., when combination vaccines are given after the birth dose); however, if monovalent HepB is used, a dose at age 4 months is not needed. Infants born to HBsAg-positive mothers should be tested for HBsAg and antibody to HBsAg after completion of the HepB series, at age 9–18 months (generally at the next well-child visit after completion of the vaccine series).

2. **Diphtheria and tetanus toxoids and acellular pertussis vaccine (DTaP).** The fourth dose of DTaP may be administered as early as age 12 months, provided 6 months have elapsed since the third dose and the child is unlikely to return at age 15–18 months. The final dose in the series should be given at age ≥4 years.

Tetanus and diphtheria toxoids and acellular pertussis vaccine (Tdap – adolescent preparation) is recommended at age 11–12 years for those who have completed the recommended childhood DTP/DTaP vaccination series and have not received a Td booster dose. Adolescents 13–18 years who missed the 11–12 year Td/Tdap booster dose should also receive a single dose of Tdap if they have completed the recommended childhood DTP/DTaP vaccination series. Subsequent **tetanus and diphtheria toxoids (Td)** are recommended every 10 years.

3. **Haemophilus influenzae type b conjugate vaccine (Hib).** Three Hib conjugate vaccines are licensed for infant use. If PRP-OMP (PedvaxHIB® or ComVax® [Merck]) is administered at ages 2 and 4 months, a dose at age 6 months is not required. DTaP/Hib combination products should not be used for primary immunization in infants at ages 2, 4 or 6 months but can be used as boosters after any Hib vaccine. The final dose in the series should be administered at age ≥12 months.

4. **Measles, mumps, and rubella vaccine (MMR).** The second dose of MMR is recommended routinely at age 4–6 years but may be administered during any visit, provided at least 4 weeks have elapsed since the first dose and both doses are administered beginning at or after age 12 months. Those who have not previously received the second dose should complete the schedule by age 11–12 years.

5. **Varicella vaccine.** Varicella vaccine is recommended at any visit at or after age 12 months for susceptible children (i.e., those who lack a reliable history of chickenpox). Susceptible persons aged ≥13 years should receive 2 doses administered at least 4 weeks apart.

6. **Meningococcal vaccine (MCV4).** Meningococcal conjugate vaccine (MCV4) should be given to all children at the 11–12 year old visit as well as to unvaccinated adolescents at high school entry (15 years of age). Other adolescents who wish to decrease their risk for meningococcal disease may also be vaccinated. All college freshmen living in dormitories should also be vaccinated, preferably with MCV4, although meningococcal polysaccharide vaccine (MPSV4) is an acceptable alternative. Vaccination against invasive meningococcal disease is recommended for children and adolescents aged ≥2 years with terminal complement deficiencies or anatomic or functional asplenia and certain other high risk groups (see *MMWR* 2005;54 [RR-7]:1-21); use MPSV4 for children aged 2–10 years and MCV4 for older children, although MPSV4 is an acceptable alternative.

7. **Pneumococcal vaccine.** The heptavalent **pneumococcal conjugate vaccine (PCV)** is recommended for all children aged 2–23 months and for certain children aged 24–59 months. The final dose in the series should be given at age ≥12 months. **Pneumococcal polysaccharide vaccine (PPV)** is recommended in addition to PCV for certain high-risk groups. See *MMWR* 2000; 49(RR-9):1-35.

8. **Influenza vaccine.** Influenza vaccine is recommended annually for children aged ≥6 months with certain risk factors (including, but not limited to, asthma, cardiac disease, sickle cell disease, human immunodeficiency virus [HIV], diabetes, and conditions that can compromise respiratory function or handling of respiratory secretions or that can increase the risk for aspiration), healthcare workers, and other persons (including household members) in close contact with persons in groups at high risk (see *MMWR* 2005;54[RR-8]:1-55). In addition, healthy children aged 6–23 months and close contacts of healthy children in this age group are at substantially increased risk for influenza-related hospitalizations. For healthy persons aged 5–49 years, the intranasally administered, live, attenuated influenza vaccine (LAIV) is an acceptable alternative to the intramuscular trivalent inactivated influenza vaccine (TIV). See *MMWR* 2005;54(RR-8):1-55. Children receiving TIV should be administered a dosage appropriate for their age (0.25 mL if aged 6–35 months or 0.5 mL if aged ≥3 years). Children aged ≤8 years who are receiving influenza vaccine for the first time should receive 2 doses (separated by at least 4 weeks for TIV and at least 6 weeks for LAIV).

9. **Hepatitis A vaccine (HepA).** HepA is recommended for all children at 1 year of age (i.e., 12–23 months). The 2 doses in the series should be administered at least 6 months apart. States, counties, and communities with existing HepA vaccination programs for children 2–18 years of age are encouraged to maintain these programs. In these areas, new efforts focused on routine vaccination of 1-year-old children should enhance, not replace, ongoing programs directed at a broader population of children. HepA is also recommended for certain high risk groups (see *MMWR* 1999; 48[RR-12]:1-37).

The Childhood and Adolescent Immunization Schedule is approved by:
Advisory Committee on Immunization Practices   www.cdc.gov/nip/acip • American Academy of Pediatrics   www.aap.org • American Academy of Family Physicians   www.aafp.org

Table A.5B Recommended immunization schedule for children and adolescents who start late or who are more than 1 month behind.

Recommended Immunization Schedule for Children and Adolescents Who Start Late or Who Are More Than 1 Month Behind

UNITED STATES · 2006

The tables below give catch-up schedules and minimum intervals between doses for children who have delayed immunizations.
There is no need to restart a vaccine series regardless of the time that has elapsed between doses. Use the chart appropriate for the child's age.

CATCH-UP SCHEDULE FOR CHILDREN AGED 4 MONTHS THROUGH 6 YEARS

Vaccine	Minimum Age for Dose 1	Minimum Interval Between Doses			
		Dose 1 to Dose 2	Dose 2 to Dose 3	Dose 3 to Dose 4	Dose 4 to Dose 5
Diphtheria, Tetanus, Pertussis	6 wks	4 weeks	4 weeks	6 months	6 months[1]
Inactivated Poliovirus	6 wks	4 weeks	4 weeks	4 weeks[2]	
Hepatitis B[3]	Birth	4 weeks	8 weeks (and 16 weeks after first dose)		
Measles, Mumps, Rubella	12 mo	4 weeks[4]			
Varicella	12 mo				
Haemophilus influenzae type b[5]	6 wks	4 weeks if first dose given at age <12 months / 8 weeks (as final dose) if first dose given at age 12-14 months / No further doses needed if first dose given at age ≥15 months	4 weeks[6] if current age <12 months / 8 weeks (as final dose)[6] if current age ≥12 months and second dose given at age <15 months / No further doses needed if previous dose given at age ≥15 mo	8 weeks (as final dose) This dose only necessary for children aged 12 months–5 years who received 3 doses before age 12 months	
Pneumococcal[7]	6 wks	4 weeks if first dose given at age <12 months and current age <24 months / 8 weeks (as final dose) if first dose given at age ≥12 months or current age 24–59 months / No further doses needed for healthy children if first dose given at age ≥24 months	4 weeks if current age <12 months / 8 weeks (as final dose) if current age ≥12 months / No further doses needed for healthy children if previous dose given at age ≥24 months	8 weeks (as final dose) This dose only necessary for children aged 12 months–5 years who received 3 doses before age 12 months	

CDC

CATCH-UP SCHEDULE FOR CHILDREN AGED 7 YEARS THROUGH 18 YEARS

Vaccine	Minimum Interval Between Doses		
	Dose 1 to Dose 2	Dose 2 to Dose 3	Dose 3 to Booster Dose
Tetanus, Diphtheria[1]	4 weeks	6 months	6 months if first dose given at age <12 months and current age <11 years; otherwise 5 years
Inactivated Poliovirus[2]	4 weeks	4 weeks	IPV[2,3]
Hepatitis B	4 weeks	8 weeks (and 16 weeks after first dose)	
Measles, Mumps, Rubella[10]	4 weeks		
Varicella[10]	4 weeks		

1. **DTaP.** The fifth dose is not necessary if the fourth dose was administered after the fourth birthday.

2. **IPV.** For children who received an all-IPV or all-oral poliovirus (OPV) series, a fourth dose is not necessary if third dose was administered at age ≥4 years. If both OPV and IPV were administered as part of a series, a total of 4 doses should be given, regardless of the child's current age.

3. **HepB.** Administer the 3-dose series to all children and adolescents <19 years of age if they were not previously vaccinated.

4. **MMR.** The second dose of MMR is recommended routinely at age 4–6 years but may be administered earlier if desired.

5. **Hib.** Vaccine is not generally recommended for children aged ≥5 years.

6. **Hib.** If current age <12 months and the first 2 doses were PRP-OMP (PedvaxHIB® or ComVax® [Merck]), the third (and final) dose should be administered at age 12–15 months and at least 8 weeks after the second dose.

7. **PCV.** Vaccine is not generally recommended for children aged ≥5 years.

8. **Td.** Adolescent tetanus, diphtheria, and pertussis vaccine (Tdap) may be substituted for any dose in a primary catch-up series or as a booster if age appropriate for Tdap. A five-year interval from the last Td dose is encouraged when Tdap is used as a booster dose. See ACIP recommendations for further information.

9. **IPV.** Vaccine is not generally recommended for persons aged ≥18 years.

10. **Varicella.** Administer the 2-dose series to all susceptible adolescents aged ≥13 years.

Report adverse reactions to vaccines through the federal Vaccine Adverse Event Reporting System. For information on reporting reactions following immunization, please visit www.vaers.hhs.gov or call the 24-hour national toll-free information line 800-822-7967. Report suspected cases of vaccine-preventable diseases to your state or local health department.

For additional information about vaccines, including precautions and contraindications for immunization and vaccine shortages, please visit the National Immunization Program Website at www.cdc.gov/nip or contact
800-CDC-INFO (800-232-4636)
(In English, En Español — 24/7)

Table A.5C Recommended adolescent immunization schedule.

Recommended Adolescent Immunization Schedule

Vaccine ▼ / Age ►	11–12 yrs	13–14 yrs	15 yrs	16–21 yrs
Hepatitis B[1]	HepB Series			
Tetanus, Diphtheria, Acellular Pertussis[2]	Tdap		Tdap	
Inactivated Poliovirus[3]		IPV		
Measles, Mumps, Rubella[4]		MMR		
Varicella[5]		Varicella		
Meningococcal[6]	MCV4	Give vaccines below broken line to all patients with risk factors. —— MCV4	MCV4	
Pneumococcal[7]		PPV		
Influenza[8]		Influenza (Yearly)		
Hepatitis A[9]		HepA Series		

Recommended routinely for all adolescents at the ages indicated.	Recommended for adolescents lacking previous vaccination or evidence of prior protection.	Recommended for adolescents with specific risk factors.

This schedule indicates the recommended ages for routine administration of currently licensed vaccines for adolescents ages 11–21 years. Any dose not given at the recommended age should be given at any subsequent visit when indicated and feasible. Providers should consult the manufacturers' package inserts for detailed recommendations. Clinically significant adverse events that follow immunization should be reported to the Vaccine Adverse Event Reporting System (VAERS). Guidance about how to obtain and complete a

1. Hepatitis B vaccine (HepB). All adolescents who have not completed a 3-dose schedule of HepB vaccine should begin (or complete) the series during any visit. The 2nd dose should be given no sooner than 4 weeks from the 1st dose and the 3rd dose no sooner than 8 weeks from the 2nd dose. Overall, there must be at least 4 months between the 1st and 3rd doses (e.g., 0, 1, 4 months; 0, 2, 4 months; or 0, 1, 6 months). If the schedule has been delayed, do not start the series over; continue from where you left off. Alternatively, unvaccinated adolescents 11–15 years of age may be given 2 doses of Recombivax HB 1.0 mL (adult formulation) spaced 4–6 months apart.

2. Tetanus and diphtheria toxoids and acellular pertussis vaccine (Tdap). Adolescents 11–12 years of age who have completed the recommended DTP/DTaP vaccination series and have not received a Td booster dose should be given a dose of Tdap. Adolescents 13–18 years who missed the 11–12-year Td/Tdap booster should receive a single dose of Tdap if they have completed the recommended childhood DTP/DTaP vaccination series. A 5-year interval between Td and Tdap is encouraged to reduce the risk of local or systemic reactions. Subsequent **tetanus and diphtheria (Td)** boosters are recommended every 10 years.

3. Inactivated poliovirus vaccine (IPV). Adolescents who previously received a combination of both oral poliovirus vaccine (OPV) and IPV but received fewer than 4 doses should complete the full 4-dose series with IPV. Other adolescents who have not completed an all-IPV schedule (begin or complete) a series of 3 doses, spaced at least 4 weeks apart. Vaccine is not indicated for persons 18 years of age and older unless they have a risk factor (e.g., pending travel to a country where polio is endemic).

4. Measles, mumps, and rubella vaccine (MMR). Adolescents who have not received at least two doses of MMR should begin (or complete) the 2-dose schedule at any visit; the two doses must be given at least 4 weeks apart.

5. Varicella vaccine. All adolescents who lack a reliable history of chickenpox or previous varicella vaccination should be given varicella vaccine. If younger than 13 years of age, give 1 dose; if 13 years of age or older, give 2 doses at least 4 weeks apart.

6. Meningococcal conjugate vaccine (MCV4). MCV4 is recommended for all children at 11–12 years of age as well as unvaccinated adolescents at 15 years of age. Other adolescents who wish to decrease their risk for meningococcal disease may also be vaccinated. In addition, all college freshmen living in dormitories should be vaccinated, preferably with MCV, although **meningococcal polysaccharide vaccine (MPSV4)** is an acceptable alternative. Vaccination against invasive meningococcal disease is recommended for adolescents with terminal complement component deficiencies or anatomic or functional asplenia and certain other high risk groups (see *MMWR* 2005;54(RR-7):1-21); use MCV4, although MPSV4 is an acceptable alternative.

7. Pneumococcal polysaccharide vaccine (PPV). PPV is recommended for adolescents with certain risk factors (e.g., chronic cardiac or pulmonary disease, chronic liver disease, diabetes mellitus, CSF leaks, candidate for or recipient of cochlear implant) as well as adolescents living in special environments (e.g., Alaska Natives and certain American Indian populations). Give a one-time revaccination to those at highest risk of fatal pneumococcal infection (see *MMWR* 2000;49(RR-9);1-35).

8. Influenza vaccine. Influenza vaccine is recommended annually for adolescents with certain risk factors (including but not limited to asthma, cardiac disease, sickle cell disease, HIV, and diabetes), healthcare workers, and other persons (including household members) in close contact with persons in groups at high risk. All other adolescents wishing to obtain immunity may also be vaccinated. For healthy adolescents, the intranasally administered **live, attenuated influenza vaccine (LAIV)** is an acceptable alternative to the intramuscular **trivalent inactivated influenza vaccine (TIV)**.

9. Hepatitis A vaccine (HepA). Hepatitis A vaccine is recommended for adolescents who lack previous vaccination or evidence of prior infection and who live in selected states and regions and for certain high-risk groups (see *MMWR* 1999;48(RR-12):1-37); consult your local public health authority. The 2 doses in the series should be given at least 6 months apart.

This "Recommended Adolescent Immunization Schedule" was adapted by the Immunization Action Coalition for the Society for Adolescent Medicine and is based on the "Recommended Childhood and Adolescent Immunization Schedule," approved by the Advisory Committee on Immunization Practices, the American Academy of Pediatrics, and the American Academy of Family Physicians, December 2005.

Table A.6A Recommended adult immunization schedule, by vaccine and medical and other indications.

Recommended Adult Immunization Schedule, by Vaccine and Medical and Other Indications
UNITED STATES, OCTOBER 2005–SEPTEMBER 2006

Vaccine ▼ / Indication ▲	Pregnancy	Congenital immunodeficiency; leukemia;[10] lymphoma; generalized malignancy; cerebrospinal fluid leaks; therapy with alkylating agents, antimetabolites, radiation, or high-dose, long-term corticosteroids	Diabetes; heart disease; chronic pulmonary disease; chronic liver disease, including chronic alcoholism	Asplenia[11] (including elective splenectomy and terminal complement component deficiencies)	Kidney failure, end-stage renal disease, recipients of hemodialysis or clotting factor concentrates	Human immunodeficiency virus (HIV) infection[12]	Healthcare workers
Tetanus, diphtheria (Td)[1]*	1-dose booster every 10 yrs						
Measles, mumps, rubella (MMR)[2]*			1 or 2 doses				
Varicella[3]*			2 doses (0, 4–8 wks)			2 doses	2 doses
Influenza[4]*	1 dose annually			1 dose annually		1 dose annually	
Pneumococcal (polysaccharide)[5,6]	1–2 doses			1–2 doses			1–2 doses
Hepatitis A[7]*			2 doses (0, 6–12 mos, or 0, 6–18 mos)				
Hepatitis B[8]*		3 doses (0, 1–2, 4–6 mos)			3 doses (0, 1–2, 4–6 mos)		
Meningococcal[9]		1 dose		1 dose		1 dose	

NOTE: These recommendations must be read along with the footnotes.
*Covered by the Vaccine Injury Compensation Program.

For all persons in this category who meet the age requirements and who lack evidence of immunity (e.g., lack documentation of vaccination or have no evidence of prior infection)

Recommended if some other risk factor is present (e.g., based on medical, occupational, lifestyle, or other indications)

Contraindicated

Recommended Adult Immunization Schedule, UNITED STATES, OCTOBER 2005–SEPTEMBER 2006

1. **Tetanus and Diphtheria (Td) vaccination.** Adults with uncertain histories of a complete primary vaccination series with diphtheria and tetanus toxoid-containing vaccines should receive a primary series using combined Td toxoid. A primary series for adults is 3 doses; administer the first 2 doses at least 4 weeks apart and the third dose 6–12 months after the second. Administer 1 dose if the person received the primary series and if the last vaccination was received ≥10 years previously. Consult ACIP statement for recommendations for administering Td as prophylaxis in wound management (www.cdc.gov/mmwr/preview/mmwrhtml/00041645.htm). The American College of Physicians Task Force on Adult Immunization supports a second option for Td use in adults: a single Td booster at age 50 years for persons who have completed the full pediatric series, including the teenage/young adult booster. A newly licensed tetanus-diphtheria-acellular pertussis vaccine is available for adults. ACIP recommendations for its use will be published.

2. **Measles, Mumps, Rubella (MMR) vaccination.** *Measles component:* adults born before 1957 can be considered immune to measles. Adults born during or after 1957 should receive ≥1 dose of MMR unless they have a medical contraindication, documentation of ≥1 dose, history of measles based on healthcare provider diagnosis, or laboratory evidence of immunity. A second dose of MMR is recommended for adults who 1) were recently exposed to measles or in an outbreak setting, 2) were previously vaccinated with killed measles vaccine, 3) were vaccinated with an unknown type of measles vaccine during 1963–1967, 4) are students in postsecondary educational institutions, 5) work in a healthcare facility, or 6) plan to travel internationally. Withhold MMR or other measles-containing vaccines from HIV-infected persons with severe immunosuppression. *Mumps component:* 1 dose of MMR vaccine should be adequate for protection for those born during or after 1957 who lack a history of mumps based on healthcare provider diagnosis or who lack laboratory evidence of immunity. *Rubella component:* administer 1 dose of MMR vaccine to women whose rubella vaccination history is unreliable or who lack laboratory evidence of immunity. For women of child-bearing age, regardless of birth year, routinely determine rubella immunity and counsel women regarding congenital rubella syndrome. Do not vaccinate women who are pregnant or might become pregnant within 4 weeks of receiving the vaccine. Women who do not have evidence of immunity should receive MMR vaccine upon completion or termination of pregnancy and before discharge from the healthcare facility.

3. **Varicella vaccination.** Varicella vaccination is recommended for all adults without evidence of immunity to varicella. Special consideration should be given to those who 1) have close contact with persons at high risk for severe disease (healthcare workers and family contacts of immunocompromised persons) or 2) are at high risk for exposure or transmission (e.g., teachers of young children; child care employees; residents and staff members of institutional settings, including correctional institutions; college students; military personnel; adolescents and adults living in households with children; nonpregnant women of childbearing age; and international travelers). Evidence of immunity to varicella in adults includes any of the following: 1) documented age-appropriate varicella vaccination (i.e., receipt of 1 dose before age 13 years or receipt of 2 doses [administered at least 4 weeks apart] after age 13 years); 2) born in the United States before 1966; 3) history of varicella disease based on healthcare provider diagnosis or self- or parental report of typical varicella disease for non-U.S.-born persons born before 1966 and all persons born during 1966–1997 [for a patient reporting a history of an atypical, mild case, healthcare providers should seek either an epidemiologic link with a typical varicella case or evidence of laboratory confirmation, if it was performed at the time of acute disease]; 4) history of herpes zoster based on healthcare provider diagnosis; or 5) laboratory evidence of immunity. Do not vaccinate women who are pregnant or might become pregnant within 4 weeks of receiving the vaccine. Assess pregnant women for evidence of varicella immunity. Women who do not have evidence of immunity should receive dose 1 of varicella vaccine upon completion or termination of pregnancy and before discharge from the healthcare facility. Dose 2 should be given 4–8 weeks after dose 1.

4. **Influenza vaccination.** *Medical indications:* chronic disorders of the cardiovascular or pulmonary systems, including asthma; chronic metabolic diseases, including diabetes mellitus, renal dysfunction, hemoglobinopathies, or immunosuppression (including immunosuppression caused by medications or by HIV); any condition (e.g., cognitive dysfunction, spinal cord injury, seizure disorder or other neuromuscular disorder) that compromises respiratory function or the handling of respiratory secretions or that can increase the risk of aspiration; and pregnancy during the influenza season. No data exist on the risk for severe or complicated influenza disease among persons with asplenia; however, influenza is a risk factor for secondary bacterial infections that can cause severe disease among persons with asplenia. *Occupational indications:* healthcare workers and employees of long-term care and assisted living facilities. *Other indications:* residents of nursing homes and other long-term care and assisted living facilities; persons likely to transmit influenza to persons at high risk (i.e., in-home household contacts and caregivers of children birth through 23 months of age, or persons of all ages with high-risk conditions); and anyone who wishes to be vaccinated.

Continued.

DEPARTMENT OF HEALTH AND HUMAN SERVICES
CENTERS FOR DISEASE CONTROL AND PREVENTION

Table A.6A   *Continued.*

Footnotes

Recommended Adult Immunization Schedule, UNITED STATES, OCTOBER 2005–SEPTEMBER 2006

For healthy nonpregnant persons aged 5–49 years without high-risk conditions who are not contacts of severely immunocompromised persons in special care units, intranasally administered influenza vaccine (FluMist*) may be administered in lieu of inactivated vaccine.

5. **Pneumococcal polysaccharide vaccination.** *Medical indications:* chronic disorders of the pulmonary system (excluding asthma); cardiovascular diseases; diabetes mellitus; chronic liver diseases, including liver disease as a result of alcohol abuse (e.g., cirrhosis); chronic renal failure or nephrotic syndrome; functional or anatomic asplenia (e.g., sickle cell disease or splenectomy [if elective splenectomy is planned, vaccinate at least 2 weeks before surgery]); immunosuppressive conditions (e.g., congenital immunodeficiency, HIV infection [vaccinate as close to diagnosis as possible when CD4 cell counts are highest], leukemia, lymphoma, multiple myeloma, Hodgkin disease, generalized malignancy, organ or bone marrow transplantation); chemotherapy with alkylating agents, antimetabolites, or high-dose, long-term corticosteroids; and cochlear implants. *Other indications:* Alaska Natives and certain American Indian populations; residents of nursing homes and other long-term care facilities.

6. **Revaccination with pneumococcal polysaccharide vaccine.** One-time revaccination after 5 years for persons with chronic renal failure or nephrotic syndrome; functional or anatomic asplenia (e.g., sickle cell disease or splenectomy); immunosuppressive conditions (e.g., congenital immunodeficiency, HIV infection, leukemia, lymphoma, multiple myeloma, Hodgkin disease, generalized malignancy, organ or bone marrow transplantation); or chemotherapy with alkylating agents, antimetabolites, or high-dose, long-term corticosteroids. For persons aged ≥65 years, one-time revaccination if they were vaccinated ≥5 years previously and were aged <65 years at the time of primary vaccination.

7. **Hepatitis A vaccination.** *Medical indications:* persons with clotting factor disorders or chronic liver disease. *Behavioral indications:* men who have sex with men or users of illegal drugs. *Occupational indications:* persons working with hepatitis A virus (HAV)-infected primates or with HAV in a research laboratory setting. *Other indications:* persons traveling to or working in countries that have high or intermediate endemicity of hepatitis A (for list of countries, visit www.cdc.gov/travel/diseases.htm#hepa) as well as any person wishing to obtain immunity. Current vaccines should be given in a 2-dose series at either 0 and 6–12 months, or 0 and 6–18 months. If the combined hepatitis A and hepatitis B vaccine is used, administer 3 doses at 0, 1, and 6 months.

8. **Hepatitis B vaccination.** *Medical indications:* hemodialysis patients (use special formulation [40 μg/mL] or two 20-μg/mL doses) or patients who receive clotting factor concentrates. *Occupational indications:* healthcare workers and public-safety workers who have exposure to blood in the workplace; and persons in training in schools of medicine, dentistry, nursing, laboratory technology, and other allied health professions. *Behavioral indications:* injection-drug users; persons with more than one sex partner in the previous 6 months; persons with a recently acquired sexually transmitted disease (STD); and men who have sex with men. *Other indications:* household contacts and sex partners of persons with chronic hepatitis B virus (HBV) infection; clients and staff of institutions for the developmentally disabled; all clients of STD clinics; inmates of correctional facilities; or international travelers who will be in countries with high or intermediate prevalence of chronic HBV infection for >6 months (for list of countries, visit www.cdc.gov/travel/diseases.htm#hepa).

9. **Meningococcal vaccination.** *Medical indications:* adults with anatomic or functional asplenia, or terminal complement component deficiencies. *Other indications:* first-year college students living in dormitories; military recruits; microbiologists who are routinely exposed to isolates of *Neisseria meningitidis*; military recruits; and persons who travel to or reside in countries in which meningococcal disease is hyperendemic or epidemic (e.g., the "meningitis belt" of sub-Saharan Africa during the dry season [Dec–June]), particularly if contact with the local populations will be prolonged. Vaccination is required by the government of Saudi Arabia for all travelers to Mecca during the annual Hajj. Meningococcal conjugate vaccine is preferred for adults meeting any of the above indications who are aged ≤55 years, although meningococcal polysaccharide vaccine (MPSV4) is an acceptable alternative. Revaccination after 5 years may be indicated for adults previously vaccinated with MPSV4 who remain at high risk for infection (e.g., persons residing in areas in which disease is epidemic).

10. **Selected conditions for which *Haemophilus influenzae* type b (Hib) vaccine may be used.** *Haemophilus influenzae* type b conjugate vaccines are licensed for children aged 6 weeks–71 months. No efficacy data are available on which to base a recommendation concerning use of Hib vaccine for older children and adults with the chronic conditions associated with an increased risk for Hib disease. However, studies suggest good immunogenicity in patients who have sickle cell disease, leukemia, or HIV infection, or have had splenectomies; administering vaccine to these patients is not contraindicated.

Approved by the Advisory Committee on Immunization Practices (ACIP).

Recommended Adult Immunization Schedule, by Vaccine and Age Group
UNITED STATES, OCTOBER 2005–SEPTEMBER 2006

Vaccine ▶ Age group ▶	19–49 years	50–64 years	≥ 65 years
Tetanus, diphtheria (Td)[1]*	1-dose booster every 10 yrs		
Measles, mumps, rubella (MMR)[2]*	1 or 2 doses	1 dose	
Varicella[3]*	2 doses (0, 4–8 wks)	2 doses (0, 4–8 wks)	
Influenza[4]*	1 dose annually	1 dose annually	
Pneumococcal (polysaccharide)[5,6]	1–2 doses		1 dose
Hepatitis A[7]*	2 doses (0, 6–12 mos, or 0, 6–18 mos)		
Hepatitis B[8]*	3 doses (0, 1–2, 4–6 mos)		
Meningococcal[9]	1 or more doses		

– – – Vaccines below broken line are for selected populations – – –

NOTE: These recommendations must be read along with the footnotes.

*Covered by the Vaccine Injury Compensation Program.

For all persons in this category who meet the age requirements and who lack evidence of immunity (e.g., lack documentation of vaccination or have no evidence of prior infection)

Recommended if some other risk factor is present (e.g., based on medical, occupational, lifestyle, or other indications)

This schedule indicates the recommended age groups and medical indications for routine administration of currently licensed vaccines for persons aged ≥19 years. Licensed combination vaccines may be used whenever any components of the combination are indicated and when the vaccine's other components are not contraindicated. For detailed recommendations, consult the manufacturers' package inserts and the complete statements from the ACIP (www.cdc.gov/nip/publications/acip-list.htm).

Report all clinically significant postvaccination reactions to the Vaccine Adverse Event Reporting System (VAERS). Reporting forms and instructions on filing a VAERS report are available by telephone, 800-822-7967, or from the VAERS website at www.vaers.hhs.gov.

Information on how to file a Vaccine Injury Compensation Program claim is available at www.hrsa.gov/osp/vicp or by telephone, 800-338-2382. To file a claim for vaccine injury, contact the U.S. Court of Federal Claims, 717 Madison Place, N.W., Washington D.C. 20005, telephone 202-357-6400.

Additional information about the vaccines listed above and contraindications for vaccination is also available at www.cdc.gov/nip or from the CDC-INFO Contact Center at 800-CDC-INFO (232-4636) in English and Spanish, 24 hours a day, 7 days a week.

DEPARTMENT OF HEALTH AND HUMAN SERVICES
CENTERS FOR DISEASE CONTROL AND PREVENTION

Vaccine Administration Record

Table A.7. Vaccine administration record.

Patient Name _____

Birthdate _____

Record # _____

Clinic Name/Address

"I have been provided a copy of the appropriate Centers for Disease Control and Prevention Vaccine Information Material(s) and have read, or have had explained to me, information about the diseases and the vaccines listed below. I have had a chance to ask questions that were answered to my satisfaction. I believe I understand the benefits and risks of the vaccines cited, and ask that the vaccine(s) listed below be given to me or to the person named above (for whom I am authorized to make this request)."

	Vaccine	Date Given m/d/y	Age	Site*	Source of Vaccine (F, S, P)**	Vaccine Manufacturer	Vaccine Lot Number	Vaccine Information Materials Publ. Date	Initials***	Parent/ Guardian Initials***
(Circle one)	DT DTP DTaP 1									
	DT DTP DTaP 2									
	DT DTP DTaP 3									
	DT DTP DTaP 4									
	DT DTP DTaP 5									
	DTP-Hib 1									
	DTP-Hib 2									
	DTP-Hib 3									
	DTP-Hib 4									
	Hib 1									
	Hib 2									
	Hib 3									
	Hib 4									
	Td 1									
	Td 2									
(Circle one)	OPV 1 IPV 1									
	OPV 2 IPV 2									
	OPV 3 IPV 3									
	OPV 4 IPV 4									
	MMR 1									
	MMR 2									
	Hep B 1									
	Hep B 2									
	Hep B 3									
	Varicella 1									
	Varicella 2									

*** Initials   Signature of Vaccine Administrator or Parent/Guardian

_____

_____

_____

(Use reverse side if more signatures are needed)

*Site Given Legend

RA = Right Arm
LA = Left Arm
RT = Right Thigh
LT = Left Thigh
O = Oral

** F = Federal, S = State, P = Private

American Academy of Pediatrics

Copyright ©1992
Rev 10/96

HE0116

Table A.8. Office review of patient immunization status.

Primary-Preventive Care Criteria Set*
The purpose of this document is to assess the adequacy of immunizations in the primary care component of practice.

Procedure:
Office review of patient immunization status

Medical Record Documentation:
The following items should be documented in the medical record:

1. Evidence that the physician(s) provides primary care for that patient
2. History or checklist that includes the patient's immunization history for the following:
   a. Diphtheria—pertussis—tetanus
   b. Tetanus—diphtheria booster
   c. Polio
   d. Rubella
   e. Hepatitis B
   f. Influenza
   g. Varicella
   h. Pneumococcus
3. An immunization history that includes a survey of high-risk factors. Examples include, but are not limited to, the following:
   a. For rubella: childbearing capability with no evidence of immunity to rubella
   b. For hepatitis: sexual activity, drug use, or occupation
   c. For influenza or pneumococcal pneumonia: age, chronic cardiopulmonary disease, metabolic disease, or immunosuppression
4. Any history of allergies
5. Initial and follow-up, or "booster," immunizations according to current guidelines

Unless otherwise indicated, each numbered and lettered item must be present.

Bibliography

American College of Obstetricians and Gynecologists. Guidelines for women's health care. Washington, DC: ACOG, 1996

American College of Obstetricians and Gynecologists. Primary and preventive care. In: Precis V: an update in obstetrics and gynecology. Washington, DC: ACOG, 1994:1–54

---

*This Criteria Set applies only to records of those patients for whom the physician provides primary care.

Contraception

Table A.9 **Percentage of woman experiencing an unintended pregnancy during the first year of typical use and the first year of perfect use of contraception and the percentage continuing use at the end of the first year, United States.**

Method	% of Woman Experiencing an Unintended Pregnancy within the First Year of Use		% of Women Continuing Use at One Year
	Typical Use	Perfect Use	
No method	85	85	
Spermicides	29	18	42
Withdrawal	27	4	43
Periodic abstinence	25		51
Calendar		9	
Ovulation method		3	
Sympto-thermal		2	
Post-ovulation		1	
Cap			
Parous women	32	26	46
Nulliparous women	16	9	57
Sponge			
Parous women	32	20	46
Nulliparous women	16	9	57
Diaphragm	16	6	57
Condom			
Female (Reality)	21	5	49
Male	15	2	53
Combined pill and minipill	8	0.3	68
Evra patch	8	0.3	68
NuvaRing	8	0.3	68
Depo-Provera	3	0.3	56
Lunelle	3	0.05	56
IUD			
Para Gard (copper T)	0.8	0.6	78
Mirena (LNG-IUS)	0.1	0.1	81
Norplant and Norplant-2	0.05	0.05	84
Female sterilization	0.5	0.5	100
Male sterilization	0.15	0.10	100

Emergency Contraceptive Pills: Treatment initiated within 72 hours after unprotected intercourse reduce the risk of pregnancy by at least 75%.
Lactation Amenorrhea Method: LAM is a highly effective, *temporary* method of contraception.
Source: Hatcher RA, et al. Contraceptive Technology. 18th ed. Ardent Media, 2004, with permission of Blackwell Publishing.

Drugs In Pregnancy

Table A.10.   Drugs in pregnancy (by risk categories).

Category X: Studies in animals or human beings have demonstrated fetal abnormalities or there is evidence of fetal risk based on human experience or both, and the risk of the use of the drug in pregnant women clearly outweighs any possible benefit. The drug is contraindicated in women who are or may become pregnant.

- Clomiphene (Clomid, Serophene)
- Danazol (Danocrine)
- Dienestrol
- Diethylstilbestrol (DES)
- Estradiol
- Estrogen-conjugated (Premarin)
- Ergotamine (Bellergal, Cafergot)
- Flurazepam (Dalmane)
- Iodinated glycerol
- Isotretinoin (Accutane)
- Leuprolide (Lupron)
- Medroxyprogesterone (Provera)
- Methotrexate
- Mifepristone (RU-486)
- Misoprostol (Cytotec)
- Norethindrone
- Norgestrel
- Oral contraceptives
- Sodium iodide
- Temazepam (Restoril)
- Triazolam (Halcion)

Category D: There is positive evidence of human fetal risk, but the benefits from use in pregnant women may be acceptable despite the risk (e.g., if the drug is needed in a life-threatening situation or for a serious disease for which safer drugs cannot be used or are ineffective).

- Alprazolam (Xanax)
- Atenolol (Tenormin)
- Azathioprine (Imuran)
- Carbamazepine (Tegretol)
- Cisplatin
- Clonazepam (Klonapin)

Continued.

Table A.10. *Continued.*

- Coumarin (Coumadin)
- Diazepam (Valium)
- Doxycycline
- Ethanol
- Hydroxyprogesterone (Delalutin)
- Iodine
- Lithium
- Lorazepam (Ativan)
- Midazolam (Versed)
- Phenobarbital
- Phenytoin (Dilantin)
- Secobarbital (Seconal)
- Tetracycline
- Valproic acid (Depakene)

Category C: Either studies in animals have revealed adverse effects on the fetus (teratogenic or embryocidal or other) and there are no controlled studies in women or studies in women and animals are not available. Drugs should be given only if the potential benefit justifies the potential risk to the fetus.

- Acetohexamide (oral hypoglycemic)
- Albuterol (Proventil, Ventolin)
- Aminophylline
- Amitriptyline (Elavil)
- Amphetamine
- Aspirin
- Bacitracin (Neosporin)
- Beclomethasone (Beconase, Beclovent)
- Betamethasone (Celestone)
- Butoconazole (Femstate)
- Captopril (Capoten)
- Chlorpromazine (Thorazine)
- Ciprofloxacin (Cipro)
- Clonidine (Catapres)
- Codeine
- Cortisone
- Desipramine (Norpramin)
- Dexamethasone (Decadron)

Table A.10.   *Continued.*

- Digitalis (Digoxin)
- Diltiazem (Cardizem)
- Diphenoxylate (Lomotyl)
- Docusate sodium (Dialose, Senokot)
- Doxepin (Sinequan)
- Droperidol (Inapsine)
- Epinephrine
- Fenflurmine (Pondimin)
- Fentanyl
- Fluconazole (Diflucan)
- Fluoxetine (Prozac)
- Fluovoxamine (Paxil)
- Guaifenesin (numerous cold medications)
- Glyburide (Diabeta)
- Haloperidol (Haldol)
- Heparin
- Hydralazine (Apresoline)
- Hydrocodone
- Hydroxyzine (Vistaril, Atarax)
- Imipramine (Tofranil)
- Isoniazid (INH)
- Ketoconazole (Nizoral)
- Labetalol (Normodyne, Trandate)
- Methocarbamol (Robaxin)
- Miconazole (Monistat)
- Mineral oil
- Morphine
- Neomycin (Cortisporin, Neosporin)
- Nicorette
- Nifedipine (Procardia, Adalat)
- Nonoxynol
- Nystatin
- Omeprazole (Prilosec)
- Pheniramine (numerous cold medications)
- Phenylephrine (numerous cold medications)
- Prednisone
- Promethazine (Phenergan)
- Propoxyphene (Darvon)
- Propranolol (Inderal)

Continued.

Table A.10. *Continued.*

- Prozac (Fluoxetine)
- Pseudephedrine (numerous cold medications)
- Quinacrine (Atabrine)
- Scopolamine
- Saccharin
- Sertraline (Zoloft)
- Simethicone (Maalox, Mylanta)
- Sulfonamides
- Spironolactone (Aldactone)
- Terconazole (Terazol)
- Terfenadine (Seldane)
- Theophylline
- Tolbutamide
- Trazodone
- Trimethoprim (Bactrim, Septra)
- Vaccines (measles, mumps, rubella, smallpox, and varicella)
- Verapamil (Calan, Isoptin)
- Zidovudine (Retrovir, AZT)

Category B: Either animal-reproduction studies have not demonstrated a fetal risk but there are no controlled studies in pregnant women or animal-reproduction studies have shown an adverse effect (other than a decrease in fertility) that was not confirmed in controlled studies in women in the first trimester (and there is no evidence of a risk in later trimesters).

- Acyclovir (Zovirax)
- Amoxicillin
- Acetaminophen (Tylenol)
- Ampicillin
- Aspartame (Nutrasweet)
- Bromocriptine (Parlodel)
- Buspirone (Buspar)
- Caffeine
- Cimetidine (Tagamet)
- Clindamycin (Cleocin)
- Clotrimazole (Lotrimin, Gyne-Lotrimin, Mycelex)
- Cromolyn sodium (Intal)
- Cyclobenzaprine (Flexeril)
- Dicyclomine (Bentyl)

Table A.10. *Continued.*

- Diphenhydramine (Benadryl, Actifed, Unisom)
- Erythromycin
- Famotidine (Pepcid)
- Hydrochlorothiazide (HCTZ)
- Ibuprofen (Motrin)
- Indomethacin (Indocin)
- Insulin
- Lidocaine (Xylocaine)
- Loperamide (Imodium)
- Meperidine (Demerol)
- Methyldopa (Aldomet)
- Metoclopramide (Reglan)
- Metronidazole (Flagyl, Metrogel)
- Naproxen (Anaprox)
- Nitrofurantoin (Macrodantin)
- Oxycodone (Trilox, Percocet)
- Penicillin
- Propofol (Diprivan)
- Ranitidine (Zantac)
- Ritodrine
- Sulfasalazine (Azulfidine)
- Terbutaline (Brethine)
- Vancomycin

Category A: Controlled studies in women fail to demonstrate a risk to the fetus in the first trimester (and there is no evidence of a risk in later trimesters), and the possibility of fetal harm appears remote.
Vitamins (A, B_{12}, C, D, folic acid, multiple)

Source: Data from Briggs GG, Freeman RK, Sumner JY, eds. *Drugs in Pregnancy and Lactation*, 7th ed. Philadelphia: Lippincott Williams & Wilkins; 2005.

Table A.11.   General instructions on medication in pregnancy.

Advise patient that no medication is 100% approved during pregnancy, but the following medications may be taken during the *first trimester* if necessary:

Emetrol as directed for nausea
Tylenol, two regular strength, 3 times daily
Neo-synephrine nasal spray, 0.25% prn at h.s.
Prenatal vitamins (Stuartnatal 1 + 1) or (Prenate 90), one daily
Cepacol mouthwash/gargle prn
Cepacol throat lozenges prn
Vitamin B_6, 50mg b.i.d. for nausea
Saline nosedrops prn
Kaopectate as directed
Allergy shots as per allergist
Metamucil once or twice daily
Mylanta, 1 tbsp up to 4 times a day
Anusol cream or suppositories twice daily.
Tums, one b.i.d or two at bedtime for indigestion or for leg cramps
Monistat 7 vaginal cream, nightly 7 nights
MOM-30cc HS if necessary—severe constipation
Glycerin Supp—rectally if necessary for immediate relief of constipation
Robitussin DM for cough as directed
Sudafed, one t.i.d.
Benadryl, 25mg q 4–6hrs p.r.n.
Phenergan 12.5–25mg po #10 or suppository, 25mg #5 1q 6 hours prn, if vitamin B_6 not effective (prescription needed)

Second and Third Trimesters: May take all of the above plus:

Actifed, one t.i.d. or at h.s.
Proctofoam-HC t.i.d. p.r.n. (prescription needed)
Anusol-HC suppository or cream b.i.d. to t.i.d.

Oral Contraceptives: You may refill oral contraceptives for up to 1 year after postpartum examination. If patient is having breakthrough bleeding for more than 3 months, discuss with M.D. If problems continue after medication change, the patient will need follow-up with an ob/gyn.

Indigestion	Tums
	Sig: One/b.i.d. or two @ bedtime for indigestion
	Mylanta
	Sig: One tbsp and up to q.i.d.
Diarrhea	Kaopectate
	Sig: As directed
Constipation	Metamucil
	Sig: Q.D. or b.i.d.
Hemorrhoids	Anusol suppositories
	Sig: b.i.d.

Table A.12.   Folic acid guidelines.

In the fall of 1992, the Centers for Disease Control and Prevention released new information concerning the importance of folic acid in the prevention of neural tube defects. The guidelines stress the need for women considering pregnancy to consume 400mcg of folic acid each day at least 1 month before conception. This can be accomplished with a diet high in dark green leafy vegetables, orange juice, fortified cereals, cooked dry beans and legumes, and liver or with a folic acid supplement. If a woman has previously delivered a child with a neural tube defect, the suggested supplementation increases to 4mg each day, which is prescribed by her physician. The guidelines also state that once a woman is pregnant the need for folic acid continues, and the Recommended Daily Allowance (RDA) for pregnancy is 800mcg each day. This level of folic acid consumption is difficult to obtain through diet alone and is best accomplished with a combination of diet and vitamin supplementation.

In Kentucky, the Division of Maternal and Child Health is developing a program to meet the needs of women seen in health department clinics. In the near future, the health departments will offer a multilevel approach to address the need for folic acid during preconception and early prenatal care. The clinics will have the option to provide B-vitamins which contain the recommended 400mcg of folic acid to the woman desiring pregnancy.

The approach includes a strong education component concerning the need for folic acid to prevent neural tube defects. All women who come to the health department for a pregnancy test and not desiring pregnancy will receive information on the importance of folic acid consumption at least one month before conception and during the first trimester of pregnancy. Women desiring pregnancy will receive the counseling on folic acid, a handout on folic acid and ways to include these foods in the diet, and the B-vitamin supplement with 400mcg of folic acid. All women receiving the health department's comprehensive prenatal program are provided with a prenatal vitamin with the recommended 800mcg of folic acid. We hope with the implementation of these new program guidelines to see a decline in the incidence of neural tube defects.

Source: Recommendations for the Use of Folic Acid to Reduce the Number of Cases of Spina Bifida and Other Neural Tube Defects September 11, 1992/41 (RR-14):001 U.S. Department of Health and Human Services Public Health Service Centers for Disease Control Atlanta, Georgia 30333.

Exercise

Table A.13. Preparticipation physical evaluation.

HISTORY FORM

DATE OF EXAM _____

Name _____ Sex_____ Age _____ Date of birth_____

Grade___ School_____ Sport(s) _____

Address _____ Phone _____

Personal physician _____

In case of emergency, contact

Name _____ Relationship _____ Phone (H) _____ (W) _____

Explain "Yes" answers below.
Circle questions you don't know the answers to.

	Yes	No
1. Has a doctor ever denied or restricted your participation in sports for any reason?	☐	☐
2. Do you have an ongoing medical condition (like diabetes or asthma)?	☐	☐
3. Are you currently taking any prescription or nonprescription (over-the-counter) medicines or pills?	☐	☐
4. Do you have allergies to medicines, pollens, foods, or stinging insects?	☐	☐
5. Have you ever passed out or nearly passed out DURING exercise?	☐	☐
6. Have you ever passed out or nearly passed out AFTER exercise?	☐	☐
7. Have you ever had discomfort, pain, or pressure in your chest during exercise?	☐	☐
8. Does your heart race or skip beats during exercise?	☐	☐
9. Has a doctor ever told you that you have (check all that apply): ☐ High blood pressure ☐ A heart murmur ☐ High cholesterol ☐ A heart infection		
10. Has a doctor ever ordered a test for your heart? (for example, ECG, echocardiogram)	☐	☐
11. Has anyone in your family died for no apparent reason?	☐	☐
12. Does anyone in your family have a heart problem?	☐	☐
13. Has any family member or relative died of heart problems or of sudden death before age 50?	☐	☐
14. Does anyone in your family have Marfan syndrome?	☐	☐
15. Have you ever spent the night in a hospital?	☐	☐
16. Have you had heart surgery?	☐	☐
17. Have you ever had an injury, like a sprain, muscle or ligament tear, or tendinitis, that caused you to miss a practice or game? If yes, circle affected area below:	☐	☐
18. Have you had any broken or fractured bones or dislocated joints? If yes, circle below:	☐	☐
19. Have you had a bone or joint injury that required x-rays, MRI, CT, surgery, injections, rehabilitation, physical therapy, a brace, a cast, or crutches? If yes, circle below:	☐	☐

Head	Neck	Shoulder	Upper arm	Elbow	Forearm	Hand/figers	Chest
Upper back	Lower back	Hip	Thigh	Knee	Calf/shin	Ankle	Foot/toes

	Yes	No
20. Have you ever had a stress fracture?	☐	☐
21. Have you been told that you have or have you had an x-ray for atlantoaxial (neck) instability?	☐	☐
22. Do you regularly use a brace or assistive device?	☐	☐
23. Has a doctor ever told you that you have asthma or allergies?	☐	☐

	Yes	No
24. Do you cough, wheeze, or have difficulty breathing during or after exercise?	☐	☐
25. Is there anyone in your family who has asthma?	☐	☐
26. Have you ever used an inhaler or taken asthma medicine?	☐	☐
27. Were you born without or are you missing a kidney, an eye, a testicle, or any other organ?	☐	☐
28. Have you had infectious mononucleosis (mono) within the last month?	☐	☐
29. Do you have any rashes, pressure sores, or other skin problems?	☐	☐
30. Have you had a herpes skin infection?	☐	☐
31. Have you ever had a head injury or concussion?	☐	☐
32. Have you been hit in the head and been confused or lost your memory?	☐	☐
33. Have you ever had a seizure?	☐	☐
34. Do you have headaches with exercise?	☐	☐
35. Have you ever had numbness, tingling, or weakness in your arms or legs after being hit or falling?	☐	☐
36. Have you ever been unable to move your arms or legs after being hit or falling?	☐	☐
37. When exercising in the heat, do you have severe muscle cramps or become ill?	☐	☐
38. Has a doctor told you that you or someone in your family has sickle cell trait or sickle cell disease?	☐	☐
39. Have you had any problems with your eyes or vision?	☐	☐
40. Do you wear glasses or contact lenses?	☐	☐
41. Do you wear protective eyewear, such as goggles or a face shield?	☐	☐
42. Are you happy with your weight?	☐	☐
43. Are you trying to gain or lose weight?	☐	☐
44. Has anyone recommended you change your weight or eating habits?	☐	☐
45. Do you limit or carefully control what you eat?	☐	☐
46. Do you have any concerns that you would like to discuss with a doctor?	☐	☐

FEMALES ONLY

	Yes	No
47. Have you ever had a menstrual period?	☐	☐

48. How old were you when you had your first menstrual period? _____

49. How many periods have you had in the last 12 months? _____

Explain "Yes" answers here: _____
_____
_____
_____
_____
_____
_____
_____
_____

I hereby state that, to the best of my knowledge, my answers to the above questions are complete and correct.

Signature of athlete _____ Signature of parent/guardian _____ Date _____

Source: © 2004 American Academy of Family Physicians, American Academy of Pediatrics, American College of Sports Medicine, American Medical Society for Sports Medicine, American Orthopaedic Society for Sports Medicine, and American Osteopathic Academy of Sports Medicine.

Table A.14. Reducing the risk of cancer with healthy food choices and physical activity.

1. Eat a variety of healthful foods, with an emphasis on plant sources.
   - Eat five or more servings of a variety of vegetables and fruits each day.
   - Choose whole grains in preference to processed (refined) grains and sugars.
   - Limit consumption of red meats, especially those high in fat and processed.
   - Choose foods that help you maintain a healthful weight.
2. Adopt a physically active lifestyle.
   - Adults: engage in at least moderate activity for 30 minutes or more on five or more days of the week; 45 minutes or more of moderate-to-vigorous activity on five or more days per week may further enhance reductions in the risk of breast and colon cancer.
   - Children and adolescents: engage in at least 60 minutes per day of moderate-to-vigorous physical activity for at least five days per week.
3. Maintain a healthful weight throughout life.
   - Balance caloric intake with physical activity.
   - Lose weight if currently overweight or obese.
4. If you drink alcoholic beverages, limit consumption.

Source: From Byers T, Nestle M, McTiernan A, et al. American Cancer Society guidelines on nutrition and physical activity for cancer prevention: reducing the risk of cancer with healthy food choices and physical activity. *CA Cancer J Clin* 2002;52:92–119.

Laboratory Reference Values

Table A.15.   Laboratory references value.

Hematology and Coagulation.			
Analyte	Specimen*	Units Used at MGH	SI Units
Activated clotting time	WB	70–180 sec	70–180 sec
Activated protein C resistance (factor V Leiden)	P	Ratio >2.1	Not applicable
Alpha$_2$-antiplasmin	P	80–130%	0.80–1.30
Antiphospholipid-antibody panel			
Partial-thromboplastin time–lupus anticoagulant screen	P	Negative	Negative
Platelet-neutralization procedure	P	Negative	Negative
Dilute viper-venom screen	P	Negative	Negative
Anticardiolipin antibody	S		
IgG		0–15 GPL units	0–15 arbitrary units
IgM		0–15 MPL units	0–15 arbitrary units
Antithrombin III	P		
Antigenic		22–39 mg/dl	220–390 mg/liter
Functional		80–130%	0.8–1.30 U/liter
Anti-Xa assay (heparin assay)	P		
Unfractionated heparin		0.3–0.7 IU/ml	0.3–0.7 kIU/liter
Low-molecular-weight heparin		0.5–1.0 IU/ml	0.5–1.0 kIU/liter
Danaparoid		0.5–0.8 IU/ml	0.5–0.8 kIU/liter
Bleeding time		2.0–9.5 min	2.0–9.5 min
Carboxyhemoglobin	WB		
Nonsmoker		0–2.3%	0–0.023
Smoker		2.1–4.2%	0.021–0.042
Clot retraction	WB	50–100%/2 hr	0.50–1.00/2 hr
Cryofibrinogen	P	Negative	Negative
D-Dimer	P	<0.5 μg/ml	<0.5 mg/liter
Differential blood count	WB		
Neutrophils		40–70%	0.40–0.70
Band forms		0–10%	0–0.10
Lymphocytes		22–44%	0.22–0.44
Monocytes		4–11%	0.04–0.11
Eosinophils		0–8%	0–0.08
Basophils		0–3%	0–0.03
Erythrocyte count	WB		
Male		4.50–5.90×10^6/mm³	4.50–5.90×10^{12}/liter
Female		4.00–5.20×10^6/mm³	4.00–5.20×10^{12}/liter
Erythrocyte lifespan	WB		
Normal survival		120 days	120 days
Chromium labeled, half-life		25–35 days	25–35 days
Erythrocyte sedimentation rate	WB		
Female		1–25 mm/hr	1–25 mm/hr
Male		0–17 mm/hr	0–17 mm/hr
Factor II, prothrombin	P	60–140%	0.60–1.40
Factor V	P	60–140%	0.60–1.40
Factor VII	P	60–140%	0.60–1.40
Factor VIII	P	50–200%	0.50–2.00
Factor IX	P	60–140%	0.60–1.40

Table A.15.   *Continued.*

Hematology and Coagulation. (Continued.)			
Analyte	**Specimen***	**Units Used at MGH**	**SI Units**
Factor X	P	60–140%	0.60–1.40
Factor XI	P	60–140%	0.60–1.40
Factor XII	P	60–140%	0.60–1.40
Factor XIII screen	P	No deficiency detected	Not applicable
Factor-inhibitor assay	P	<0.5 Bethesda unit	<0.5 Bethesda unit
Ferritin	S		
Male		30–300 ng/ml	30–300 µg/liter
Female		10–200 ng/ml	10–200 µg/liter
Fibrin and fibrinogen-degradation products	P	<2.5 µg/ml	<2.5 mg/liter
Fibrinogen	P	150–400 mg/dl	1.50–4.00 g/liter
Folate (folic acid)	S, P		
Normal		3.1–17.5 ng/ml	7.0–39.7 nmol/liter
Borderline deficient		2.2–3.0 ng/ml	5.0–6.8 nmol/liter
Deficient		<2.2 ng/ml	<5.0 nmol/liter
Excess		>17.5 ng/ml	>39.7 nmol/liter
Glucose-6-phosphate dehydrogenase, erythrocyte	WB	No gross deficiency	Not applicable
Ham's test (acidified serum test)	WB	Negative	Negative
Haptoglobin	S	16–199 mg/dl	0.16–1.99 g/liter
Hematocrit	WB		
Male		41.0–53.0%	0.41–0.53
Female		36.0–46.0%	0.36–0.46
Hemoglobin			
Plasma	P	1–5 mg/dl	0.01–0.05 g/liter
Whole blood			
Male	WB	13.5–17.5 g/dl	8.4–10.9 mmol/liter
Female	WB	12.0–16.0 g/dl	7.4–9.9 mmol/liter
Hemoglobin electrophoresis	WB		
Hemoglobin A		95–98%	0.95–0.98
Hemoglobin A_2		1.5–3.5%	0.015–0.035
Hemoglobin F		0–2.0%	0–0.02
Hemoglobins other than A, A_2, or F		Absent	Absent
Heparin-induced thrombocytopenia antibody	P	Negative	Negative
Homocysteine	P	0–12 µmol/liter	0–12 µmol/liter
Iron	S	30–160 µg/dl	5.4–28.7 µmol/liter
Iron-binding capacity	S	228–428 µg/dl	40.8–76.7 µmol/liter
Leukocyte count (WBC)	WB	4.5–11.0×10³/mm³	4.5–11×10⁹/liter
Mean corpuscular hemoglobin (MCH)	WB	26.0–34.0 pg/cell	26.0–34.0 pg/cell
Mean corpuscular hemoglobin concentration (MCHC)	WB	31.0–37.0 g/dl	310–370 g/liter
Mean corpuscular volume (MCV)	WB	80–100 µm³	80–100 fl
Methemoglobin	WB	≤1% of total hemoglobin	
Osmotic fragility of erythrocytes	WB	No increased hemolysis as compared with normal control	Not applicable
Partial-thromboplastin time, activated	P	22.1–35.1 sec	22.1–35.1 sec
Plasminogen	P		
Antigenic		8.4–14.0 mg/dl	84–140 mg/liter
Functional		80–130%	0.80–1.30

Continued.

Table A.15. *Continued.*

Hematology and Coagulation. (Continued.)			
Analyte	Specimen*	Units Used at MGH	SI Units
Plasminogen activator inhibitor 1	P	4–43 ng/ml	4–43 µg/liter
Platelet aggregation	PRP	>65% aggregation in response to adenosine diphosphate, epinephrine, collagen, ristocetin, and arachidonic acid	Not applicable
Platelet count	WB	150–350×10³/mm³	150–350×10⁹/liter
Prekallikrein assay	P	60–140%	0.60–1.40
Prekallikrein screen	P	Deficiency not detected	Not applicable
Protein C	P		
Total antigen		70–140%	0.70–1.40
Functional		70–140%	0.70–1.40
Protein S	P		
Total antigen		70–140%	0.70–1.40
Functional		70–140%	0.70–1.40
Free antigen		70–140%	0.70–1.40
Prothrombin-gene mutation G20210A	WB	Not present	Not applicable
Prothrombin time	P	11.1–13.1 sec	11.1–13.1 sec
Protoporphyrin, free erythrocyte	WB	16–36 µg/dl red cells	0.28–0.64 µmol/liter red cells
Red-cell distribution width	WB	11.5–14.5%	0.115–0.145
Reptilase time	P	16–24 sec	16–24 sec
Reticulocyte count	WB	0.5–2.5% red cells	0.005–0.025 red cells
Reticulocyte hemoglobin content	WB	>26 pg/cell	>26 pg/cell
Ristocetin cofactor (functional von Willebrand factor)	P		
Blood group O		75% mean of normal	0.75 mean of normal
Blood group A		105% mean of normal	1.05 mean of normal
Blood group B		115% mean of normal	1.15 mean of normal
Blood group AB		125% mean of normal	1.25 mean of normal
Schilling test, orally administered vitamin B₁₂ excreted in urine	U	7–40%	Not applicable
Sickle-cell test	WB	Negative	Negative
Sucrose hemolysis	WB	<10%	<0.1
Thrombin time	P	16–24 sec	16–24 sec
Transferrin receptor	S, P	9.6–29.6 nmol/liter	9.6–29.6 nmol/liter
Viscosity	P	1.7–2.1	1.7–2.1
	S	1.4–1.8	1.4–1.8
Vitamin B₁₂	S, P		
Normal		>250 pg/ml	>185 pmol/liter
Borderline		125–250 pg/ml	92–185 pmol/liter
Deficient		<125 pg/ml	<92 pmol/liter
von Willebrand factor (vWF) antigen (factor VIII:R antigen)	P		
Blood group O		75% mean of normal	0.75 mean of normal
Blood group A		105% mean of normal	1.05 mean of normal
Blood group B		115% mean of normal	1.15 mean of normal
Blood group AB		125% mean of normal	1.25 mean of normal
von Willebrand factor multimers	P	Normal distribution	Normal distribution
White cells: see Leukocytes			

Table A.15. *Continued.*

Immunology.			
Analyte	**Specimen***	**Units Used at MGH**	**SI Units**
Autoantibodies			
Antiadrenal antibody	S	Negative at 1:10 dilution	Not applicable
Anti–double-stranded (native) DNA	S	Negative at 1:10 dilution	Not applicable
Anti–glomerular basement membrane antibody	S		
Qualitative		Negative	Negative
Quantitative		<5 U/ml	<5 kU/liter
Antigranulocyte antibody	S	Negative	Not applicable
Anti–Jo-1 antibody	S	Negative	Not applicable
Anti-La antibody	S	Negative	Not applicable
Antimitochondrial antibody	S	Negative	Not applicable
Antineutrophil cytoplasmic autoantibody, cytoplasmic (c-ANCA)	S		
Qualitative		Negative	Negative
Quantitative (antibody to proteinase 3)		<2.8 U/ml	<2.8 kU/liter
Antineutrophil cytoplasmic autoantibody, perinuclear (p-ANCA)	S		
Qualitative		Negative	Negative
Quantitative (antibody to myeloperoxidase)		<1.4 U/ml	<1.4 kU/liter
Antinuclear antibody	S	Negative at 1:40 dilution	Not applicable
Anti–parietal-cell antibody	S	Negative at 1:20 dilution	Not applicable
Anti-Ro antibody	S	Negative	Not applicable
Antiplatelet antibody	S	Negative	Not applicable
Anti-RNP antibody	S	Negative	Not applicable
Anti–Scl-70 antibody	S	Negative	Not applicable
Anti-Smith antibody	S	Negative	Not applicable
Anti–smooth-muscle antibody	S	Negative at 1:20 dilution	Not applicable
Antithyroglobulin	S	Negative	Not applicable
Antithyroid antibody	S	<0.3 IU/ml	<0.3 kIU/liter
Bence Jones protein	S	None detected	Not applicable
Qualitative	U	None detected in 50-fold concentrated specimen	Not applicable
Quantitative	U		
Kappa		<2.5 mg/dl	<0.03 g/liter
Lambda		<5.0 mg/dl	<0.05 g/liter
Beta$_2$-microglobulin	S	<0.27 mg/dl	<2.7 mg/liter
	U	<120 µg/day	<120 µg/day
C1-esterase–inhibitor protein	S		
Antigenic		12.4–24.5 mg/dl	0.12–0.25 g/liter
Functional		Present	Present
C-reactive protein	S		
Routine		0.08–3.10 mg/liter	0.08–3.10 mg/liter
High-sensitivity		0.02–8.00 mg/liter	0.02–8.00 mg/liter
Complement			
C3	S	86–184 mg/dl	0.86–1.84 g/liter
C4	S	20–58 mg/dl	0.20–0.58 g/liter
Total complement, enzyme immunoassay	S	63–145 U/ml	63–145 kU/liter
Factor B	S	17–42 mg/dl	0.17–0.42 g/liter

Continued.

Table A.15. *Continued.*

Immunology. **(Continued.)**			
Analyte	**Specimen***	**Units Used at MGH**	**SI Units**
Cryoproteins	S	Negative	Not applicable
Immunofixation	S	Negative	Not applicable
Immunoglobulin			
IgA	S	60–309 mg/dl	0.60–3.09 g/liter
IgD	S	0–14 mg/dl	0–140 mg/liter
IgE	S	10–179 IU/ml	24–430 µg/liter
IgG	S	614–1295 mg/dl	6.14–12.95 g/liter
IgG1	S	270–1740 mg/dl	2.7–17.4 g/liter
IgG2	S	30–630 mg/dl	0.3–6.3 g/liter
IgG3	S	13–320 mg/dl	0.13–3.20 g/liter
IgG4	S	11–620 mg/dl	0.11–6.20 g/liter
IgM	S	53–334 mg/dl	0.53–3.34 g/liter
Joint-fluid crystal	JF	Negative	Not applicable
Joint-fluid mucin	JF	Only type I mucin present	Not applicable
LE-cell test	WB	Negative	Negative
Rheumatoid factor	S, JF	<30.0 IU/ml	<30 kIU/liter
Serum protein electrophoresis	S	Normal pattern	Not applicable

Clinical Chemistry.			
Analyte	**Specimen***	**Units Used at MGH**	**SI Units**
Acetoacetate	P	<1 mg/dl	<100 µmol/liter
Albumin	S	3.5–5.5 g/dl	35–55 g/liter
Aldolase	S	0–6 U/liter	0–100 nkat/liter
Alpha$_1$-antitrypsin	S	85–213 mg/dl	0.8–2.1 g/liter
Alpha-fetoprotein	S	<15 ng/ml	<15 µg/liter
Aminotransferases	S		
Aspartate (AST, SGOT)		0–35 U/liter	0–0.58 µkat/liter
Alanine (ALT, SGPT)		0–35 U/liter	0–0.58 µkat/liter
Ammonia, as NH_3	P	10–80 µg/dl	6–47 µmol/liter
Amylase	S	60–180 U/liter	0.8–3.2 µkat/liter
Angiotensin-converting enzyme (ACE)	S	<40 U/liter	<670 nkat/liter
Anion gap	S	7–16 mmol/liter	7–16 mmol/liter
Apolipoprotein	S		
Apolipoprotein A-1		119–240 mg/dl	1.2–2.4 g/liter
Apolipoprotein B		52–163 mg/dl	0.52–1.63 g/liter
Apolipoprotein B:apolipoprotein A-1		0.35–0.98	0.35–0.98
Arterial blood gases, sea level	WB, arterial		
Bicarbonate (HCO_3^-)		21–30 mEq/liter	21–28 mmol/liter
Partial pressure of carbon dioxide (PCO_2)		35–45 mm Hg	4.7–5.9 kPa
pH		7.38–7.44	7.38–7.44
Partial pressure of oxygen (PO_2)		80–100 mg Hg	11–13 kPa
β-Hydroxybutyrate	P	<3 mg/dl	<300 µmol/liter

Table A.15. *Continued.*

Clinical Chemistry. (Continued.)			
Analyte	**Specimen☆**	**Units Used at MGH**	**SI Units**
Beta₂-microglobulin	S	1.2–2.8 mg/liter	1.2–2.8 mg/liter
	U	≤200 µg/liter	≤200 µg/liter
Bilirubin	S		
Total		0.3–1.0 mg/dl	5.1–17.0 µmol/liter
Direct		0.1–0.3 mg/dl	1.7–5.1 µmol/liter
Indirect		0.2–0.7 mg/dl	3.4–12.0 µmol/liter
Brain-type natriuretic peptide (BNP)	P	<167 pg/ml (age- and sex-dependent)	<167 ng/liter (age- and sex-dependent)
Calcium	S	9.0–10.5 mg/dl	2.2–2.6 mmol/liter
Calcium, ionized	WB	4.5–5.6 mg/dl	1.1–1.4 mmol/liter
CA 15-3	S	0–30 U/ml	0–30 kU/liter
CA 19-9	S	0–37 U/ml	0–37 kU/liter
CA 27-29	S	0–32 U/ml	0–32 kU/liter
CA 125	S	0–35 U/ml	0–35 kU/liter
Calcitonin	S		
Male		3–26 pg/ml	3–26 ng/liter
Female		2–17 pg/ml	2–17 ng/liter
Carbon dioxide			
Content, sea level	P	21–30 mEq/liter	21–30 mmol/liter
Partial pressure (PCO₂), sea level	WB, arterial	35–45 mm Hg	4.7–5.9 kPa
Carbon monoxide content	WB		Symptoms with 20% saturation of hemoglobin
Carcinoembryonic antigen (CEA)	S	0–3.4 ng/ml	0–3.4 µg/liter
Ceruloplasmin	S	27–37 mg/dl	270–370 mg/liter
Cholinesterase	S	5–12 U/ml	5–12 kU/liter
Chloride	S	98–106 mEq/liter	98–106 mmol/liter
Cholesterol	P		
Low-density lipoprotein (LDL) cholesterol			
Optimal		<100 mg/dl	<2.59 mmol/liter
Near or above normal		100–129 mg/dl	2.59–3.34 mmol/liter
Borderline high		130–159 mg/dl	3.36–4.11 mmol/liter
High		160–189 mg/dl	4.13–4.88 mmol/liter
Very high		≥190 mg/dl	≥4.91 mmol/liter
High-density lipoprotein (HDL) cholesterol			
Low		<40 mg/dl	<1.03 mmol/liter
High		≥60 mg/dl	≥1.55 mmol/liter
Total cholesterol			
Desirable		<200 mg/dl	<5.17 mmol/liter
Borderline high		200–239 mg/dl	5.17–6.18 mmol/liter
High		≥240 mg/dl	≥6.18 mmol/liter
Copper	S	70–140 µg/dl	11–22 µmol/liter
	U	3–35 µg/24 hr	0.047–0.55 µmol/24 hr
Coproporphyrins, types I and III	U	100–300 µg/24 hr	150–460 µmol/24 hr
C-peptide	S	0.5–2.0 ng/ml	0.17–0.66 nmol/liter

Continued.

Table A.15. *Continued.*

Clinical Chemistry. (Continued.)			
Analyte	Specimen*	Units Used at MGH	SI Units
Creatine kinase	S		
Total			
Female		40–150 U/liter	0.67–2.50 μkat/liter
Male		60–400 U/liter	1.00–6.67 μkat/liter
MB isoenzyme	S	0–7 ng/ml	0–7 μg/liter
Relative index†	S	Method-dependent	Method-dependent
Creatinine	S	<1.5 mg/dl	<133 μmol/liter
Erythropoietin	S	5–36 IU/liter	5–36 IU/liter
Fatty acids, free (nonesterified)	P	<8–25 mg/dl	0.28–0.89 mmol/liter
Fibrinogen and fibrinogen-degradation products: see under Hematology and Coagulation			
Folic acid	RC	150–450 ng/ml/cells	340–1020 nmol/liter/cells
γ-Glutamyltransferase	S	1–94 U/liter	1–94 U/liter
Glucose	P		
Fasting			
Normal		75–115 mg/dl	4.2–6.4 mmol/liter
Diabetes mellitus		>125 mg/dl	>7.0 mmol/liter
2 Hr postprandial	P	120 mg/dl	<6.7 mmol/liter
Hemoglobin A_{1c}	WB	3.8–6.4%	0.038–0.064 hemoglobin fraction
Homocysteine	P	4–12 μmol/liter	4–12 μmol/liter
Hydroxyproline	U	0–1.3 mg/24 hr	0–10 μmol/24 hr
Iron	S	50–150 μg/dl	9–27 μmol/liter
Iron-binding capacity	S	250–370 μg/dl	45–66 μmol/liter
Iron-binding capacity, saturation	S	20–45%	0.2–0.45
Ketone (acetone)	S, U	Negative	Negative
Lactate	P, venous	5–15 mg/dl	0.6–1.7 mmol/liter
Lactate dehydrogenase	S	100–190 U/liter	1.7–3.2 μkat/liter
Lactate dehydrogenase isoenzymes	S		
Fraction 1 (of total)		14–26%	0.14–0.25
Fraction 2		29–39%	0.29–0.39
Fraction 3		20–26%	0.20–0.25
Fraction 4		8–16%	0.08–0.16
Fraction 5		6–16%	0.06–0.16
Lead (adult)	S	<10–20 μg/dl	<0.5–1 μmol/liter
Lipase	S	0–160 U/liter	0–2.66 μkat/liter
Lipids, triglyceride: see Triglycerides			
Lipoprotein(a)	S	0–30 mg/dl	0–300 mg/liter
Magnesium	S	1.8–3.0 mg/dl	0.8–1.2 mmol/liter
Mercury	WB	0.6–59 μg/liter	3.0–294 nmol/liter
	U, 24 hr	<20 μg/liter	<99.8 nmol/liter
Microalbumin	U		
24-hr		<20 mg/liter or <31 mg/24 hr	<0.02 g/liter or <0.031 g/24 hr
Spot, morning		<0.03 mg albumin/mg creatinine	<0.03 g albumin/g creatinine

Table A.15. *Continued.*

Clinical Chemistry. (Continued.)			
Analyte	**Specimen***	**Units Used at MGH**	**SI Units**
Myoglobin	S		
Male			19–92 µg/liter
Female			12–76 µg/liter
5'-Nucleotidase	S	0–11 U/liter	0.02–0.18 µkat/liter
Osmolality	P	285–295 mOsm/kg serum water	285–295 mmol/kg serum water
	U	300–900 mOsm/kg	300–900 mmol/kg
Oxygen			
Content, sea level	WB, arterial	17–21 vol%	
	WB, venous (arm)	10–16 vol%	
Saturation, sea level	WB, arterial	97%	0.97 mol/mol
	WB, venous (arm)	60–85%	0.60–0.85 mol/mol
Partial pressure (PO$_2$)	WB	80–100 mm Hg	11–13 kPa
pH	WB	7.38–7.44	
Parathyroid hormone–related peptide	S	<1.3 pmol/liter	<1.3 pmol/liter
Phosphatase			
Acid	S	0–5.5 U/liter	0.90 nkat/liter
Alkaline	S	30–120 U/liter	0.5–2.0 nkat/liter
Phosphorus, inorganic	S	3–4.5 mg/dl	1.0–1.4 mmol/liter
Porphobilinogen	U	None	None
Potassium	S	3.5–5.0 mEq/liter	3.5–5.0 mmol/liter
Prealbumin	S	19.5–35.8 mg/dl	195–358 mg/liter
Prostate-specific antigen (PSA)	S		
Female		<0.5 ng/ml	<0.5 µg/liter
Male			
≤40 yr		0–2.0 ng/ml	0–2.0 µg/liter
>40 yr		0–4.0 ng/ml	0–4.0 µg/liter
Prostate-specific antigen (PSA), free (men 45–75 yr with PSA values between 4 and 20 ng/ml)		>25% associated with benign prostatic hyperplasia	>0.25 associated with benign prostatic hyperplasia
Protein			
Total	S	5.5–8.0 g/dl	55–80 g/liter
Fractions	S		
Albumin		3.5–5.5 g/dl (50–60%)	35–55 g/liter
Alpha$_1$		0.2–0.4 g/dl (4.2–7.2%)	2–4 g/liter
Alpha$_2$		0.5–0.9 g/dl (6.8–12%)	5–9 g/liter
Beta		0.6–1.1 g/dl (9.3–15%)	6–11 g/liter
Gamma		0.7–1.7 g/dl (13–23%)	7–17 g/liter
Globulin		2.0–3.5 g/dl (40–50%)	20–35 g/liter
Pyruvate	P, venous	0.5–1.5 mg/dl	60–170 µmol/liter
Sodium	S	136–145 mEq/liter	136–145 mmol/liter
Transferrin	S	230–390 mg/dl	2.3–3.9 g/liter
Triglycerides	S	<160 mg/dl	<1.8 mmol/liter
Troponin			
I	S	0–0.4 ng/ml	0–0.4 µg/liter
T	S	0–0.1 ng/ml	0–0.1 µg/liter

Continued.

Table A.15.   *Continued.*

Clinical Chemistry. **(Continued.)**			
Analyte	**Specimen***	**Units Used at MGH**	**SI Units**
Urea nitrogen	S	10–20 mg/dl	3.6–7.1 mmol/liter
Uric acid	S		
Male		2.5–8.0 mg/dl	150–480 µmol/liter
Female		1.5–6.0 mg/dl	90–360 µmol/liter
Urobilinogen	U	1–3.5 mg/24 hr	1.7–5.9 µmol/24 hr
Vitamin A	S	20–100 µg/dl	0.7–3.5 µmol/liter
Vitamin B₁ (thiamine)	S	0–2 µg/dl	0–75 nmol/liter
Vitamin B₂ (riboflavin)	S	4–24 µg/dl	106–638 nmol/liter
Vitamin B₆	P	5–30 ng/ml	20–121 nmol/liter
Vitamin C (ascorbic acid)	S	0.4–1.0 mg/dl	23–57 µmol/liter
Vitamin D₃ (1,25-dihydroxyvitamin D)	S	25–45 pg/ml	60–108 pmol/liter
Vitamin D₃ (25-hydroxyvitamin D)	P	10–68 ng/ml	24.9–169.5 nmol/liter
Vitamin E	S	5–18 µg/ml	12–42 µmol/liter
Vitamin K	S	0.13–1.19 ng/ml	0.29–2.64 nmol/liter

Metabolic and Endocrine Tests.			
Analyte	**Specimen***	**Units Used at MGH**	**SI Units**
Adrenocorticotropin (ACTH)	P	6.0–76.0 pg/ml	1.3–16.7 pmol/liter
Aldosterone			
Supine, normal-sodium diet	S, P	2–9 ng/dl	55–250 pmol/liter
Upright, normal-sodium diet	S, P	2–5 times supine value with normal-sodium diet	
Supine, low-sodium diet	S, P	2–5 times supine value with normal-sodium diet	
Random, low-sodium diet	U	2.3–21.0 µg/24 hr	6.38–58.25 nmol/24 hr
Androstenedione	S	50–250 ng/dl	1.75–8.73 nmol/liter
Cortisol			
Fasting, 8 a.m.–noon	S	5–25 µg/dl	138–690 nmol/liter
Noon–8 p.m.		5–15 µg/dl	138–414 nmol/liter
8 p.m.–8 a.m.		0–10 µg/dl	0–276 nmol/liter
Cortisol, free	U	20–70 µg/24 hr	55–193 nmol/24 hr
Dehydroepiandrosterone (DHEA)			
Male	S	180–1250 ng/dl	6.24–41.6 nmol/liter
Female		130–980 ng/dl	4.5–34.0 nmol/liter
Dehydroepiandrosterone (DHEA) sulfate	S		
Male		10–619 µg/dl	100–6190 µg/liter
Female (premenopausal)		12–535 µg/dl	120–5350 µg/liter
Female (postmenopausal)		30–260 µg/dl	300–2600 µg/liter
Deoxycorticosterone (DOC)	S	2–19 ng/dl	61–576 nmol/liter
11-Deoxycortisol (8 a.m.)	S	12–158 ng/dl	0.34–4.56 nmol/liter
Dopamine	P	<87 pg/ml	<475 pmol/liter
	U	65–400 µg/day	425–2610 nmol/day

Table A.15. *Continued.*

Metabolic and Endocrine Tests. (Continued.)			
Analyte	**Specimen***	**Units Used at MGH**	**SI Units**
Epinephrine			
Supine (30 min)	P	<50 pg/ml	<273 pmol/liter
Sitting	P	<60 pg/ml	<328 pmol/liter
Standing (30 min)	P	<900 pg/ml	<4914 pmol/liter
	U	0–20 µg/day	0–109 nmol/day
Estradiol	S, P		
Female			
Menstruating			
Follicular phase		<20–145 pg/ml	184–532 pmol/liter
Mid-cycle peak		112–443 pg/ml	411–1626 pmol/liter
Luteal phase		<20–241 pg/ml	184–885 pmol/liter
Postmenopausal		<59 pg/ml	217 pmol/liter
Male		<20 pg/ml	184 pmol/liter
Estrone	S, P		
Female			
Menstruating			
Follicular phase		1.5–15.0 pg/ml	55–555 pmol/liter
Luteal phase		1.5–20.0 pg/ml	55–740 pmol/liter
Postmenopausal		1.5–5.5 pg/ml	55–204 pmol/liter
Male		1.5–6.5 pg/ml	55–240 pmol/liter
Follicle-stimulating hormone (FSH)	S, P		
Female			
Menstruating			
Follicular phase		3.0–20.0 mIU/ml	3.0–20.0 IU/liter
Ovulatory phase		9.0–26.0 mIU/ml	9.0–26.0 IU/liter
Luteal phase		1.0–12.0 mIU/ml	1.0–12.0 IU/liter
Postmenopausal		18.0–153.0 mIU/ml	18.0–153.0 IU/liter
Male		1.0–12.0 mIU/ml	1.0–12.0 IU/liter
Fructosamine	S	1.61–2.68 mmol/liter	1.61–2.68 mmol/liter
Gastrin	S	<100 pg/ml	<100 ng/liter
Glucagon	P	20–100 pg/ml	20–100 ng/liter
Growth hormone (resting)	S	0.5–17.0 ng/ml	0.5–17.0 µg/liter
Human chorionic gonadotropin (hCG) (nonpregnant women)	S	<5 mIU/ml	<5 IU/liter
17-Hydroxyprogesterone	S		
Male		5–250 ng/dl	0.15 nmol/liter
Female			
Menstruating			
Follicular phase		20–100 ng/dl	0.6–3.0 nmol/liter
Mid-cycle peak		100–250 ng/dl	3.0–7.5 nmol/liter
Luteal phase		100–500 ng/dl	3.0–15 nmol/liter
Postmenopausal		≤70 ng/dl	≤2.1 nmol/liter
5-Hydroxyindoleacetic acid (5-HIAA)	U	<6 mg/24 hr	<31 µmol/24 hr
Insulin	S, P	2–20 µU/ml	14.35–143.50 pmol/liter
17-Ketosteroids	U	3–12 mg/24 hr	10–42 µmol/24 hr

Continued.

Table A.15. *Continued.*

Metabolic and Endocrine Tests. **(Continued.)**			
Analyte	Specimen*	Units Used at MGH	SI Units
Luteinizing hormone (LH)	S, P		
Female			
Menstruating			
Follicular phase		2.0–15.0 mIU/ml	2.0–15.0 IU/liter
Ovulatory phase		22.0–105.0 mIU/ml	22.0–105.0 IU/liter
Luteal phase		0.6–19.0 mIU/ml	0.6–19.0 IU/liter
Postmenopausal		16.0–64.0 mIU/ml	16.0–64.0 IU/liter
Male		2.0–12.0 mIU/ml	2.0–12.0 IU/liter
Metanephrine	P U	<0.5 nmol/liter 0.05–1.20 µg/mg creatinine	<0.5 nmol/liter 0.03–0.69 mmol/mol creatinine
Norepinephrine	U	15–80 µg/24 hr	89–473 nmol/24 hr
Norepinephrine	P		
Supine (30 min)		<110–410 pg/ml	650–2423 pmol/liter
Sitting		120–680 pg/ml	709–4019 pmol/liter
Standing (30 min)		125–700 pg/ml	739–4137 pmol/liter
Parathyroid hormone	S	10–60 pg/ml	10–60 ng/liter
Pregnanetriol	U	Age- and sex-dependent	Age- and sex-dependent
Progesterone	S, P		
Menstruating female			
Follicular		<0.2 ng/ml	<0.6 nmol/liter
Midluteal		3–20 ng/ml	9.54–63.6 nmol/liter
Male		<0.2–1.4 ng/ml	<0.60–4.45 nmol/liter
Prolactin	S		
Female		0–20 ng/ml	0–20 µg/liter
Male		0–15 ng/ml	0–15 µg/liter
Serotonin	WB Platelets	50–200 ng/ml 125–500 ng/10⁹ platelets	0.28–1.14 µmol/liter 0.7–2.8 amol/platelet
Sex hormone–binding globulin	S		
Male		13–71 nmol/liter	13–71 nmol/liter
Female		18–114 nmol/liter	18–114 nmol/liter
Somatostatin	P	<25 pg/ml	<25 ng/liter
Somatomedin C (insulin-like growth factor I [IGF-I])	S		
16–24 yr		182–780 ng/ml	182–780 µg/liter
25–39 yr		114–492 ng/ml	114–492 µg/liter
40–54 yr		90–360 ng/ml	90–360 µg/liter
>54 yr		71–290 ng/ml	71–290 µg/liter
Testosterone	S		
Total, morning			
Female		6–86 ng/dl	0.21–2.98 nmol/liter
Male		270–1070 ng/dl	9.36–37.10 nmol/liter
Unbound, morning			
Female		0.2–3.1 pg/ml	6.9–107.5 pmol/liter
Male		12.0–40.0 pg/ml	416–1387 pmol/liter

Table A.15. *Continued.*

Metabolic and Endocrine Tests. **(Continued.)**			
Analyte	Specimen☆	Units Used at MGH	SI Units
Thyroglobulin	S	0–60 ng/ml	0–60 µg/liter
Thyroid-binding globulin	S	16–24 µg/ml	206–309 nmol/liter
Thyroid-stimulating hormone	S	0.5–4.7 µU/ml	0.5–4.7 µU/liter
Thyroxine	S		
Total (T_4)		4.5–10.9 µg/dl	58–140 nmol/liter
Free (fT_4)		0.8–2.7 ng/dl	10.3–35.0 pmol/liter
Triiodothyronine	S		
Total (T_3)		60–181 ng/dl	0.92–2.78 nmol/liter
Free (fT_3)		1.4–4.4 pg/ml	0.22–6.78 pmol/liter
Vanillylmandelic acid (VMA)	U	0.15–1.20 mg/24 hr	7.6–37.9 µmol/24 hr
Vasoactive intestinal polypeptide (VIP)	P	<75 pg/ml	<75 ng/liter

Therapeutic-Drug Monitoring and Toxicology.				
Drug	**Therapeutic Level**		**Toxic Level**	
	Units Used at MGH	SI Units	Units Used at MGH	SI Units
Acetaminophen	10–30 µg/ml	66–199 µmol/liter	>200 µg/ml	>1324 µmol/liter
Amikacin				
Peak	25–35 µg/ml	43–60 µmol/liter	>35 µg/ml	>60 µmol/liter
Trough	4–8 µg/ml	6.8–13.7 µmol/liter	>10 µg/ml	>17 µmol/liter
Amitriptyline	120–250 ng/ml	433–903 nmol/liter	>500 ng/ml	>1805 nmol/liter
Amphetamine	20–30 ng/ml	148–222 nmol/liter	>200 ng/ml	>1480 nmol/liter
Barbiturates, most short-acting			>20 mg/liter	>88 µmol/liter
Bromide			>1250 µg/ml	>15.6 mmol/liter
Carbamazepine	6–12 µg/ml	26–51 µmol/liter	>15 µg/ml	>63 µmol/liter
Chlordiazepoxide	700–1000 ng/ml	2.34–3.34 µmol/liter	>5000 ng/ml	>16.7 µmol/liter
Clonazepam	15–60 ng/ml	48–190 nmol/liter	>80 ng/ml	>254 nmol/liter
Clozapine	200–350 ng/ml	0.6–1.0 µmol/liter		
Cocaine			>1000 ng/ml	>3300 nmol/liter
Cyclosporine	Varies with time after dose and type of transplantation, with ranges of 100–400 ng/ml	Varies with time after dose and type of transplantation, with ranges of 83–333 nmol/liter	Varies with time after dose and type of transplantation	Varies with time after dose and type of transplantation
Desipramine	75–300 ng/ml	281–1125 nmol/liter	>400 ng/ml	>1500 nmol/liter
Diazepam	100–1000 ng/ml	0.35–3.51 µmol/liter	>5000 ng/ml	>17.55 µmol/liter
Digoxin	0.8–2.0 ng/ml	1.0–2.6 nmol/liter	>2.5 ng/ml	>3.2 nmol/liter
Doxepin	30–150 ng/ml	107–537 nmol/liter	>500 ng/ml	>1790 nmol/liter
Ethanol			>300 mg/dl	>65 mmol/liter
Behavioral changes			>20 mg/dl	>4.3 mmol/liter
Clinical intoxication			>100 mg/dl	>1 g/liter

Continued.

Table A.15. *Continued.*

Therapeutic-Drug Monitoring and Toxicology. **(Continued.)**				
Drug	**Therapeutic Level**		**Toxic Level**	
	Units Used at MGH	SI Units	Units Used at MGH	SI Units
Ethosuximide	40–100 μg/ml	283–708 μmol/liter	>150 μg/ml	>1062 μmol/liter
Flecainide	0.2–1.0 μg/ml	0.5–2.4 μmol/liter	>1.0 μg/ml	>2.4 μmol/liter
Gentamicin				
Peak	8–10 μg/ml	16.7–20.9 μmol/liter	>10 μg/ml	>21.0 μmol/liter
Trough	<2–4 μg/ml	<4.2–8.4 μmol/liter	>4 μg/ml	>8.4 μmol/liter
Ibuprofen	10–50 μg/ml	49–243 μmol/liter	100–700 μg/ml	485–3395 μmol/liter
Imipramine	125–250 ng/ml	446–893 nmol/liter	>500 ng/ml	>1784 nmol/liter
Lidocaine	1.5–6.0 μg/ml	6.4–26 μmol/liter		
Central nervous system or cardio-vascular depression			6–8 μg/ml	26–34.2 μmol/liter
Seizures, obtundation, decreased cardiac output			>8 μg/ml	>34.2 μmol/liter
Lithium	0.6–1.2 mEq/liter	0.6–1.2 nmol/liter	>2 mEq/liter	>2 mmol/liter
Methadone	100–400 ng/ml	0.32–1.29 μmol/liter	>2000 ng/ml	>6.46 μmol/liter
Methotrexate	Variable	Variable		
1–2 wk after low dose			>9.1 ng/ml	>20 nmol/liter
48 hr after high dose			>227 ng/ml	>0.5 μmol/liter
Morphine	10–80 ng/ml	35–280 nmol/liter	>200 ng/ml	>700 nmol/liter
Nortriptyline	50–170 ng/ml	190–646 nmol/liter	>500 ng/ml	>1.9 μmol/liter
Phenobarbital	10–40 μg/ml	43–170 μmol/liter		
Slowness, ataxia, nystagmus			35–80 μg/ml	151–345 μmol/liter
Coma with reflexes			65–117 μg/ml	280–504 μmol/liter
Coma without reflexes			>100 μg/ml	>430 μmol/liter
Phenytoin	10–20 μg/ml	40–79 μmol/liter	>20 μg/ml	>79 μmol/liter
Procainamide	4–10 μg/ml	17–42 μmol/liter	>10–12 μg/ml	>42–51 μmol/liter
Quinidine	2–5 μg/ml	6–15 μmol/liter	>6 μg/ml	>18 μmol/liter
Salicylates	150–300 μg/ml	1086–2172 μmol/liter	>300 μg/ml	>2172 μmol/liter
Theophylline	8–20 μg/ml	44–111 μmol/liter	>20 μg/ml	>110 μmol/liter
Thiocyanate				
After nitroprusside infusion	6–29 μg/ml	10⁻–499 μmol/liter	>120 μg/ml	>2064 μmol/liter
Nonsmoker	1–4 μg/ml	17–69 μmol/liter		
Smoker	3–12 μg/ml	52–206 μmol/liter		
Tobramycin				
Peak	8–10 μg/ml	17–21 μmol/liter	>10 μg/ml	>21 μmol/liter
Trough	<4 μg/ml	<9 μmol/liter	>4 μg/ml	>9 μmol/liter
Valproic acid	50–150 μg/ml	347–1040 μmol/liter	>150 μg/ml	>1040 μmol/liter
Vancomycin				
Peak	18–26 μg/ml	12–18 μmol/liter	>80–100 μg/ml	>55–69 μmol/liter
Trough	5–10 μg/ml	3–7 μmol/liter		

Table A.15. *Continued.*

Urine Analysis.		
Analyte	**Units Used at MGH**	**SI Units**
Acidity, titratable	20–40 mEq/24 hr	20–40 mmol/24 hr
Ammonia	30–50 mEq/24 hr	30–50 mmol/24 hr
Amylase	4–400 U/liter	0.07–7.67 nkat/liter
Amylase:creatinine clearance ratio‡	1–5	1–5
Calcium (with dietary calcium 10 mEq/24 hr or 200 mg/24 hr)	<300 mg/24 hr	<7.5 mmol/24 hr
Creatine, as creatinine		
Female	<100 mg/24 hr	<760 μmol/24 hr
Male	<50 mg/24 hr	<380 μmol/24 hr
Creatinine	1.0–1.6 g/24 hr	8.8–14 mmol/24 hr
Eosinophils	<100 eosinophils/ml	<100 eosinophils/ml
Glucose, true (oxidase method)	50–300 mg/24 hr	0.3–1.7 mmol/24 hr
Microalbumin	0–2.0 mg/dl	0–0.02 g/liter
Oxalate	2–60 mg/24 hr	228–684 μmol/24 hr
pH	5.0–9.0	5.0–9.0
Phosphate (phosphorus)	400–1300 mg/24 hr (varies with intake)	12.9–42.0 mmol/24 hr (varies with intake)
Potassium	25–100 mEq/24 hr (varies with intake)	25–100 mmol/24 hr (varies with intake)
Protein	<150 mg/24 hr	<0.15 g/24 hr
Sediment		
Bacteria	Negative	Negative
Bladder cells	Negative	Negative
Broad casts	Negative	Negative
Crystals	Negative	Negative
Epithelial-cell casts	Negative	Negative
Granular casts	Negative	Negative
Hyaline casts	0–5/low-power field	0–5/low-power field
Red-cell casts	Negative	Negative
Red cells	0–2/high-power field	0–2/high-power field
Squamous cells	Negative	Negative
Tubular cells	Negative	Negative
Waxy casts	Negative	Negative
White cells	0–2/high-power field	0–2/high-power field
White-cell casts	Negative	Negative
Sodium	100–260 mEq/24 hr (varies with intake)	100–260 mmol/24 hr (varies with intake)
Specific gravity	1.001–1.035	1.001–1.035
Urea nitrogen	6–17 g/24 hr	214–607 mmol/24 hr
Uric acid (with normal diet)	250–800 mg/24 hr	1.49–4.76 mmol/24 hr

Continued.

Table A.15. *Continued.*

Microbiology.

Specimen	Routinely Cultured For	Also Reported	Normal Flora
Throat	Group A beta-hemolytic streptococci, pyogenic groups C and G beta-hemolytic streptococci, *Arcanobacterium haemolyticum*	If complete throat culture is requested: *Haemophilus influenzae, Staphylococcus aureus, Streptococcus pneumoniae, Neisseria meningitidis,* and yeast	Alpha-hemolytic streptococci, non-hemolytic streptococci, diphtheroids, coagulase-negative staphylococci, saprophytic neisseria
Sputum	Pneumococci, *H. influenzae*, beta-hemolytic streptococci, *Staph. aureus,* Moraxella (*Branhamella*) *catarrhalis*, gram-negative bacilli	Presence or absence of normal throat flora	Little or no normal throat flora, if specimen carefully collected
Urine	Aerobic bacteria and yeast: "abundant" if >10⁵ colony-forming units/ml, "moderate" if 10⁴–10⁵ colony-forming units/ml	"Few" if 10^3–10^4 colony-forming units/ml, "rare" if 10^2–10^3 colony-forming units/ml (either may indicate clinically significant bacteriuria if accompanied by pyuria, clinical symptoms, or both)	No mixed bacterial species (i.e., not more than one of the following: lactobacilli, non–beta-hemolytic streptococci, diphtheroids, coagulase-negative staphylococci, or *Gardnerella vaginalis*) if specimen carefully collected
Blood	Aerobic bacteria, anerobic bacteria, yeasts		None; common contaminants: aerobic diphtheroids, anaerobic diphtheroids, coagulase-negative staphylococci
Cerebrospinal fluid and other fluids	Aerobic bacteria, anaerobic bacteria, yeasts (including cryptococcus)	Any organism isolated	None
Stool	Enteric pathogens: salmonella, shigella, campylobacter, plesiomonas, and aeromonas when predominant	Moderate or abundant yeast or *Staph. aureus*; presence or absence of normal gram-negative enteric flora; if special cultures requested, yersinia, *Vibrio cholerae, V. parahemolyticus,* or hemorrhagic strains of *Escherichia coli* (O157)	Enterobacteriaceae, streptococci, pseudomonas, small numbers of staphylococci and yeast (and anaerobes that are not routinely cultured)
Wounds	Aerobic bacteria, anaerobic bacteria, yeasts		
Cervical or vaginal	Gonococci, group A beta-hemolytic streptococci, pyogenic groups C and G beta-hemolytic streptococci, *Staph. aureus* (Gram's stain for diagnosis of bacterial vaginosis according to Nugent score)	Yeasts and enteric gram-negative rods if present in large numbers	

* WB denotes whole blood, P plasma, S serum, PRP platelet-rich plasma, U urine, and JF joint fluid, and RC red cells.
† The creatine kinase relative index is calculated as [MB isoenzyme (in nanograms per milliliter) ÷ total creatine kinase (in units per liter)]×100.
‡ The amylase:creatinine clearance ratio is calculated as [amylase clearance ÷ creatinine clearance]×100.

For further information, see Kratz A, Sluss PM, Januzzi JL, Lewandrowski KB. Laboratory values of clinical importance. In: Kasper DL, Braunwald E, Fauci AS, Hauser SL, Longo DL, Jameson JL, eds. Harrison's principles of internal medicine. 16th ed. New York: McGraw-Hill, 2004:A1-A15.
Copyright © 2004 Massachusetts Medical Society.

Index